Dedication
Richard Johanson 1957–2002

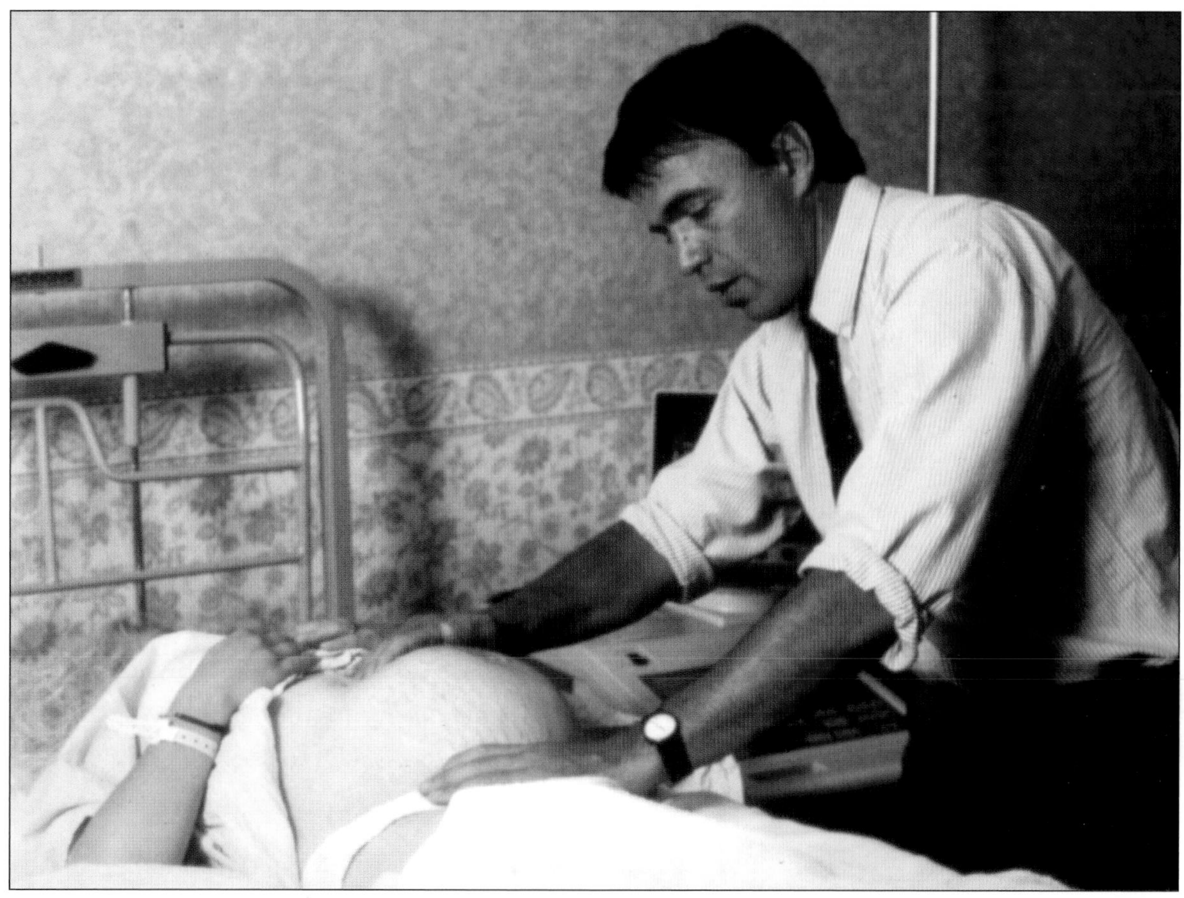

This book is dedicated to the memory of Richard Johanson, who died on 20 February 2002, before he could see this work come to fruition.

'It's never too late to be what you might have been'

George Eliot

This quotation had meaning for Richard – it was posted on his study wall.

Richard had two major aims in obstetrics – to avoid unnecessary intervention but to apply urgent skilled intervention when needed and he had a gift for both. He wanted interventions to be based on the best evidence available and for there to be good audit to check that the correct processes were being followed. His experience in Stoke and overseas had given him the skills to achieve these aims. His drive was for simple emergency protocols to save the lives of mothers and babies. This led to his leadership in practice and education in labour ward emergencies.

Initially he organised structured training for life-threatening obstetric emergencies in the West Midlands and in 1997 he and Charles Cox were the inspiration for developing the 'Managing Obstetric Emergencies and Trauma' (MOET) course, aimed at senior obstetricians and anaesthetists. A modified MOET course was taken overseas where he introduced ideas and protocols with tact and efficiency.

He worked closely with midwives in research and in the implementation of labour ward guidelines. He organised national meetings dealing with childbirth and worked with the National Childbirth Trust and Baby Lifeline, again to promote safer childbirth without over-medicalisation. The foundation of his research charity 'Childbirth without Fear' aims to continue to improve the care of women during childbirth.

Richard will be remembered by many, particularly by his trainees. His boundless enthusiasm and generosity with his time, ideas and academic work meant that there was a queue to work with him. The publication problem would be solved and the trainee would have a nationally respected mentor who continued to take an interest in their career.

Perhaps instinctively feeling that time was precious led him to achieve so much so quickly. Much of it was due to the intellectual sparking between him and his anaesthetist wife, Charlotte. They demonstrated the teamwork that is part of the philosophy of MOET.

> *'To see a human being reveal really exceptional qualities one must be able to observe his activities over many years. If these activities are completely unselfish; if the idea motivating them is unique in its magnanimity; if it is quite certain that they have never looked for any reward; and if in addition they have left visible traces on the world – then one may say, without fear of error, that one is in the presence of an unforgettable character.'*

[Jean Giono, from a short story called *The Man Who Planted Trees*]

THE

COURS

Managing Obstetric Emergencies and Trauma

Third edition

EDITED BY

Sara Paterson-Brown
AND
Charlotte Howell

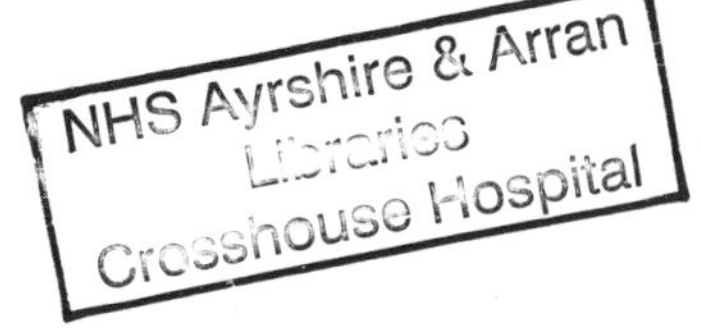

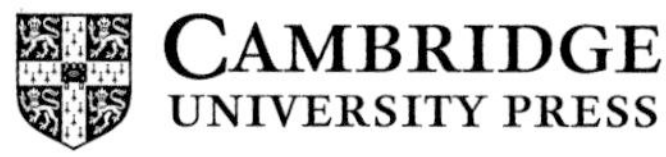

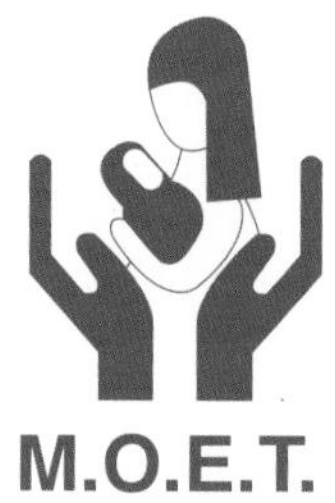

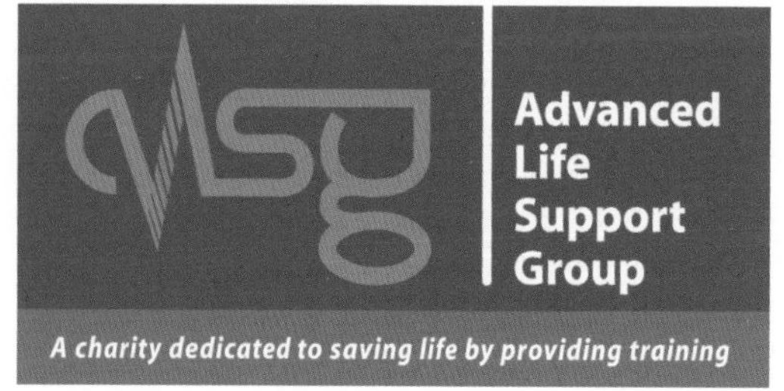

CAMBRIDGE
UNIVERSITY PRESS

CAMBRIDGE UNIVERSITY PRESS
Cambridge, New York, Melbourne, Madrid, Cape Town, Singapore,
São Paulo, Delhi, Mexico City

Cambridge University Press
The Edinburgh Building, Cambridge CB2 8RU, UK

Published in the United States of America by Cambridge University Press, New York

www.cambridge.org
Information on this title: www.cambridge.org/9781107675346

First edition published 2002
Second edition published 2007
Third edition published 2014

Printed in Singapore by C.O.S Printers Pte Ltd

A catalogue record for this publication is available from the British Library

ISBN: 978-1-107-67534-6 (Paperback).

Every effort has been made in preparing this book to provide accurate and up-to-date information which is in accord with accepted standards and practice at the time of publication. Although case histories are drawn from actual cases, every effort has been made to disguise the identities of the individuals involved. Nevertheless, the authors, editors and publishers can make no warranties that the information contained herein is totally free from error, not least because clinical standards are constantly changing through research and regulation. The authors, editors and publishers therefore disclaim all liability for direct or consequential damages resulting from the use of material contained in this book. Readers are strongly advised to pay careful attention to information provided by the manufacturer of any drugs or equipment that they plan to use.

Contents

		Page
	Working Group	vii
	About the authors	ix
	Acknowledgements	xii
	Abbreviations	xiii
Section 1 Introduction		**1**
1	Introduction	3
2	Saving mothers' lives: lessons from the Confidential Enquiries	7
3	Structured approach to emergencies in the obstetric patient	17
Section 2 Recognition		**23**
4	Recognising the seriously sick patient	25
5	Shock	39
6	Sepsis	51
7	Intravenous access and fluid replacement	65
Section 3 Resuscitation		**83**
8	Airway management and ventilation	85
9	Cardiopulmonary resuscitation in the nonpregnant and pregnant patient	109
10	Amniotic fluid embolism	121
11	Pulmonary thromboembolism	129
12	Resuscitation of the baby at birth	139
Section 4 Trauma		**157**
13	Introduction to trauma	159
14	Domestic abuse	163
15	Thoracic emergencies	171
16	Abdominal trauma in pregnancy	179
17	The unconscious patient	189
18	Spine and spinal cord injuries	201
19	Musculoskeletal trauma	213
20	Burns	221

Section 5 Other medical and surgical emergencies **227**

21 Abdominal emergencies in pregnancy 229

22 Cardiac, diabetic and neurological emergencies in pregnancy 241

23 Perinatal psychiatric illness 267

Section 6 Obstetric emergencies **275**

24 Pre-eclampsia and eclampsia 277

25 Major obstetric haemorrhage 297

26 Caesarean section 313

27 Placenta accreta and retained placenta 325

28 Uterine inversion 333

29 Ruptured uterus 339

30 Ventouse and forceps delivery 347

31 Shoulder dystocia 369

32 Umbilical cord prolapse 383

33 Face presentation 389

34 Breech delivery and external cephalic version 395

35 Twin pregnancy 411

36 Complex perineal and anal sphincter trauma 417

37 Symphysiotomy and destructive procedures 429

38 Anaesthetic complications in obstetrics 437

Section 7 Triage and transfer **451**

39 Triage 453

40 Transfer 459

Section 8 Human issues **467**

41 Human factors 469

42 Consent matters 481

Index 493

Working Group

Virginia Beckett

Alastair Campbell

Charles Cox

Johan Creemers

Kara Dent

John Elton

Diana Fothergill

Simon Grant

Brigid Hayden

Kim Hinshaw

Charlotte Howell

Shirin Irani

Geraldine Masson

Douglas Mein

Sara Paterson-Brown

Felicity Plaat

Bheemasenachar Prasad

Rahul Sen

Paul Sharpe

About the authors

Contributors to the third edition

Charles Cox	Consultant Obstetrician and Gynaecologist, Wolverhampton
Johan Creemers	Consultant Obstetrician and Gynaecologist, Netherlands
James Drife	Professor of Obstetrics and Gynaecology, Leeds
John Elton	Consultant Anaesthetist, Coventry
Peter-Marc Fortune	Paediatric Intensive Care, Manchester
Diana Fothergill	Consultant Obstetrician and Gynaecologist, Sheffield
Simon Grant	Consultant Obstetrician and Gynaecologist, Bristol
Brigid Hayden	Consultant Obstetrician and Gynaecologist, Bolton
Carol Henshaw	Consultant in Perinatal Mental Health, Liverpool
Kim Hinshaw	Consultant Obstetrician and Gynaecologist, Sunderland
Charlotte Howell	Consultant Anaesthetist, Stoke-on-Trent
Shirin Irani	Consultant Obstetrician and Gynaecologist, Birmingham
Geraldine Masson	Consultant Obstetrician and Gynaecologist, Stoke-on-Trent
Douglas Mein	Consultant Anaesthetist, New Zealand
Jane Mooney	Medical Editor, ALSG, Manchester
Fidelma O'Mahoney	Consultant Obstetrician and Gynaecologist, Stoke
Sara Paterson-Brown	Consultant Obstetrician and Gynaecologist, London
Simon Paterson-Brown	Consultant General Surgeon, Edinburgh
Barbara Phillips	Medical Editor, ALSG, Manchester
Felicity Plaat	Consultant Anaesthetist, London
Bheemasenachar Prasad	Consultant Anaesthetist, Perth, Australia
Rahul Sen	Consultant Obstetrician and Gynaecologist, Australia
Paul Sharpe	Consultant Anaesthetist, Leicester
Derek Tuffnell	Consultant Obstetrician and Gynaecologist, Bradford
Sarah Vause	Consultant Obstetrician and Gynaecologist, Manchester
J Wardrope	Consultant in Emergency Medicine, Sheffield
Sue Wieteska	CEO ALSG, Manchester
Jonathan Wyllie	Consultant Neonatologist, Middlesbrough

Additional contributors to the second edition

Kavita Goswami	Consultant Obstetrician and Gynaecologist, Coventry
Kate Grady	Consultant Anaesthetist, Manchester
Elaine Metcalfe	ALSG, Manchester
Margaret Oates	Consultant Perinatal Psychiatrist, Nottingham
Poonam Pradhan	Consultant Obstetrician and Gynaecologist, Birmingham
Abdul Sultan	Consultant Obstetrician and Gynaecologist, Croydon
Gargeswari Sunanda	Consultant Obstetrician and Gynaecologist, Birmingham
Ranee Thaker	Consultant Obstetrician and Gynaecologist, Croydon
Steve Walkinshaw	Consultant in Fetomaternal Medicine, Liverpool
Catherine Wykes	Consultant Obstetrician and Gynaecologist, Brighton

Additional contributors to the first edition

The late Professor Richard Johanson

Nick Coleman	Consultant Anaesthetist, Stoke-on-Trent
Mona Khadra	Specialist Registrar in Obstetrics, John Radcliffe Hospital, Oxford
David Griffiths	Consultant Obstetrician and Gynaecologist, Swindon
Harmini Sidhu	Consultant Obstetrician and Gynaecologist, Craigavon
Peter Young	Consultant Obstetrician and Gynaecologist, Stoke on Trent

Contact details and website information

ALSG: www.alsg.org
BestBETS: www.bestbets.org

For details on ALSG courses visit the website or contact:

Advanced Life Support Group
ALSG Centre for Training and Development
29–31 Ellesmere Street
Swinton, Manchester
M27 0LA
Tel: +44 (0) 161 794 1999
Fax: +44 (0) 161 794 9111
Email: enquiries@alsg.org

Updates

The material within this book will be updated on a 5-yearly cycle. However, practice and advice may change in the interim period. We will post any changes on the ALSG website, so we advise that you visit the website regularly to check for updates (url: www.alsg.org – go to the MOET page). The website will provide you with a new page to download and replace the existing page in your book.

Online feedback

It is important to ALSG that the contact with our providers continues after a course is completed. We now contact everyone 6 months after the course has taken place, asking for online feedback. This information is then used whenever the course is updated, to ensure that MOET provides optimum training to its participants.

Acknowledgements

A great many people have put a lot of hard work into the production of this book and the accompanying course. The editors would like to thank all the contributors for their efforts and all the MOET providers and instructors who took the time to send their comments during the development of the text and the course.

Some of the material used in this text is from other Advanced Life Support Group (ALSG) publications, in particular from the books *Advanced Paediatric Life Support: The Practical Approach* (Wiley-Blackwell Publishing), *Safe Transfer and Retrieval: The Practical Approach* (Wiley-Blackwell Publishing) and *Major Incident Medical Management and Support: The Practical Approach in the Hospital* (Wiley-Blackwell Publishing). We would also like to thank Bios Scientific Publishers for permission to reproduce material from the book *Managing Obstetric Emergencies.*

Chapter 31 Shoulder dystocia was derived from the chapter on shoulder dystocia written by Onsy Louca and Richard Johanson for the *Yearbook of Obstetrics and Gynaecology* Volume 6. We acknowledge comments from Barbara Franks.

The chapters on resuscitation have been informed by the new international guidelines produced by an evidence-based process from the collaboration of many international experts under the umbrella of the International Liaison Committee on Resuscitation (ILCOR) 2010.

We acknowledge and sincerely thank Barbara Phillips and Jane Mooney for their work in the preparation of this manuscript. Our grateful appreciation goes to Claire Dunn in the RCOG publishing team.

We would like to thank Helen Carruthers and Kate Wieteska for their work on many of the line drawings within the text. We would also like to thank Arrow (Figure 7.1), the Northern Neonatal Network (Figures 12.1–12.3), South Tees Foundation Trust Maternity (Figure 4.1) and the Resuscitation Council UK (Algorithms 9.1–9.3 and 12.1).

Finally, we would like to thank, in advance, those of you who will attend the Managing Obstetric Emergencies and Trauma (MOET) course; no doubt you will have much constructive critique to offer and we welcome your feedback.

Abbreviations

ABG	arterial blood gases
ACE	angiotensin-converting enzyme
AED	automated external defibrillator
AFE	amniotic fluid embolism
ALS	advanced life support
ALSG	Advanced Life Support Group
ALSO	Advanced Life Support in Obstetrics
ALT	alanine aminotransferase
AMPLE	allergies; medication; previous medical history; last meal; events and environments related to the injury
APTT	activated partial thromboplastin time
ARDS	adult respiratory distress syndrome
AS	anal sphincter
AST	aspartate aminotransferase
AVPU	**a**lert; responding to **v**oice; only responding to **p**ain; **u**nresponsive
BLS	basic life support
BMI	body mass index
BP	blood pressure
CC	chest compressions
CEMACH	Confidential Enquiry into Maternal and Child Health
CEMD	Confidential Enquiries into Maternal Deaths
CESDI	Confidential Enquiry into Stillbirths and Deaths in Infancy
CI	confidence interval
CMACE	Centre for Maternal and Child Enquiries
CMV	cytomegalovirus
CNST	Clinical Negligence Scheme for Trusts
CPP	cerebral perfusion pressure
CPR	cardiopulmonary resuscitation
CRP	C-reactive protein
CRT	capillary refill time

CS	caesarean section
CSE	combined spinal/epidural anaesthesia
CSF	cerebrospinal fluid
CT	computed tomography
CTG	cardiotocography
CTPA	computed tomography pulmonary angiogram
CVP	central venous pressure
CVVH	continuous venovenous haemofiltration
CXR	chest radiograph
DIC	disseminated intravascular coagulation
DPL	diagnostic peritoneal lavage
DVT	deep vein thrombosis
EAS	external anal sphincter
ECG	electrocardiogram
ECMO	extracorporeal membrane oxygen
ECV	external cephalic version
ESICM	European Society of Intensive Care Medicine
EWS	early warning score
FAST	focused assessment sonography in trauma
FBC	full blood count
FDPs	fibrin/fibrinogen degradation products
F_ECO_2	end tidal carbon dioxide
FFP	fresh frozen plasma
FHR	fetal heart rate
GCS	Glasgow Coma Scale
GIC	Generic Instructor Course
GMC	General Medical Council
GTT	glucose tolerance test
Hb	haemoglobin
HbA_1C	glycated haemoglobin
hCG	human chorionic gonadotrophin
HDU	high-dependency unit
HELLP	haemolysis; elevated liver enzymes; low platelets
HAS	Human Albumin Solution

HOCM	hypertrophic obstructive cardiomyopathy
IAS	internal anal sphincter
ICP	intracranial pressure
ICU	intensive care unit
ILCOR	International Liaison Committee on Resuscitation
IO	intraosseous
IPPV	intermittent positive pressure ventilation
ISF	International Sepsis Forum
IV	intravenous
LDH	lactate dehydrogenase
LDL	low-density lipoprotein
LFT	liver function test
LMA	laryngeal mask airway
LMWH	low-molecular-weight heparin
LSCS	lower segment caesarean section
MAP	mean arterial pressure
MEOWS	modified early obstetric warning system
MI	myocardial infarction
MIST	mechanism of injury; injuries already identified; symptoms and signs; treatment already received
MMR	maternal mortality rate
MOET	Managing Obstetric Emergencies and Trauma
MRI	magnetic resonance imaging
mRNA	messenger RNA
MRSA	methicillin-resistant *Staphylococcus aureus*
MSSU	mid-stream sample of urine
MSV	Mauriceau–Smellie–Viet
NICE	National Institute for Health and Clinical Excellence
NNT	number needed to treat
OASIS	obstetric anal sphincter injuries
ONS	Office for National Statistics
OR	odds ratio
OVD	operative vaginal delivery
PaO_2	Arterial concentration of oxygen

PCI	percutaneous coronary intervention
PDS	polydiaxanone
PE	pulmonary embolism
PEA	pulseless electrical activity
PET	pre-eclamptic toxaemia
PIH	pregnancy-induced hypertension
PND	postnatal depression
PPH	postpartum haemorrhage
PRECOG	Pre-eclampsia Community Guideline
PT	prothrombin time
PVL	Panton–Valentine leucocydin
RCOG	Royal College of Obstetricians and Gynaecologists
rhAPC	recombinant human activated protein C
ROSC	return of spontaneous circulation
RR	relative risk
SADS	sudden adult death syndrome
SBAR	situation; background; assessment; recommendation
SCCM	Society of Critical Care Medicine
SHOTS	Serious Hazards of Transfusion Scheme
SIRS	systemic inflammatory response syndrome
SI	Système International d'unités
SSRIs	selective serotonin reuptake inhibitors
U&E	urea and electrolytes
UKOSS	United Kingdom Obstetric Surveillance System
V/Q	ventilation/perfusion
VE	vaginal examination
VF	ventricular fibrillation
VT	ventricular tachycardia
VTE	venous thromboembolism
WBC	white blood cell
WHO	World Health Organization

SECTION 1

Introduction

CHAPTER 1

Introduction

Throughout both the developed and the developing world, maternal mortality continues to present a serious challenge. Globally, there is estimated to be one maternal death every minute. This course will provide you with a system for managing the seriously ill and seriously injured. The system is designed to be simple and easy to remember when life-threatening emergencies arise and is known as 'the structured approach'. The structured approach is based on the ABC of resuscitation and is practised throughout all areas of medicine and the emergency services. The concept is familiar to the lay person and known even to school children. The structured approach has led to the development of courses that attend to the resuscitation needs of all patients, from neonates to children, adults and now for those with the altered physiology and anatomy of pregnancy.

This manual, the Managing Obstetric Emergencies and Trauma (MOET) online material and practical course are divided into sections that provide a structured revision in recognition, resuscitation and treatment of emergencies in pregnancy. This includes trauma, medical and surgical emergencies and obstetric emergencies and is aimed at obstetricians, anaesthetists, emergency physicians and midwives. The structured approach is applied to resuscitation and is taught didactically as a drill. Subsequently, what has been learned is applied to the recognition and management of the seriously ill and injured pregnant patient. Although trauma management is not widely taught to obstetricians, trauma occurs to their patients and those in other specialties will consider them the experts on the management of the injured pregnant woman.

The physiological adjustments of pregnancy affect the response of the mother to illness and injury. These changes mean that resuscitation should be tailored to the pregnant patient and this manual, and the MOET course, teaches how this is achieved.

The MOET course began in 2001 and runs under the auspices of the Advanced Life Support Group (ALSG). Its aim is to provide the knowledge, practical skills and procedures necessary to save the mother and fetus in life-threatening circumstances. The course runs in six countries and, since its inception, over 3300 providers and 430 instructors have been trained. Course information and links for candidates and faculty are available from the ALSG website (www.alsg.org).

This text is essential pre-course reading for the MOET course and also provides a valuable reference for all obstetricians and anaesthetists.

In more recent years, and in acknowledgement of the challenging study leave climate in the UK, a precourse online learning component (Box 1.1) has been devised and piloted (www.alsg.org/vle). This reinforces the current text and provides an interactive method of delivering the knowledge components of the course. It prepares participants for the practical application of knowledge during the face-to-face course.

Box 1.1 Content of the MOET online learning package

- Structured approach to MOET
- Cardiopulmonary resuscitation
- Resuscitation and perimortem C-section
- Airway management and breathing
- Structured approach to trauma
- Abdominal and pelvic trauma
- Hypertensive diseases of pregnancy
- Massive obstetric haemorrhage
- Complications of delivery
- Domestic abuse and perinatal psychiatric illness
- Shock
- Patient with headache and confusion
- Jehovah's witnesses
- Triage
- Drug calculations

The face-to-face course (Box 1.2) offers participants the opportunity to further reinforce their pre-course learning and also to have hands-on practice of essential skills. Interactive sessions and workshops explore a variety of acute medical emergencies that have been identified by the eighth Report of the Confidential Enquiries into Maternal Deaths in the UK, produced by the Centre for Maternal and Child Enquiries (CMACE), as leading causes of death in pregnancy. Simulations allow candidates to put knowledge and skills together and to practise and learn within a safe environment. In this, they are supported with structured debriefing by instructors and their fellow candidates. Continuous assessment on key skills and an end-of-course assessment on both a simulation and a multiple choice paper indicates those candidates that have achieved the required standard to be a 'MOET provider'.

Those candidates who demonstrate the potential to be an instructor are invited to undertake a structured training programme. The Generic Instructor Course (GIC) prepares instructors to deliver lectures, skills teaching, small group discussions, simulations and also to carry out assessments. This is then reinforced with support and assessment by experienced instructors when new instructors teach on MOET courses on the first two occasions. Instructors then teach on three courses over each 2-year period to maintain their status.

As priorities for training change, the MOET course is continually improved following feedback from course directors, instructors and candidates and from important trend information from major reports, e.g. MBRRACE. This ensures that it remains fit-for-purpose and focuses on the current leading causes of maternal death.

Box 1.2 Content of the MOET face-to-face course

Lectures and demonstrations

- Structured approach to MOET
- Cardiopulmonary resuscitation demonstration
- Shock
- Trauma review
- Newborn resuscitation
- Nonstandard procedures in modern obstetrics
- Medical emergencies

Workshops, skill stations and simulations

- Airway management
- Basic life support (BLS) and automated external defibrillator (AED) use
- Surgical airway
- Newborn resuscitation and vascular access
- Trauma moulage
- Instrumental delivery
- Vaginal breech delivery
- Failed ventouse leading to forceps delivery
- Acute abdominal emergencies
- Obstetric triage
- Eclampsia and Haemolysis, elevated liver enzymes, and lowered platelets (HELLP)
- Anaesthetic complications
- Massive obstetric haemorrhage
- Advanced surgical techniques
- Version techniques for delivery of twin II
- Uterine inversion
- Shoulder dystocia
- Headache and confusion

CHAPTER 2

Saving mothers' lives: lessons from the Confidential Enquiries

Introduction

Much of the wisdom in this book has been learned the hard way, some of it in the hardest way of all. When a woman dies as a result of an obstetric complication, the only good thing that can come out of the tragedy is that appropriate lessons are learned. For over 50 years, England and Wales have had a system in place to analyse all maternal deaths, identify the causes and highlight avoidable factors.

The Confidential Enquiries into Maternal Deaths (CEMD) have become so familiar to UK obstetricians and midwives that we can hardly imagine life without them. The UK, however, is one of only a few countries with a national system in which experienced clinicians scrutinise cases in detail to work out whether death could be prevented when a similar emergency happens again and, if so, how.

CEMD recommendations carry considerable weight at both political and clinical levels. This chapter will describe the system that produces these recommendations and will then focus on lessons relevant to emergencies and trauma – including those learned in the early years of the Enquiry, which are all too easily forgotten.

How the Enquiries work

The CEMD for England and Wales began collecting data in 1952 and has published reports every 3 years since 1957. Similar enquiries began in Northern Ireland in 1956 and in Scotland in 1965. Since 1985, the CEMD has covered the whole of the UK and, in 2003, it became part of the Confidential Enquiry into Maternal and Child Health (CEMACH), subsequently CMACE.

In 2012 CMACE joined the programme of MBRRACE-UK ('Mothers and Babies – Reducing Risk through Audit and Confidential Enquiries across the UK'), a collaboration based in the National Perinatal Epidemiology Unit in Oxford. Maternal deaths in the UK should now be notified to the MBRRACE-UK office by ringing 01865 289715.

From the outset, confidentiality was recognised to be essential if staff were to give an honest account of events without fear of litigation or disciplinary action. In this, and in other essentials, the approach initiated in the 1950s is still used today. The process summarised here applies to England, but is similar in the other UK countries.

Regional reporting

When a maternal death occurs, a form is sent to all the professionals involved to obtain anonymous factual information and reflective comments. The form, together with an anonymised copy of the woman's medical records, is returned to the MBRRACE-UK office.

Expert assessment

To ensure confidentiality, the report is kept under lock and key. All cases (still anonymised) are reviewed by Expert Assessors, who are senior clinicians in obstetrics, midwifery, anaesthetics, pathology, perinatal psychiatry, cardiology, neurology, infectious diseases, emergency medicine, general practice and intensive care. They look for emerging patterns and lessons for clinical colleagues, managers and politicians. Public health messages are particularly important and denominator data are obtained from the Office for National Statistics (ONS).

Reports

A report is published every year and includes surveillance information as well as topic-specific chapters, each of which appears on a triennial basis. Chapters are drafted by a writing committee, including the Expert Assessors of the four UK countries and other relevant experts in the topic area, and discussed by the whole editorial panel, which includes epidemiologists. Individual chapters are reviewed by outside experts. Once the final report is sent to the printers, any information linked to the identity of the women concerned is destroyed. The published report is available to the public, a fact that surprises doctors in countries that have a less open approach.

A challenge for any report is to ensure that people read it. Recent CEMD reports have been entitled *Saving Mothers' Lives* (and before that *Why Mothers Die* with an emotive cover picture) and launched with a press conference. They are bestsellers in the Royal College of Obstetricians and Gynaecologists (RCOG) bookshop, partly because examination candidates know that they are essential reading. Their messages, however, also need to be heard by other specialties and this is more difficult to achieve.

Lessons from the past

Effective intervention

Before the CEMD started, maternal mortality had dropped dramatically in the UK, from 400/100 000 in 1935 to 66/100 000 in 1952–54. The most rapid fall had occurred during the Second World War, contradicting the idea that social conditions are the major factor determining the safety of pregnancy. The reasons for the fall were the introduction of effective treatments as follows:

- antibiotics: puerperal sepsis was the leading cause of maternal death in the 1930s, despite the widespread use of aseptic precautions; when sulphonamides were introduced in 1937 the effect on death rates was spectacular

- blood transfusion became safe during the 1940s
- ergometrine, for the treatment and prevention of postpartum haemorrhage, was introduced in the 1940s.

In the 1930s, Britain had a well-developed medical infrastructure, so that when effective treatments finally became available their effects were rapidly felt.

Obstetric injury

In the first CEMD report, covering 1952–54, obstetric injury was the second cause of death after hypertensive disease (Table 2.1). It did not, however, warrant its own chapter and Table 2.1 is drawn from the Appendix to that report.

Table 2.1 Number of maternal deaths from obstetric injury, 1952–54

Cause	Deaths (*n*)
Prolonged labour	63
Disproportion or malposition of the fetus	23
Other trauma	55
Other complications of childbirth	66
Total	197

Nowadays, we can hardly imagine a woman dying of prolonged labour and we can only guess at what the terms 'other trauma' and 'other complications' conceal (Table 2.1). In the 1950s, the caesarean section (CS) rate was less than 3% and maternity care was quite different from that of today. The 1955–57 report included 33 deaths from ruptured uterus, mostly due to intrauterine manipulations. In 1958–60, there were 43 deaths from obstructed labour, of whom 18 were delivered in the patient's own home and 14 in a general practitioner maternity home. These reports are a useful corrective to the idea that the 1950s were a golden age of non-medicalised childbirth.

Obstetric injury today

In 2006–08 there were, for the first time, no deaths from genital tract trauma and the chapter dealing with these cases was discontinued. Nevertheless, the report commented that, 'Genital tract tears were implicated in two women who died of postpartum haemorrhage.' The risk of trauma has not disappeared and, indeed, high vaginal tears have become more difficult to deal with because of the current prevalence of obesity. The CEMD recommends that a surgeon faced with life-threatening haemorrhage should routinely ask a colleague to come and help.

Recent lessons

Who is at risk?

The CEMD identifies groups at increased risk of complications and with increased awareness death rates have fallen among, for example, ethnic minority women and those with a history of thromboembolism. Recognition of risk factors early in pregnancy is essential.

Age

In the 2006–08 CEMD report, the maternal mortality rate (MMR) was constant up to age 34, but doubled after age 35 and trebled after 40 years of age. The average age of childbearing in the UK has risen and in 2008 it was 29.3 years with 20% of births being to women aged 35 years or over.

Obesity

In the 2006–08 report, 22% of the women who died were overweight – with a body mass index (BMI) of 25–29.9 – and 27% were obese (with a BMI >30).

Socio-economic classification

In 2006–08, the MMR among unemployed women was 60.2 compared with 14.9 for manual workers and 6.5 among women classified as 'managerial and professional'. Attention should also be focused on women who book late or are poor attenders for antenatal care.

Ethnicity

Black women have higher maternal mortality rates than white women in all countries for which data are available. In the UK, Black African and Black Caribbean women have the same increased risk – almost four times that of white women – although the increase is less among other ethnic groups (Table 2.2). Women recently arrived from overseas often have communication difficulties and are at particular risk.

Table 2.2 Estimated maternal mortality rates by ethnic group, UK, 2006–08

Ethnic group	Deaths (*n*)	Rate/100 000	Relative risk
Black African	25	32.8	3.9
Black Caribbean	8	31.9	3.8
Pakistani	13	14.3	1.7
Indian	8	12.5	1.5
Bangladeshi	2	6.1	0.7
Chinese	2	15.1	1.8
Other	8	8.0	0.9
White	156	8.5	1.0

Direct deaths

Hypertensive disease

The number of deaths from pre-eclampsia is a fraction of what it was in 1952–54 (Table 2.3), but in recent years improvement has stalled. There were 20 deaths in 1991–93 and 19 deaths in 2006–08. For the past four triennia, thanks to guidelines on fluid management, none of the deaths has been due to pulmonary or cerebral oedema, but there is a continuing problem with failure to control systolic hypertension. In each of the last three triennia nine women have died from intracranial haemorrhage. Among the recommendations in 2006–08 were the following:

- epigastric pain in the second half of pregnancy should be considered to be the result of pre-eclampsia until proved otherwise
- systolic blood pressure (BP) of 150 mg or above requires effective antihypertensive treatment; if systolic BP is very high – >180 mmHg – this is a medical emergency
- women with severe pre-eclampsia need effective team care, based on clear communication and effective understanding.

Some of these recommendations are directed at non-obstetricians but, unfortunately, maternity staff do not always recognise the need for effective control of BP.

Table 2.3 The changes in direct deaths reported to the CEMD

Cause	1952–54 (England and Wales)	2006–08 (UK)
Hypertensive disease	246	19
Obstetric injury	197	0
Haemorrhage	188	8
Abortion	153	0
Thromboembolism	138	18
Anaesthesia	49	7
Sepsis	42	26

Haemorrhage

Over the past 33 years, deaths from haemorrhage have risen and fallen in a strangely regular pattern (Table 2.4) that may represent relaxation and tightening of standards. For example, the peak in 1988–90 included cases where doctors had ignored the recommendation that CS for placenta praevia should be carried out by a consultant.

It is important, however, to see these numbers in context. Haemorrhage is by far the commonest life-threatening complication of childbirth: surveys of severe morbidity show that haemorrhage of >2.5l occurs once in about 300 births. Therefore over a 3-year period with more than 2 million births in the UK, several thousand cases are treated successfully.

In 2006–08 the total of nine deaths included two cases of abruption, two of placenta praevia and five of postpartum haemorrhage (PPH). In three of these five cases, the main cause was lack of observation in the postpartum period. Regular observations are essential and Modified Early Obstetric Warning system (MEOWS) charts recommended. The RCOG has published guidelines on the management of PPH.

Every triennium, one or more deaths occur in women who refuse blood transfusion and guidelines have been issued about the management of such patients. Placenta praevia associated with a uterine scar is particularly dangerous and all women with a previous CS should have a scan for placental localisation in the second trimester and, if low-lying, again at 32 weeks.

Table 2.4 Deaths from haemorrhage reported in CEMD reports, 1976–78 to 2000–02

Triennium							1900			2000
76–78	79–81	82–84	85–87	88–91	91–93	94–96	97–99	00–02	03–05	06–08
Deaths (*n*)										
24	14	9	10	22	15	12	7	17	14	9

Thromboembolism

Thromboembolism has been the leading direct cause of maternal death in the UK since 1985, but recently, the number of deaths fell dramatically – from 41 in 2003–05 to only 18 in 2006–08. In the 1990s, a fall occurred after the RCOG published recommendations on thromboprophylaxis at CS. Deaths during pregnancy and after vaginal delivery, however, continued to rise and these were targeted by a further RCOG guideline in 2004. These categories fell sharply in 2006–08, the first full triennium after the new guideline was published.

This fall shows the value of well-focused guidelines, but further improvement could still be achieved. The most important risk factor for thromboembolism is obesity and the revised guidance includes weight-specific dosage advice on thromboprophylaxis. Risk assessment early in pregnancy is the key to reducing mortality further; this message needs to be heard in gynaecology wards and early pregnancy assessment units as well as in maternity units.

The value of individualised care also needs to be emphasised. The 2006–08 report stresses that vulnerable women, for example, those with a learning disability, may not be able to follow instructions about self-injection and will require particular care.

Chest symptoms appearing for the first time in pregnancy or the puerperium need careful assessment, particularly in at-risk women. This lesson needs to get across to other specialties.

Ectopic pregnancy

Deaths from ectopic pregnancy still show no sign of falling. Atypical presentation is common and the CEMD has repeatedly drawn attention to gastrointestinal symptoms which may mimic food poisoning. The 2006–08 report recommended that all women of reproductive age presenting to an Emergency Department with gastrointestinal symptoms should have a pregnancy test. Women from ethnic minorities are over-represented among deaths from ectopic pregnancy, possibly because of communication difficulties.

Abortion

The Abortion Act of 1967 eliminated deaths from criminal abortion, which in the 1950s caused about 30 deaths a year. In 2006–08 two deaths from sepsis were associated with legal termination of pregnancy, one after medical and one after surgical termination. Neither woman had received prophylactic antibiotics, which are recommended in RCOG guidelines. Haemorrhage after spontaneous miscarriage accounted for five deaths. Three of these occurred in the mid-trimester, associated with a placenta implanted over a CS scar. This again emphasises the importance of placental localisation.

Amniotic fluid embolism

The number of deaths from amniotic fluid embolism has remained constant for 20 years. The condition is not always fatal, however, and useful information may be gained when the woman survives. All cases, whether fatal or not, should be reported to the UK Obstetric Surveillance System (UKOSS) at the National Perinatal Epidemiology Unit in Oxford.

Sepsis

In 1982–84, there were only nine deaths from this cause and none were due to puerperal sepsis. Since then, deaths from sepsis have risen steadily. In 2006–08 it became the leading direct cause of maternal death with 26 deaths. Thirteen of these were due to the Group A beta-haemolytic streptococcus (*Streptococcus pyogenes*), compared with eight in 2003–05 and three in 2000-02. This organism is easily spread in the community, and all 13 women who died in 2006–08 either had, or worked with, young children. Women need to be informed about hygiene, which means washing their hands **before**, as well as after, going to the toilet or changing sanitary towels.

Sepsis is often insidious in onset and can progress very quickly. If it is suspected, urgent referral to hospital is necessary. In hospital, high-dose broad-spectrum antibiotics should be started immediately, without waiting for the results of investigations. In 2012, in response to the rise in deaths, the RCOG published new guidelines on bacterial sepsis during and after pregnancy.

Anaesthesia

Deaths from anaesthesia fell steadily during the 1970s, due to a move to regional anaesthesia and better training of anaesthetists. Since 1985, however, the number has been constant at about two per year. In view of the rising CS rate this represents an improvement of sorts, but it is concerning that in 2006–08 failed tracheal intubation was again the cause of two of the seven anaesthetic deaths. The report recommends that effective management of failed tracheal intubation is a core anaesthetic skill that should be rehearsed and assessed regularly.

Indirect deaths

Indirect deaths have outnumbered direct deaths in the UK since 1994–96 (Table 2.5). In that triennium, birth and death registrations were linked by the Office for National Statistics (ONS), leading to better ascertainment.

Table 2.5 The rise in indirect deaths: maternal deaths notified to the CEMD 1991–2008

	1991–93	1994–96	1997–99	2000–02	2003–05	2006–08
Direct	129	134	106	106	132	107
Indirect	100	134	136	155	163	154
Total	229	268	242	261	295	261

From 2000–02 onwards, CEMACH Regional Managers were involved in collecting data and this improved ascertainment further. Better identification of cases, however, is only one reason for the rise in indirect deaths, the other being a rise in risk factors such as smoking, obesity and older age at childbearing.

Cardiac disease

Deaths from cardiac disease have been rising and this is now the leading cause of maternal death in the UK, with 53 deaths in 2006–08. Only four were due to congenital heart disease and there were no deaths from rheumatic heart disease. The leading causes were sudden adult death syndrome, myocardial infarction, dissection of the thoracic aorta and cardiomyopathy (most commonly peripartum cardiomyopathy). Half of the women who died from cardiac disease had a BMI of 30 or more. The main learning point from all these cases was that there must be a low threshold for investigation of pregnant or recently delivered women who complain of chest pain, especially if they have risk factors such as hypertension.

Psychiatric disease

Psychiatric disease is common in pregnancy and after delivery. In 2006–08 there were 29 deaths from suicide during pregnancy or within six months afterwards. Sixteen of these occurred more than 42 days after delivery and so would be missed by the standard definition of maternal death. Suicide is usually by violent means and, unlike most causes of maternal death, shows no social class gradient. Most women who die by suicide have a history of serious affective disorder, which has a high risk of recurrence after delivery.

Previous psychiatric history must be identified in early pregnancy and the risk managed proactively.

Other indirect deaths

Of the many causes of indirect death, the leading category is central nervous system disease, including 14 deaths from epilepsy. Women may stop taking their medication when they become pregnant and medical diseases in pregnancy may be inadequately supervised because responsibility falls between the GP, midwife, obstetrician and physician. Good communication among carers is essential.

Coincidental deaths

The most common causes of coincidental death in 2006–08 were road traffic accidents (17 deaths) and murder (11 deaths). The report recommends that all pregnant women should be advised to wear a three-point seat belt in a motor vehicle and that routine enquiry about domestic abuse should be made at booking or during pregnancy. All women should be seen alone at least once in pregnancy. If an injury, like a black eye, is noticed, staff should ask sympathetically – but directly – how it was caused and should be prepared to offer support.

Substandard care

Standards are rising all the time, but the assessors are realistic when assessing whether or not care was substandard. The proportion of direct deaths with substandard care has risen slightly over the last 12 years, but among indirect deaths it has more than doubled. In 2006–08, major substandard care was present in 44% of direct and 31% of indirect deaths. The main causes included: lack of clinical knowledge and skills; failure to identify very sick women and lack of senior support.

In recent years, hospitals have undertaken their own investigations of serious untoward incidents and these reports have been made available to the Enquiry. Their quality was highly variable and the report commented that some were, 'Not worth the paper they were written on and a few [were] actually whitewashes or cover-ups for unacceptable situations.' Learning lessons from maternal deaths is not easy when they occur in your own hospital.

The international dimension

There are over 500 000 maternal deaths annually worldwide, of which 99% are in developing countries. The leading causes are shown in Table 2.6.

The underlying problems include: lack of access to contraception; lack of primary care or transport facilities and inadequate equipment and staffing in district hospitals. The United Nations has made reduction of maternal mortality one of its Millennium Development

Goals. The worldwide proportion of births with a trained attendant has risen to 61%, but much remains to be done.

The UK CEMD is globally respected as an example of good practice and the Director and Assessors have assisted several countries – for example South Africa, Moldova and Kazakhstan – to set up their own enquiries adapted from the UK model.

Table 2.6 Causes of maternal deaths worldwide
(Source: World Health Organization)

Cause	Percentage (%)
Haemorrhage	25
Sepsis	15
Unsafe abortion	13
Pre-eclampsia/eclampsia	12
Obstructed labour	8
Other direct causes	8
Indirect causes	20

Summary

- The common assumption that safe childbirth is a side effect of national prosperity is wrong.
- Complications such as haemorrhage, pre-eclampsia or malpresentation cannot be prevented but they can be treated promptly and effectively.
- It is often forgotten that women's lives are routinely saved on a daily basis throughout the UK. When a death does occur, the public expects exhaustive analysis. Sometimes this reinforces old lessons, but often, new lessons emerge.
- One conclusion is clear from reviewing CEMD reports from the past 50 years: when vigilance is relaxed, people die.

Further reading

1 Centre for Maternal and Child Enquiries (CMACE). Saving Mothers' Lives: reviewing maternal deaths to make motherhood safer: 2006–8. The Eighth Report on Confidential Enquiries into Maternal Deaths in the United Kingdom. *Br J Obstet Gynaecol* 2011;118(Suppl. 1):1–203.

CHAPTER 3

Structured approach to emergencies in the obstetric patient

Objectives

On successfully completing this topic, you will be able to:

- identify the correct sequence to be followed in assessing and managing seriously ill or seriously injured patients
- understand the concept of the primary and secondary surveys.

Introduction

The structured approach refers to the 'ABCDE' approach to lifesaving. The aim of the structured approach is to provide a system of assessment and management that is effective, and simple to remember, in the heat of an emergency. It can be applied to any patient with a threat to life, be that from illness or injury. Assessment is divided into primary survey and secondary survey. The approach is the same for all: adults, children, the elderly and pregnant women.

Primary survey

The system follows a simple ABCDE approach, with resuscitation taking place as problems are identified, i.e. a process of simultaneous evaluation and resuscitation.

Airway

Assess whether the airway is open and, if not, open the airway using simple manoeuvres, such as head tilt and chin lift, followed by more complex actions (as detailed in Chapter 8) where necessary. Manoeuvres to secure the patient's airway should not cause harm, or further harm, to the cervical spine. Therefore, if an injury to the cervical spine is suspected in caring for the airway, the cervical spine must be immobilised.

Breathing

Look, listen and feel for respiration, using supplementary oxygen and ventilatory support as required.

Circulation

Assess the circulation by checking perfusion, heart rate and blood pressure. Volume replacement and haemorrhage control may be needed (see Chapters 5 and 7).

Disability

Assessment and support of the functioning of the neurological system.

Exposure

Adequately expose the patient to make a full assessment, taking care to avoid cooling and potential hypothermia by adjusting the environment.

The primary survey uncovers immediately life-threatening problems by priority, i.e. in the order in which they will most quickly kill. The medical sequence in the ABCDE approach is that an Airway problem will kill the patient more quickly than a Breathing problem, which in turn will kill a patient more quickly than a Circulation problem, which in turn will kill a patient more quickly than a Disability (neurological) problem.

Resuscitation

The resuscitation phase is carried out at the same time as the primary survey. Life-threatening conditions are managed as they are identified. Do not move on to the next stage of the primary survey until a problem, once found, has been corrected. If the patient's condition deteriorates, go back and reassess, starting again with ABCD.

Secondary survey

The secondary survey is a comprehensive assessment, which takes place after life-threatening problems have been found and treated (primary survey) and uncovers problems that are not immediately life-threatening.

The secondary survey is performed once the patient is stable. The secondary survey might not take place until after surgery, if surgery has been necessary as part of the resuscitation phase. The secondary survey is a top-to-toe process, as follows:

- scalp and vault of skull
- face and base of skull
- neck and cervical spine
- chest
- abdomen

- pelvis
- remainder of spine and limbs
- neurological examination
- rectal and vaginal examinations, if indicated
- examination of wounds caused by injury – Note: do not remove foreign objects from penetrating wounds, they may be tamponading a bleeding vessel.

If the Glasgow Coma Score has not been evaluated in the primary survey it should be performed during the secondary survey (see Chapter 17).

Assessment of the collapsed patient using the ABC approach

First, speak loudly to the patient: 'Hello, how are you Mrs Tilt?'

The response gives you several pieces of clinical information. To be able to respond verbally, the patient must:

- have circulating oxygenated blood (i.e. has not had a cardiopulmonary arrest)
- have a reasonably patent airway
- have a reasonable tidal volume to phonate
- have reasonable cerebral perfusion to comprehend and answer

If the patient does not respond then we cannot make the above assumptions.

Management of the apparently lifeless (unresponsive) patient

The approach to an apparently lifeless patient is the cardiopulmonary resuscitation drill, which starts with opening the airway and assessing breathing, then proceeding to CPR as necessary (see Chapter 9 for details).

Management of the seriously injured patient

In the seriously injured patient who has signs of life, the following approach is taken. If possible, during the primary survey and resuscitation, seek as much history as possible (from the patient and/or witnesses), including:

- history of the acute illness
- mechanism, speed, height of fall
- pre-existing medical problems, medications
- details of pregnancy where appropriate.

Consider management in three phases:

1. Primary survey and resuscitation: identify life-threatening problems and deal with these problems as they are identified. In trauma, if there is visible catastrophic haemorrhage (usually, this will be at the scene), stemming the loss of blood takes early precedence in resuscitation.

2. Secondary survey: top to toe, back to front examination.
3. Definitive care: specific management.

Management of the pregnant woman

In the pregnant woman, the sequence should be as follows:

1. Primary survey and resuscitation: identify life-threatening problems and deal with these problems as they are identified.
2. Assess fetal wellbeing and viability: may require delivery.
3. Secondary survey: top to toe, back to front examination.
4. Definitive care: specific management.

Continuous re-evaluation is very important to identify new life-threatening problems as they arise.

Monitoring (applied during primary survey):

- pulse oximetry
- heart rate/electrocardiogram (ECG)
- blood pressure: noninvasive or invasive
- respiratory rate
- F_ECO_2 (end tidal CO_2) monitoring is appropriate in an intubated patient
- urine output: as a measure of adequate perfusion and fluid resuscitation
- fetal heart monitoring where appropriate.

The pulse oximeter's limitations are that the patient must be well perfused to get a reading and ambient light and dyes, such as nail polish or circulating methaemoglobin, cause erroneous readings. A fall in oxygen saturation is a late sign of an airway, breathing or even a circulation problem.

Assess fetal wellbeing and viability

Use ultrasound to:

- detect fetal heart and check rate
- ascertain the number of babies and their positions
- locate the position of the placenta and the amount of liquor
- look for retroplacental bleeding and haematoma
- detect an abnormal position of the fetus and free fluid in the abdominal cavity, suggesting rupture of the uterus
- detect damage to other structures

- check for free fluid and blood in the abdominal cavity.

Adequately resuscitating the mother will improve the outcome for the baby.

Adjuncts to assessment:

- urinary catheter
- nasogastric tube: contraindicated if there is a suspected fracture of the base of the skull
- essential radiographs during the primary survey and resuscitation are chest, pelvis and lateral cervical spine.

Definitive care

Definitive care takes place under the supervision of relevant specialists. It is of utmost importance to the patient's continued quality of life.

Summary

- A systematic approach of Primary Survey, Resuscitation, Secondary Survey and Definitive Care enables the clinician to give the best patient care possible in complex situations.

SECTION 2

Recognition

CHAPTER 4

Recognising the seriously sick patient

Objectives

On successfully completing this topic, you will be able to:

- identify the current causes of maternal mortality and problems in their detection and treatment
- understand a systematic approach to monitoring using early warning charts to aid recognition of women at risk
- recognise 'red flag' symptoms and their need for urgent responses by the obstetric team and other specialties.

Introduction

In March 2011, the CMACE report for the triennium 2006–08 once again highlighted substandard care as a common contributory factor in the deaths reported. The lack of clinical knowledge across the professions at both senior and junior levels, the failure to recognise signs and symptoms of potentially life-threatening conditions and the delay in acting on findings and seeking help from appropriate specialists are all of particular concern. Attention is therefore focusing on ways to improve the recognition of, and responses to, signs of the deteriorating condition of patients.

The diagnosis of a severe life-threatening condition in a pregnant or recently pregnant woman may be difficult if the presentation is insidious or atypical. There is a potential for any woman to be at risk of physiological deterioration and this cannot always be predicted.

The early detection of severe illness in mothers remains a challenge to all professionals involved in their care. The relative rarity of such events combined with the normal changes in physiology associated with pregnancy and childbirth compounds the problem and reinforces the need for multiprofessional working.

The lessons that apply to all health professionals dealing with pregnant women can be summarised as follows:

- understand the normal changes of pregnancy in order to be able to recognise the pathological changes of serious illness – it is important to be able to distinguish between common discomforts of pregnancy and the signs of serious illness so that these signs are not ignored
- focus on getting simple things right – high-quality history taking, physical examination, meticulous recording of basic observations and findings by both doctors and midwives
- ensuring good communication and referrals between professionals.

Modified early-warning systems

It is recognised that pregnancy and labour are normal physiological events; however, regular observations of vital signs are an integral part of care, and will aid the recognition of changes in a woman's condition. Modified early-warning scoring systems improve the detection of life-threatening illness.

All women who enter an acute hospital setting should have their observations recorded on a MEOWS chart (NICE guideline 50). There is a minimum dataset of observations suggested at each assessment. The minimum recommended frequency of observations as an inpatient is 12 hourly. It has been suggested that intrapartum care observations should be recorded on a MEOWS chart (Figure 4.1). Women should retain the same MEOWS chart when moving from one clinical area to another, so that physiological trends can be observed.

These charts have been widely modified by the addition of other data and there is a balance to be struck between having too much information and not enough clarity. Practitioners are recommended to be familiar with the system in use at their hospital.

The use of MEOWS charts prompts early referral to an appropriate practitioner who can undertake a full review, order appropriate investigations, resuscitate and treat as required. Scores outside the normal range for pregnancy are recorded in the coloured zones of the chart and trigger a response from medical staff.

The following set of observations is required at each assessment:

- temperature
- respiratory rate
- BP: use the correct cuff size for the woman's arm; check electronic recordings of BP manually at least once
- pulse: if the woman is peripherally vasoconstricted as in haemorrhage, the pulse oximetry probe may not detect the pulse accurately; pulse properties such as volume and regularity cannot be assessed easily; nail varnish affects waveform accuracy
- conscious level: AVPU score (alert, voice, painful, unresponsive).

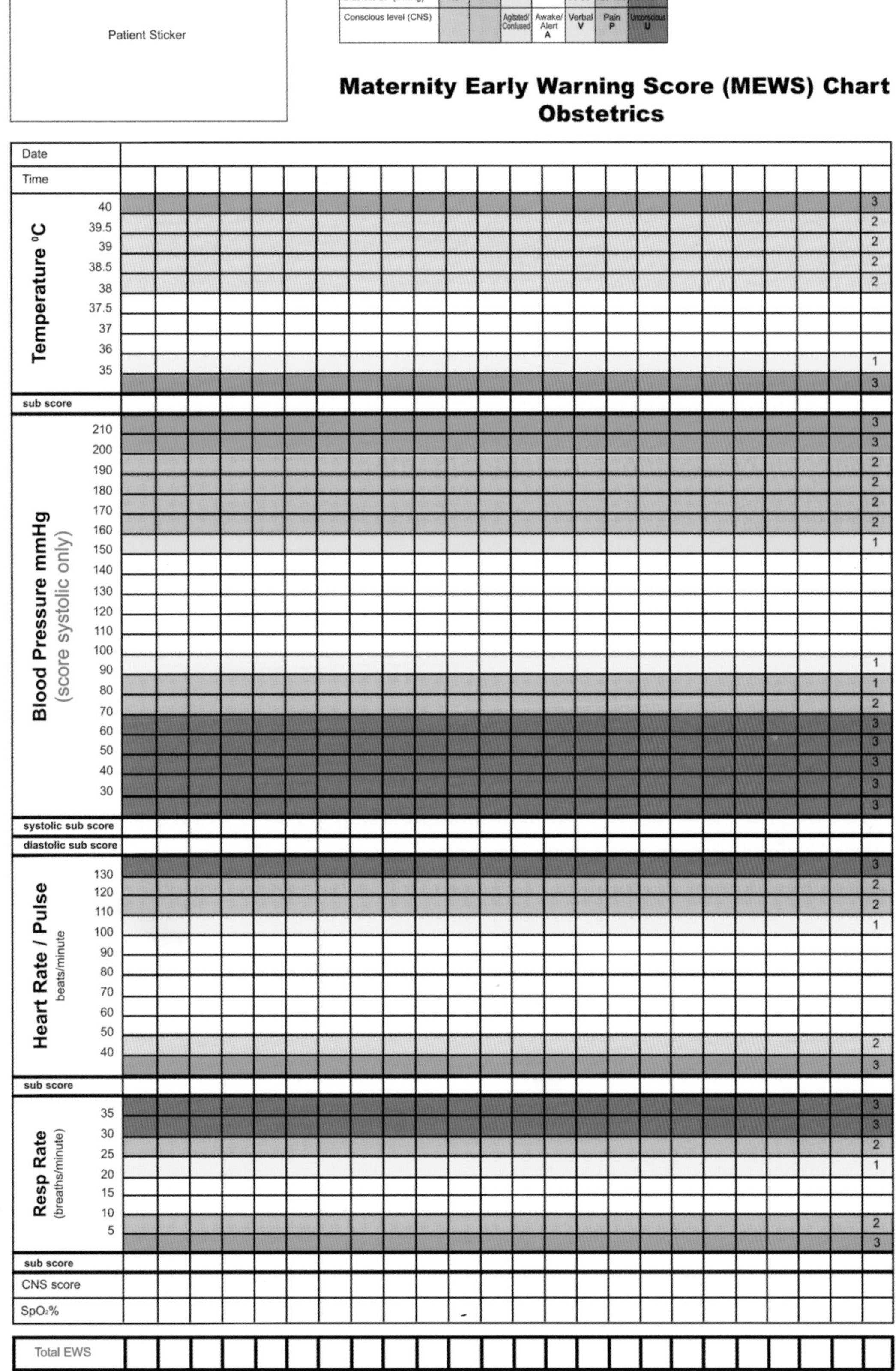

Patient Sticker

Score	3	2	1	0	1	2	3
Diastolic BP (mmHg)	<40				90-99	100-109	≥110
Conscious level (CNS)			Agitated/ Confused	Awake/ Alert A	Verbal V	Pain P	Unconscious U

South Tees Hospitals NHS
NHS Trust

Maternity Early Warning Score (MEWS) Chart Obstetrics

		Score
Date		
Time		
Temperature °C	40	3
	39.5	2
	39	2
	38.5	2
	38	2
	37.5	
	37	
	36	
	35	1
		3
sub score		
Blood Pressure mmHg (score systolic only)	210	3
	200	3
	190	2
	180	2
	170	2
	160	2
	150	1
	140	
	130	
	120	
	110	
	100	
	90	1
	80	1
	70	2
	60	3
	50	3
	40	3
	30	3
		3
systolic sub score		
diastolic sub score		
Heart Rate / Pulse beats/minute	130	3
	120	2
	110	2
	100	1
	90	
	80	
	70	
	60	
	50	
	40	2
		3
sub score		
Resp Rate (breaths/minute)	35	3
	30	3
	25	2
	20	1
	15	
	10	
	5	2
		3
sub score		
CNS score		
SpO_2%		
Total EWS		

MICC0756 MEWS/OBS February 09

Figure 4.1 An example of a MEOWS chart (reproduced with kind permission from South Tees Foundation Trust Maternity)

Additional observations which may be required:

- pulse oximetry should be in place if the woman is unwell, or has an increase or decrease in her respiratory rate, or has a medical/obstetric condition that necessitates use; all women who TRIGGER require oxygen saturation monitoring (normal value should be 95% or over when breathing air); if receiving oxygen therapy, record flow in l/min O_2 in use
- urine output: detail of input and output must be recorded on a separate fluid balance chart; optimum urine output is 1 ml/kg/h and the minimum acceptable urine output 0.5ml/kg/h (excepting in fulminating pre-eclampsia – see Chapter 24)
- looks unwell: an overall clinical judgement of woman's appearance
- pain score: postoperative only
- lochia: postnatal.

Frequency of observations is determined by:

- risk status
- diagnosis
- reason for admission
- initial observations on admission.

TRIGGERING means there is a requirement for an urgent review by the medical team.

While awaiting review there are a number of actions that can be carried out by the midwifery staff. There should also be an escalation policy whereby midwifery staff can escalate the request to a more senior doctor if the response is felt to be too slow or otherwise inadequate.

The SBAR tool is recommended to improve communication between team members (Box 4.1):

- situation
- background
- assessment
- recommendation.

Box 4.1

Example in the context of a woman triggering on the MEOWS with high BP:

Situation:	State the current problem giving the observation findings and state which ones are triggering. If raised systolic or diastolic, report any prodromal signs, such as headache, nausea, vomiting or upper epigastric pain.
Background:	Relevant information from the history of this patient, such as essential hypertension, current medication, recent blood results.
Assessment:	Midwife's interpretation of findings.
Recommendation:	Be clear about your expectations for the clinician, that the woman requires a bedside review in less than 10 minutes.

Immediate midwifery measures continued:

If rapid deterioration occurs, assess ABCD and act accordingly (see resuscitation chapters). Otherwise:

- increase observation frequency
- monitor pulse oximetry and give O_2 via face mask if required
- if antenatal, apply left lateral tilt 15–30° and commence cardiotocography (CTG)
- check intravenous lines
- check the drug chart and ensure medications have been administered, report time of delay of any drugs especially antihypertensive medications
- ensure you have senior midwife help and consider location of the woman
- arrangements may need to be made to transfer patient
- consider optimum positioning, sitting upright or lowering bed head
- ensure a safe environment by appropriate use of cot sides
- ensure outstanding laboratory results are obtained
- bring ECG machine, Haemaccue, arterial blood gas syringes and blood bottles to bedside to prepare for further investigations
- maintain contemporaneous record in notes detailing plan of care
- ask patient about any signs or changes she perceives, and ensure adequate documentation
- explain the plan of care to the woman and relatives.

Escalation procedure if obstetrician is unable to review in 10 minutes

Options would include contacting more senior obstetrician or anaesthetic team, or consider early obstetric consultant and anaesthetic consultant involvement.

If a senior registrar has deputised a more junior obstetrician to attend, then the midwife and/or senior colleague need to assess whether this is an appropriate level of clinician attending and consider escalation as above.

It is important to care for the woman in the most appropriate clinical area. If this is not possible, then a delay in transfer must not delay immediate investigations such as ECG, arterial blood gases or ordering of a CXR. Full review of the woman continues including repeated ABCD assessment and treatment, notes review, history taking and examination.

Contact clinical manager on call for assistance if required.

Clinical symptoms that may represent underlying serious illness including red flag symptoms (from *Saving Mothers' Lives* 2011):

- pyrexia
- breathlessness
- headache
- abdominal pain, diarrhoea and vomiting
- anxiety and distress.

Pyrexia

Absence of pyrexia does not exclude sepsis, as paracetamol and other antipyretics may temporarily suppress the pyrexia; equally, absence of pyrexia in the presence of sepsis is worrying.

Red flag symptoms (see also Chapter 6):

- pyrexia >38°C
- pulse rate sustained >100 bpm
- respiratory rate >20 breaths per minute
- abdominal or chest pain
- diarrhoea and/or vomiting
- reduced or absent fetal movements or fetal heart rate
- spontaneous rupture of membranes or significant vaginal discharge

- uterine or renal angle pain or tenderness
- generally not well, or unusually distressed or anxious.

Breathlessness

This common symptom of pregnancy can arise in any trimester, is gradual in onset and is usually noticed by the woman when she is talking or at rest. Differential diagnoses for breathlessness in the pregnant woman are shown in Table 4.1. In pregnancy, there is a 40–50% increase in minute ventilation, mostly owing to an increase in tidal volume rather than respiratory rate and this leads to the subjective awareness. A mild fully compensated respiratory alkalosis is therefore normal in pregnancy (arterial pH 7.44).

Remember:

- breathlessness as a symptom may be respiratory, cardiac or relate to a metabolic disturbance such as diabetic ketoacidosis
- breathlessness may represent an exacerbation of pre-existing respiratory or cardiac disease, or new-onset cardiac or respiratory disease.

Red flag features are:

- breathlessness of sudden onset
- breathlessness associated with chest pain
- orthopnoea; paroxysmal nocturnal dyspnoea.

Headache

This is a common problem in pregnancy. It is one of the most difficult symptoms to manage, as it can neither be seen, examined nor measured. Most of the time it will have a benign cause, but there are a wide variety of dangerous diagnoses presenting with headache or confusion as the predominant feature (see Chapter 22).

Red flag features include:

- sudden onset
- associated neck stiffness
- described as 'the worst headache ever'
- any neurological sign on examination.

Abdominal pain and diarrhoea

In early pregnancy, the key diagnosis to exclude is an ectopic pregnancy. Vaginal bleeding may be absent. Fainting and dizziness would not usually occur with gastroenteritis unless there is significant dehydration, but is seen with hypovolaemia from blood loss. A pregnancy test is essential to rule out pregnancy in women of childbearing age with abdominal pain.

Abdominal pain and diarrhoea can also be symptoms of intra-abdominal sepsis. See also Chapter 21 on abdominal emergencies.

Table 4.1 Differential diagnosis of breathlessness in pregnancy (not comprehensive)

Condition	Signs	Symptoms	Investigations	Treatment
Asthma	Expiratory wheeze	Cough, wheeze often nocturnal/seasonal. May be a known condition or first presentation	Usually none, CXR and blood gas if severe	Oxygen, bronchodilators, steroids, theophylline
Pulmonary embolus	See Chapter 11	Sudden onset, pleuritic pain, haemoptysis	CXR, CTPA or VQ scan, ECG, blood gas	Oxygen, anticoagulation, surgery if severe
Pneumonia	Tachypnoea, bronchial breathing, crepitations, fever	Cough, fever, unwell Increased susceptibility to viral pneumonia	CXR, CRP, WBC, blood gas	Oxygen, antibiotics, antivirals
Pulmonary oedema	Tachypnoea, inspiratory crepitations, raised JVP	Orthopnoea, paroxysmal nocturnal dyspnoea, frothy pink sputum, ? chest pain, ? known heart disease	CXR, blood gas, ECG, echocardiogram	Oxygen, diuretics, inotropic support if needed
Pulmonary hypertension	Loud second sound on heart auscultation	Breathing worse on exertion	CXR, ECG, echocardiogram	Cardiac support
Diabetic ketoacidosis	Signs of dehydration, Kussmaul breathing	No respiratory symptoms except tachypnoea, ketotic odour	Blood glucose, blood gas	Normal saline, infusion, insulin, see Chapter 22

Anxiety and distress

Symptoms of anxiety can be due to serious medical conditions but are sometimes attributed to 'baby blues' meaning serious pathology can go unrecognised. A full set of observations should be taken if there is an elevated level of anxiety and the MEOWS chart completed. In addition, guidance from *Saving Mothers' Lives* (2011) suggests that the questions in Box 4.2 are considered.

Box 4.2

- Is there is a clear pathway to symptom production?
- Is there is a known previous psychiatric history and is it relevant now?
- Do the symptoms represent a marked change from normal function?
- Are the only psychological symptoms behavioural and nonspecific e.g. distress and agitation?

Complete the MEOWS chart also when symptoms may not be communicated clearly because the woman does not speak English or is from an ethnic minority group.

If there is uncertainty about the woman's condition, the mental state exam should be performed.

Summary

- There should be systematic measurements of vital signs, which should be plotted on a MEOWS chart.
- There should be an understanding of the triggering of escalation with medical review.
- Deterioration can be rapid and understanding worrying symptoms and signs should raise vigilance.
- In order to reduce the maternal mortality rate from serious illness occurring in pregnancy, labour and the puerperium, a high level of awareness of clinical signs followed by prompt, informed emergency management by senior clinicians is required.

Further reading

1 Centre for Maternal and Child Enquiries (CMACE). Saving Mothers' Lives: reviewing maternal deaths to make motherhood safer: 2006–8. The Eighth Report on Confidential Enquiries into Maternal Deaths in the United Kingdom. *Br J Obstet Gynaecol.* 2011; 118(Suppl. 1):1–203.

APPENDIX 4A

Blood gas interpretation

Current intensive care practice is to measure both arterial blood gases and lactate together

Arterial blood gas is useful to determine physiological disturbance and monitor the effects of therapy. Modern analysers are usually able to measure the blood lactate, a product of anaerobic metabolism and marker of the state of the microcirculation. In all kinds of shock, elevated blood lactate levels can be used to predict mortality, and in septic shock the development of multiple organ failure is predicted more reliably than by basic observations. Failure to respond to therapy is associated with a higher mortality. Even haemodynamically stable patients with raised lactate levels, a condition referred to as compensated shock, are at increased risk of death. Lactate measurements >4 mmol/l can be taken as a marker of severe illness and used as a trigger to start resuscitation (see sepsis Chapter 6).

Interpretation

Normal values for both the nonpregnant and the pregnant state are in Table 4A.1 below. The key physiological fact is that increased acidity of the blood reaching the brain stem increases respiratory rate and volume promptly. Change in pH reaching the kidneys triggers a slower response in terms of variation in excretion of hydrogen ions and retention of bicarbonate. To interpret a blood gas, review the following:

- check the pH value to determine the direction of primary change (acidosis or alkalosis), compensation is always incomplete
- check $PaCO_2$, which is determined by breathing (alveolar ventilation): a low PCO_2 (hyperventilation) indicates a respiratory alkalosis or respiratory compensation for a metabolic acidosis; a raised PCO_2 (hypoventilation) indicates respiratory acidosis – note that PCO_2 does not rise to compensate for a metabolic alkalosis
- check standard bicarbonate (the bicarbonate value adjusted to what it would have been if the PCO_2 were normal): if the standard bicarbonate is raised then there is either a metabolic alkalosis or metabolic compensation for a respiratory acidosis; if the standard bicarbonate is low then there is either a metabolic acidosis or metabolic compensation for a respiratory alkalosis
- check base excess, if it is negative then there is a metabolic acidosis; if it is positive then a metabolic alkalosis

- check PaO_2 (normal values 11–13kPa): if it is low, then the patient is hypoxaemic. If the patient was receiving oxygen then the PaO_2 would be expected to be approximately FIO_2 (inspired oxygen fraction) minus 5 (in kPa). If the measured arterial PaO_2 is significantly lower, the patient has a gas exchange problem in the lungs; check how much inspired oxygen the patient is receiving.

Table 4A.1 Blood gases in nonpregnant and pregnant women

	pH	pCO_2	St bicarb	Base excess	
Normal values	7.34–7.44	4.7–6.0 kPa	21–27 mmol/l	–2 to +2 mmol/l	
Values in pregnancy	7.40–7.46 *increased*	3.7–4.2 kPa *decreased*	18–21 mmol/l *decreased*		
Respiratory acidosis	↓	↑	↑	+ve	Hypoventilation leading eventually to compensatory renal retention of bicarbonate
Respiratory alkalosis	↑	↓	↓	–ve	Hyperventilation leading to renal excretion of bicarbonate
Metabolic acidosis	↓	↓	↓	–ve	Excess metabolic acid leading to respiratory hyperventilation to compensate Raised lactate in most types of shock
Metabolic alkalosis	↑		↑	+ve	Excess metabolic alkali but no respiratory compensation

Radiology in the pregnant woman

Imaging, using ionising radiation, is often part of the management of seriously ill patients. Patients and healthcare workers are concerned that the doses of radiation used may be harmful to the fetus. Units of radiation are measured in the UK in the SI units of grays and sieverts. The unit ***gray*** measures the *absorbed dose* of radiation (*D*), absorbed by *any* material. The unit ***sievert*** measures the *equivalent dose* of radiation (*H*), supposed to have a damaging effect equivalent to the same dose of gamma rays.

Both the gray (Gy) and the sievert (Sv) are SI-derived units, defined as a unit of energy (joule) per unit of mass (kilogramme):

$$1\,\text{Gy} = 1\,\text{Sv} = 1\,\text{J/kg}$$

The naturally occurring background dose of radiation in the UK is less than 2 mSv. The lethal dose of radiation needed to kill 50% of fetuses is 1 Gy. For adults it is 3–5 Gy. The risk of radiation causing malignancy or developmental damage depends on the dose and the age of development of the fetus. Data from the Centre for Disease Control and Prevention estimate that in fetuses between the ages of 8–15 weeks there may be a reduction in IQ scores and severe mental impairment with doses of radiation between 50 and 500 mGy.

Table 4A.2 Approximate fetal doses from conventional X-ray examinations – data from the UK, 1998 (Dr C. Nelson Piercy)

Examination	Mean (mGy)	Maximum (mGy)
Abdomen	1.4	4.2
Chest	< 0.01	<0.01
Intravenous urogram: lumbar spine	1.7	10
Pelvis	1.1	4.0
Skull: thoracic spine	<0.01	<0.01
Head CT	<0.005	<0.005
Chest CT	0.06	1.0
Abdomen CT	8.0	49
Pelvis CT	25	80
Perfusion scan		0.8
Ventilation scan		0.1
CTPA/Helical CT		0.13

It can be seen from Table 4A.2 that the majority of imaging techniques required for seriously ill patients deliver acceptably small doses of radiation to the fetus.

Imaging in pregnant women should be carefully discussed with the radiology teams, but rarely denied on the basis of risk to the fetus in a serious maternal illness.

ALGORITHM 5.1 Shock

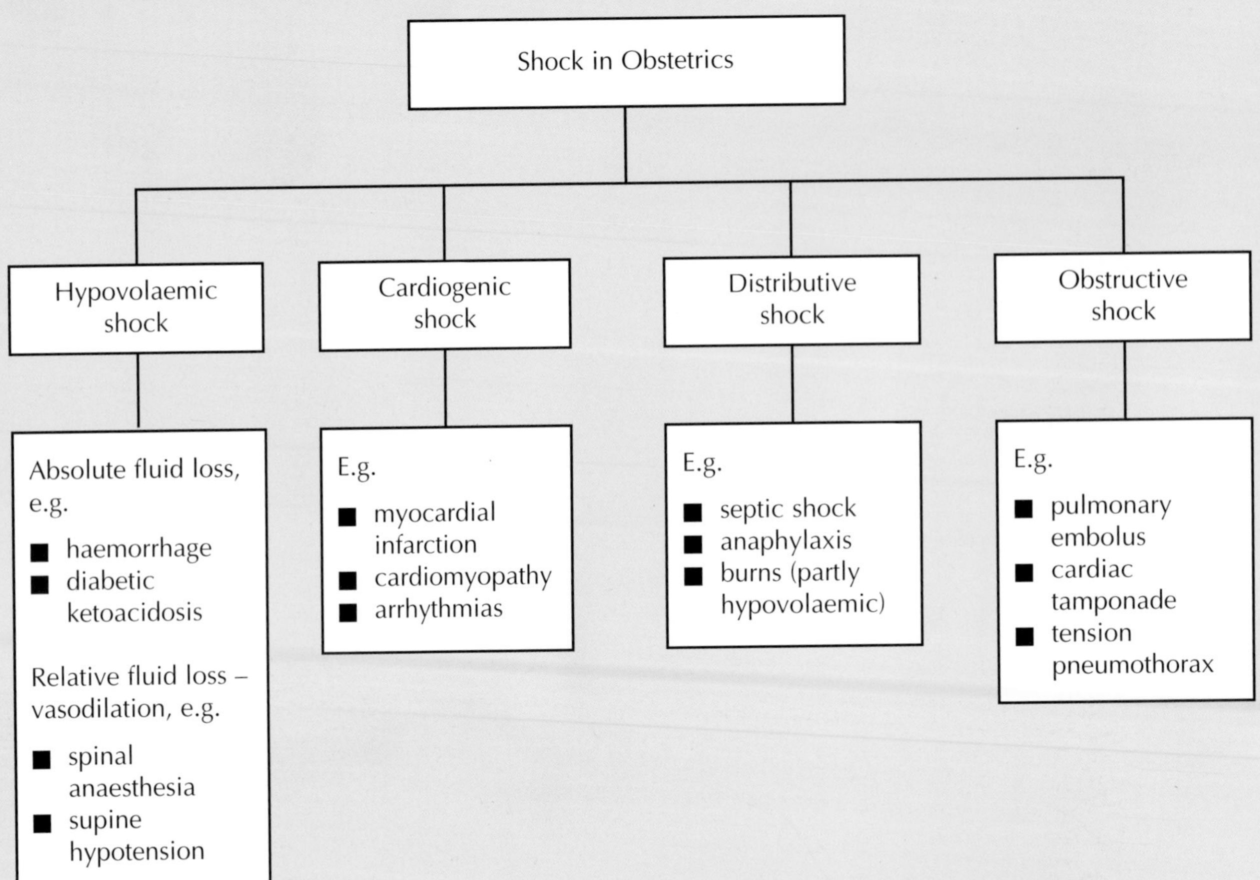

CHAPTER 5

Shock

Objectives

On successfully completing this topic, you will be able to:

- define and recognise shock
- discuss the principles of treatment of hypovolaemic shock
- understand the physiological changes to the cardiovascular system in pregnancy and how they affect the presentation of hypovolaemia
- identify other shock syndromes and understand their management.

Introduction

Definition and general pathophysiology of shock

The pathophysiological basis of all forms of shock is the inability of cells to obtain or utilise adequate oxygen and nutrients to meet their metabolic demands and dispose of their waste products.

While certain haemodynamic disturbances are considered to characterise different forms of shock, there is evidence that there is a significant overlap of these haemodynamic characteristics. Bedside clinical examination to arrive at a definitive diagnosis is helpful in that only half of patients present with shock. A high index of suspicion, a multidisciplinary team approach and focused investigations are important to diagnose and treat these life-threatening conditions promptly.

Shock caused by the inability of cells to receive oxygen represents a failure of cardiovascular adaptation to systemic challenges, for example, blood loss or sepsis. The challenge has, in effect, overwhelmed the emergency responses of the body. This results in decreased cellular perfusion due to either a drop in cardiac output or a drop in perfusion pressure, or both. Tissue perfusion is dependent on both adequate flow (cardiac output) and a good perfusion pressure (blood pressure).

Cardiac output is the product of stroke volume, i.e. blood pumped out of the heart each beat, and heart rate.

Stroke volume is dependent on preload (filling status), cardiac contractility (pumping strength) and the afterload (vascular resistance) against which the myocardium has to pump. Hence, shock could result if any of the above components suffer compromise and is broadly classified depending on whether this compromise is evident.

During normal homeostasis, organ perfusion is regulated by local metabolic and microcirculatory factors within a wide range of arterial pressure. This is called autoregulation. The flow of blood into the organ, beyond these arterial pressure limits of autoregulation, is primarily determined by the pressure differential between the arterial and venous systems. Local factors no longer play an important part in regulating blood flow to the organs.

There is a hierarchy in the set limits for autoregulation among different organs. The lower limit of autoregulation is set at a lower level for organs supporting vital functions, i.e. blood supply will be maintained to vital organs at a lower limit of blood pressure than nonvital organs. This is a protective adaptation, to preserve life in times of adversity. Unfortunately for the fetus, the uterine, hence placental, blood supply is nonessential in the face of a life-threatening challenge to the mother.

In shocked states, blood is preferentially supplied to the brain and the heart at the expense of perfusion elsewhere. The identification of which organs are deprived of perfusion gives the clinician vital clues during clinical examination to diagnose and quantify the degree of shock. This compensatory adaptation involves the shutting down of blood flow to the feto-placental unit, so that blood loss in the mother may first be reflected by fetal distress. Along with other signs of shock in pregnancy, fetal monitoring gives the clinician another sensitive indicator for monitoring the mother's wellbeing.

Types of shock: specific pathophysiology

Shock can be classified into four types, as follows:

- hypovolaemic shock
- cardiogenic shock
- distributive shock
- obstructive shock.

In order to differentiate between these types of shock, clues can be gained from the history, careful examination, selected additional tests and the response to treatment.

Hypovolaemic shock: insufficient preload

- absolute loss of fluid: haemorrhage or fluid loss, e.g. diabetic ketoacidosis
- relative loss of fluid: vasodilatation, e.g. spinal/epidural anaesthesia.

Absolute hypovolaemia – blood loss, fluid loss

This form of shock is due to a drop in the effective circulating volume resulting in a decrease in venous return. This causes a drop in stroke volume. There is a compensatory increase in heart rate to preserve cardiac output and also a compensatory increase in vascular resistance. This results in vasoconstriction, due to endogenous catecholamine release, as a compensation for hypovolaemia, thereby causing the diastolic pressure to rise to maintain perfusion pressure for vital organs, i.e. a narrowed pulse pressure. Compensatory fluid shifts occur from the extravascular space into the vascular compartment, resulting in intracellular dehydration and a sensation of thirst.

Circulatory volumes with reference to haemorrhage

During pregnancy we see an increase in plasma volume and red cell volume to make a total increase in circulating blood volume of approximately 40%. This means the volume increases from 70 ml/kg to 100 ml/kg, or 4900 ml to 7000 ml in a 70 kg woman. It is this expansion in circulating volume that allows the pregnant woman to lose 1200–1500 ml of blood before showing any signs of hypovolaemia (35% of her circulating blood volume) and, therefore, to compensate extremely well for blood loss. It is also the reason why we sometimes underestimate the severity of blood loss, occasionally even until the point of maternal collapse.

Relative hypovolaemia – vasodilatation due to regional anaesthesia

The effect of local anaesthetic on the sympathetic nervous control of blood vessels results in the hypotension seen with regional anaesthesia. In this circumstance, initially, a tachycardia is seen, accompanying a fall in diastolic pressure as the circulation has lost the compensatory mechanism mentioned above due to nerve blockade. Systolic blood pressure will then fall as a relatively early sign compared with blood loss, as mentioned above. Further ascent of the block will result in an apparent paradoxical fall in heart rate, caused by blockade of the sympathetic supply to the heart. This leaves the vagal nerve supply to the heart unopposed, hence the apparently inappropriate bradycardia seen.

The above paragraph explains why women under regional anaesthesia are very dependent on the attendants paying close attention, as their own physiological responses to crisis have been overridden.

Postural supine hypotension

In the heavily pregnant woman in a supine position, the uterus may lie on the vena cava and reduce the venous return to the heart. Vena caval and aortic compression may reduce cardiac output by up to 30%. This is known as supine hypotension syndrome.

Hypotension due to any other cause is exacerbated by vena caval obstruction. To prevent this, the heavily pregnant woman should be lying in the lateral position, or tilted 30° to the left, or have the uterus manually displaced to the left, to reduce the pressure on the inferior vena cava (Figure 5.1).

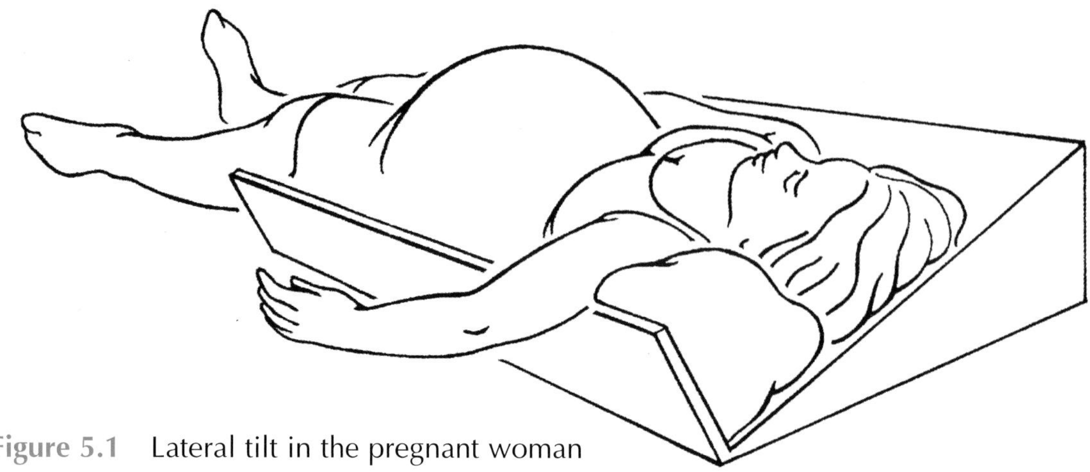

Figure 5.1 Lateral tilt in the pregnant woman

To prompt uterine tilt early in the process of resuscitation, remember:

'Hello. How are you Mrs Tilt?'

This effect is marked in the situation of relative hypovolaemia caused by regional blockade, where compensatory vasoconstriction in response to hypovolaemia is restricted, apart from the upper limbs, due to blockade of the sympathetic nervous system.

Cardiogenic shock – reduced cardiac contractility

The causes of cardiogenic shock include:

- ischaemic heart disease
- cardiomyopathy
- arrhythmias.

In this form of shock, patients may present with chest pain, shortness of breath and orthopnoea. The features overlap many of the signs seen in hypovolaemic shock, e.g. tachycardia, cool peripheries and sweating. The distinguishing features include orthopnoea and presence of signs of pulmonary congestion, such as a raised jugular venous pressure and basal pulmonary crackles. Cyanosis is more likely to be a feature.

Distributive shock – abnormal vascular resistance and fluid distribution

The following pathologies can result in distributive shock:

- septic shock
- anaphylaxis
- burns.

Septic shock

In this form of shock (see also Chapter 6), the patients have signs and symptoms of systemic inflammation along with the features of the disease causing the sepsis. The primary process causing the shock in this condition is profound vasodilatation and hence these patients sometimes have warm peripheries, particularly early in the process, despite being in shock. There is a compensatory tachycardia and increase in cardiac output to maintain perfusion pressure.

Varying degrees of organ dysfunction are seen, depending on the duration and degree of sepsis. The very sick septic patient will progress to vasoconstriction, with cold extremities, in the advanced stages.

Anaphylactic shock

Anaphylaxis is a severe, life-threatening, generalised, systemic, hypersensitivity reaction to a trigger agent in which histamine, serotonin and other vasoactive substances are released. Anaphylactic and anaphylactoid reactions are indistinguishable and managed in the same way. They have a different immunological mechanism. Anaphylactic reactions usually begin within 5–10 minutes of exposure to the drug or other allergen and the full reaction usually evolves within 30 minutes.

Serial serum tryptase estimations are helpful in the diagnosis of anaphylaxis. Tryptase enzyme is released from mast cells and it parallels histamine release. Peak concentrations well above 20 ng/ml indicate true anaphylaxis/anaphylactic reaction. The peak value of tryptase in the serum occurs between 30 minutes to 6 hours after an anaphylactic reaction. It is very important to take samples at the time of the acute event, both early and delayed, as the rise and fall of tryptase will be used in making the diagnosis. Later investigation, after the acute event, will involve skin testing. The value of skin tests, and especially the prick test, has been shown in extensive studies. This demonstrates the presence of specific IgE antibodies.

There are estimated to be 500 severe reactions in the UK each year. The estimated intraoperative incidence is between one in 3500 and 20 000 per year. History of atopy is present in less than 50% of patients.

All drugs can cause anaphylaxis. Intravenous drugs cause reactions more commonly than oral preparations and the most frequent trigger agents are anaesthetic muscle relaxants and antibiotics. *Latex sensitivity* is more common in the pregnant than the nonpregnant female population and in a patient with latex allergy, repeated vaginal examination with gloves containing latex, and other exposure to latex can lead to anaphylaxis.

The clinical pathology here is characterised by profound vasodilatation and fluid leakage due to the release of the vasoactive mediators, hence the classification as distributive shock as there is no overt loss of fluid. As the condition progresses, there is a massive leakage of fluid from the intravascular compartment into the tissues, which is seen externally as severe tissue swelling, particularly, obvious facial swelling. Internally, this results in laryngeal and pulmonary oedema, leading to respiratory collapse. The leakage of intravascular fluid and the vasodilatation results in cardiovascular collapse. Morbidity and mortality are related to cerebral hypoxia as a consequence of inadequate resuscitation.

Burns

The direct effect of the burn trauma causes fluid loss leading to hypovolaemic shock. In addition, the inflammatory mediators released cause a massive leak of fluid into the tissues resulting in a problem of distribution. This topic is discussed further in Chapter 20.

Obstructive shock

Obstructive shock can result from the following:

- massive pulmonary embolism (Chapter 11)
- cardiac tamponade (Chapter 15)
- tension pneumothorax (Chapter 15).

This form of shock is due to a reduction in venous return to the heart. Patients, if conscious, are very dyspnoeic and are invariably sitting upright gasping for breath. Extreme tachycardia is a compensatory mechanism for compromised cardiac output. There will also be associated features of the pathology causing the obstruction of blood flow.

Types of shock: clinical issues and clinical management

The signs and symptoms seen in the various forms of shock are primarily due to organ dysfunction resulting from inadequate tissue perfusion. The presentation is also partly influenced by the pathology causing the shock syndrome.

Hypovolaemic shock

This is the most common form of shock encountered on the labour ward.

The signs of hypovolaemia are:

- increase in heart rate
- cold, pale, sweaty, cyanosed skin with delayed capillary refill
- alteration of mental state
- fall in urine output
- narrowed pulse pressure
- hypotension (late sign).

Increase in heart rate

An increase in the heart rate is an early compensation for hypovolaemia or vasodilatation, both of which can cause hypotension and shock. A maternal heart rate of greater than 100 beats/minute should be considered sinister, until proven otherwise. Most, but not all, women will demonstrate a tachycardia if bleeding significantly, but paradoxical bradycardia has also been observed; cervical stimulation from both blood clots or peritoneal irritation can stimulate the parasympathetic nervous system.

Skin, capillary refill, mental state and urine output

The skin, kidneys and brain can be thought of as 'end organs' that reflect the adequacy of perfusion to tissues.

Capillary refill time (CRT)

This is an indication of skin perfusion. It can be assessed by compressing a fingernail, or pressing on the sternum, for 5 seconds. The test is normal if colour returns within 2 seconds of releasing compression (i.e. a CRT of less than 2 seconds – the time taken to say the words 'capillary refill'). If the patient is in a cold environment, CRT, especially peripherally, will be unreliable.

Mental state

If the woman is conscious and talking sensibly, she is not only breathing through an open airway, she is perfusing her cerebral cortex with sufficient oxygenated blood (50% of the normal cardiac output). Increasing hypovolaemia and subsequent cerebral hypoxia cause alterations in the level of consciousness. These alterations may begin with agitation and, if untreated, may proceed through confusion and aggression to eventual unresponsiveness and death.

Narrowed pulse pressure

This is caused by an increase in diastolic blood pressure, that reflects vasoconstriction occurring due to endogenous catecholamine release as a compensation for hypovolaemia.

Systolic hypotension

The sign most commonly referred to in the context of shock, hypotension, is a very late sign, developing only when significant blood loss has occurred. Successful outcome for the patient depends on the early recognition of shock, restoration of volume and control of haemorrhage.

Recognition of hypovolaemia

Maternal blood loss can be categorised into four classes of increasing severity, as shown in Table 5.1 and graphically in Figure 5.2.

To remember the different percentages in these classes of blood loss, think of the way of scoring in a tennis match!

Figure 5.2 illustrates the various clinical signs seen in ongoing acute blood loss suffered by a pregnant mother related to the volume lost. The point where the pulse rate is a higher number than the systolic blood pressure is clearly a very serious warning sign.

Pitfalls in the recognition of shock in pregnancy

Some common pitfalls are listed here:

- some pregnant women do not mount a tachycardia, or can even produce a bradycardia, which is very misleading and makes the recognition of serious haemorrhage very difficult (see explanation above)

- women with pacemakers have a fixed upper heart rate
- athletes may have a very slow baseline heart rate
- women on beta-blockers are relatively unable to mount a tachycardia
- haemoglobin level may be a useful measure of acute blood loss, but only after there has been fluid resuscitation.

In the very acute phases of loss, the haemoglobin measurement will not change. However, the rapid movement of fluid from the extracellular space into the intravascular compartment in compensation for the loss, or the provision of intravenous fluids to restore circulating volume, will result in a fall in haematocrit. It is always worth tracking the haematocrit if there is any suspicion of haemorrhage, as this may be the only indicator of a slow steady bleed. If the haematocrit has fallen quickly with early signs of hypovolaemia, this is suggestive of very severe loss.

Table 5.1 Severity of blood loss during maternal haemorrhage

Class	Loss of circulating volume %	Amount in a 70 kg pregnant woman	Signs and symptoms
I	0–15	<1000	Fully compensated due to blood diversion from the splanchnic pool. No symptoms. Minimal tachycardia is likely to be the only abnormal sign. No treatment needed in otherwise healthy woman as long as the bleeding has stopped.
II	15–30	1000–2000	Peripheral vasoconstriction maintains systolic blood pressure. The woman may be aware of increased heart rate and may display agitation or aggression. Narrowed pulse pressure and tachypnoea are the keys to early detection, as heart rate is only modestly increased and systolic blood pressure remains normal. Peripheral vasoconstriction maintains blood pressure. Requires crystalloid fluid replacement.
III	30–40	2000–2700	Cardiovascular system shows signs of decompensation. The woman will look unwell. Tachycardia, tachypnoea, changes in mental status, fall in systolic blood pressure. Will require crystalloid, colloid and blood transfusion.
IV	>40	>2700	Immediately life threatening. Tachycardia, fall in blood pressure, altered mental status, evidence of negligible urine output. Loss of >50% results in loss of consciousness, requiring immediate surgery as well as massive transfusion.

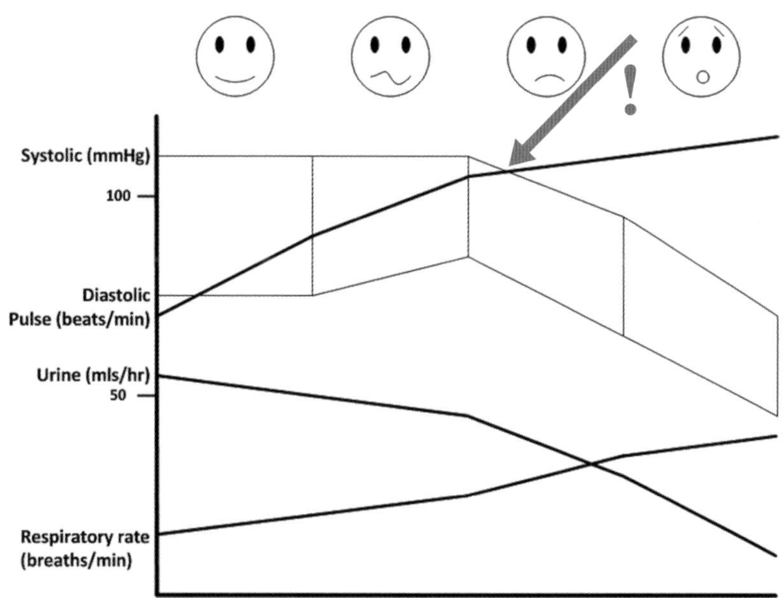

Figure 5.2 Clinical parameters following increasing blood loss in the pregnant and post-partum woman

Principles of treatment

Hypovolaemic shock

Primary survey and resuscitation according to the ABC principles. See Chapter 8 for the management of A and B.

C – Circulation:

Diagnosis of hypovolaemic shock must be promptly followed by:

- restoration of adequate circulating volume (see Chapter 7 for intravenous fluids)
- stopping the bleeding (see Chapter 25 for major obstetric haemorrhage).

Consider haemorrhage to be of two types:

- compressible
- noncompressible.

Compressible haemorrhage is controllable by direct pressure, limb elevation, packing, or by reduction and immobilisation of fractures or, in obstetric situations, compression of the uterus.

Noncompressible haemorrhage may be found in a body cavity (chest, abdomen, pelvis or retroperitoneum). See Chapters 15, 16 and 19 for haemorrhage in trauma.

Septic shock

Septic shock is a recognised complication of delivery, where the source of infection will be the genital tract, but could occur with any source of infection, for example, a urinary tract or chest infection.

The mechanism of shock is one of vasodilatation caused by bacterial toxins. Septic patients have a metabolic acidosis, detectable on sampling of arterial or venous blood.

In trauma patients, sepsis is unlikely to cause shock at presentation. It is most likely to occur in patients with penetrating abdominal injuries and in whom the peritoneal cavity has been contaminated by intestinal contents.

The key to management is a high degree of suspicion, rapid diagnosis and urgent treatment, as perinatal sepsis is a rapidly progressive disease. See Chapter 6 for further information on maternal septic shock.

Cardiogenic shock

Myocardial dysfunction may occur, following myocardial infarction or cardiomyopathy, resulting in cardiogenic shock.

In trauma, patients can develop cardiogenic shock due to myocardial contusion. Tension pneumothorax can cause profound shock that is not directly due to a myocardial problem, but has similar symptoms. Massive pulmonary embolism can present with features of acute right heart failure caused by an increase in the afterload on the right ventricle.

There is a significant overlap in the signs and symptoms between these forms of shock and hypovolaemic shock. One distinguishing feature is the extreme air hunger and orthopnoea seen in patients suffering cardiogenic shock. Listening to the chest may give clues of congestion due to increased pressure in the pulmonary circulation.

Patients in shock due to suspected coronary disease, pulmonary embolism and cardiomyopathy should be referred to medical and critical care teams early. These patients have a high mortality and should be looked after by a multidisciplinary team in critical care units. Treatment may include early recourse to ventilation, vasopressors and inotropes.

Anaphylactic shock: symptoms and treatment

The diagnosis is made on clinical grounds.

Symptoms can include:

- pruritus, erythema, flushing, urticaria, angio-oedema
- nausea, diarrhoea, vomiting
- stridor due to laryngeal oedema
- wheeze due to bronchospasm
- alteration in mental state; extreme anxiety or panic, then loss of consciousness due to respiratory distress and cardiovascular collapse.

Management:

- stop administration of drug(s)/blood product likely to have caused anaphylaxis
- resuscitation as for any collapse following ABC principles
- the key treatment therapies are *oxygen, adrenaline* and *fluids*.

1 Adrenaline/epinephrine – 0.5 mg (0.5 ml of 1:1000) intramuscularly every 5 minutes until improvement in pulse and blood pressure. Intravenous adrenaline may be used by experienced (anaesthetic) staff in a monitored patient 50 microgram boluses (0.5 ml of 1:10 000) in divided doses titrated against response. Give at a rate of 0.1 mg/minute and stop when a response has been obtained.
2 Intravascular volume expansion with crystalloid e.g. Hartmann's solution. Large volumes are often required.
3 Antihistamines: chlorphenamine 10 mg by slow intravenous infusion.
4 Corticosteroids: hydrocortisone 200 mg intravenously.

Continually reassess airway, breathing and circulation.
In the case of airway oedema, it may be appropriate to give 5 ml adrenaline 1:1000 by nebuliser. Early intubation may be required for severe stridor, or respiratory collapse. Delay may increase the difficulty of the intubation.

- Consider bronchodilators if there is persistent bronchospasm, e.g. salbutamol, 2.5 mg via oxygen-driven nebuliser, or 250 microgram intravenously slowly, or aminophylline 250 mg slowly intravenously, or magnesium sulphate 2 g intravenously over 20 minutes.
- Consider catecholamine infusion if blood pressure still low: adrenaline (epinephrine) 0.05–0.10 microgram/kg/min (approximately 4–8 microgram/min); 4 mg adrenaline in 50 ml 5% dextrose solution 5–10 ml/h.
- Summon intensive care help and plan to insert arterial line and central venous line and transfer to a critical care unit.
- Check fetal heart and continuously monitor by CTG and consider timing and method of delivery. A severe reaction will often necessitate an urgent delivery if the mother's condition cannot be stabilised.

Following the incident, serial clotted blood samples should be sent looking for mast cell tryptase as evidence of histamine release (immediate, 2 hours and 24 hours) and liaise with the hospital laboratory. The patient will require referral to a specialist allergy centre.

Summary

- Hypovolaemia is the cause of shock in most obstetric and trauma patients.
- A high index of suspicion is essential during assessment to ensure early recognition and prompt resuscitation.
- In haemorrhagic shock, management requires replacement of lost volume and immediate control of haemorrhage either by direct compression, splintage or, where necessary, by urgent surgery.
- Other forms of shock require equal vigilance and early resuscitative measures to restore circulation and tissue perfusion.

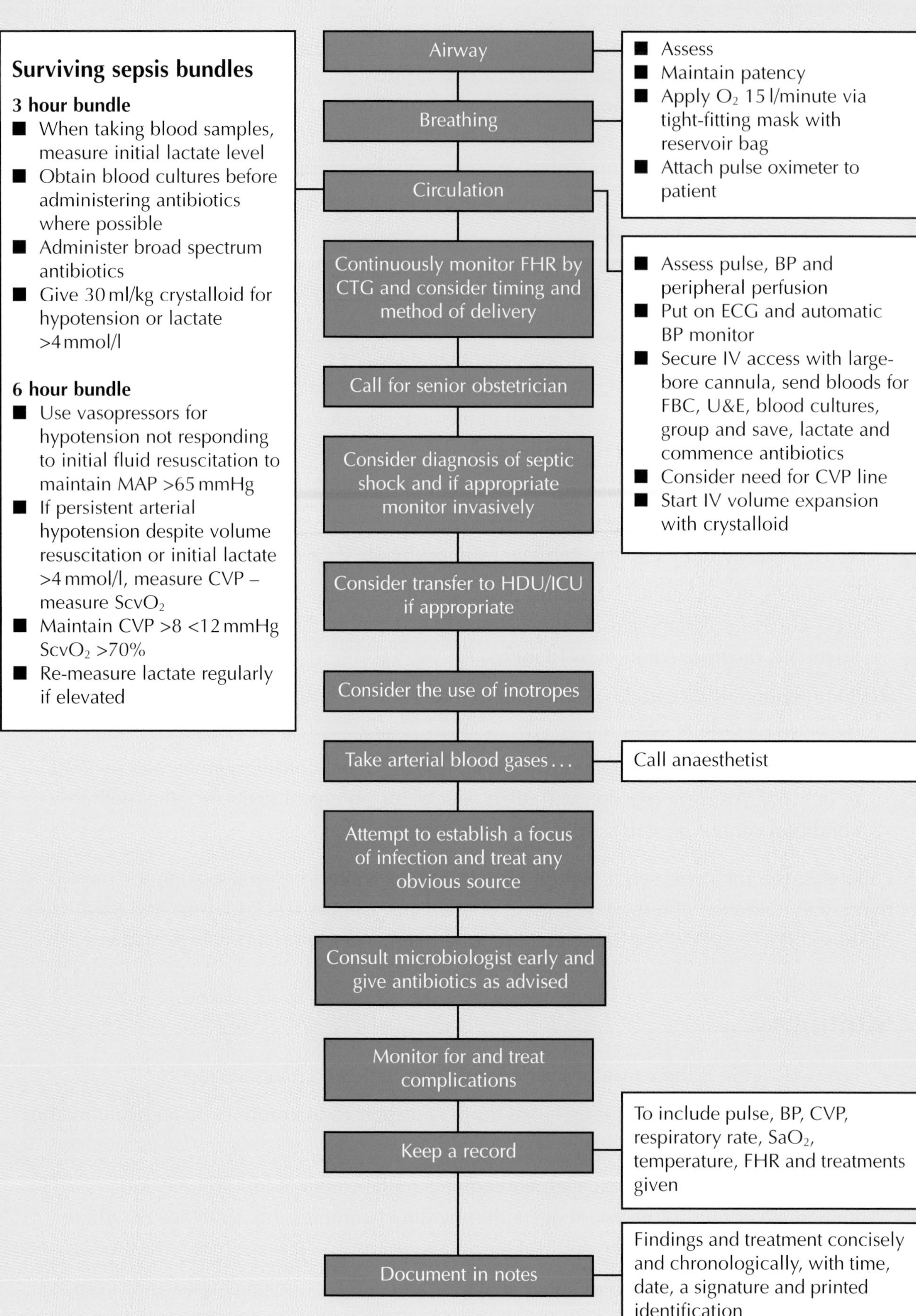

Surviving Sepsis campaign: http://www.survivingsepsis.org

CHAPTER 6

Sepsis

Objectives

On successfully completing this topic, you will be able to:

- discuss the pathophysiology of sepsis
- identify the septic patient
- commence supportive management
- arrange appropriate investigations and referral.

Terminologies

Different terminologies have been used to describe the various manifestations of sepsis; a brief account of these will help in understanding the syndrome. Sepsis, severe sepsis and septic shock are terms used to identify the continuum of the clinical response to severe infection (Figure 6.1).

Introduction and incidence

Sepsis is one of the five major causes of maternal morbidity and mortality worldwide. It accounts for 10% of maternal mortality in the developed world. This figure is higher in the developing world as septic abortions are seen more frequently. Pregnant women tend to be young and healthy. Only 0–4% of pregnant women who develop bacteraemia develop septic shock and of these, 2–3% die.

There are specific opportunities to improve the management of the condition. Clinical trials involving new therapeutic interventions have demonstrated, for the first time in 20 years, improved survival in patients with severe sepsis and septic shock. Improvements in mortality can be made by:

- having a high index of suspicion to allow earlier identification/diagnosis of sepsis
- adopting agreed standards of care for timely investigation and treatment.

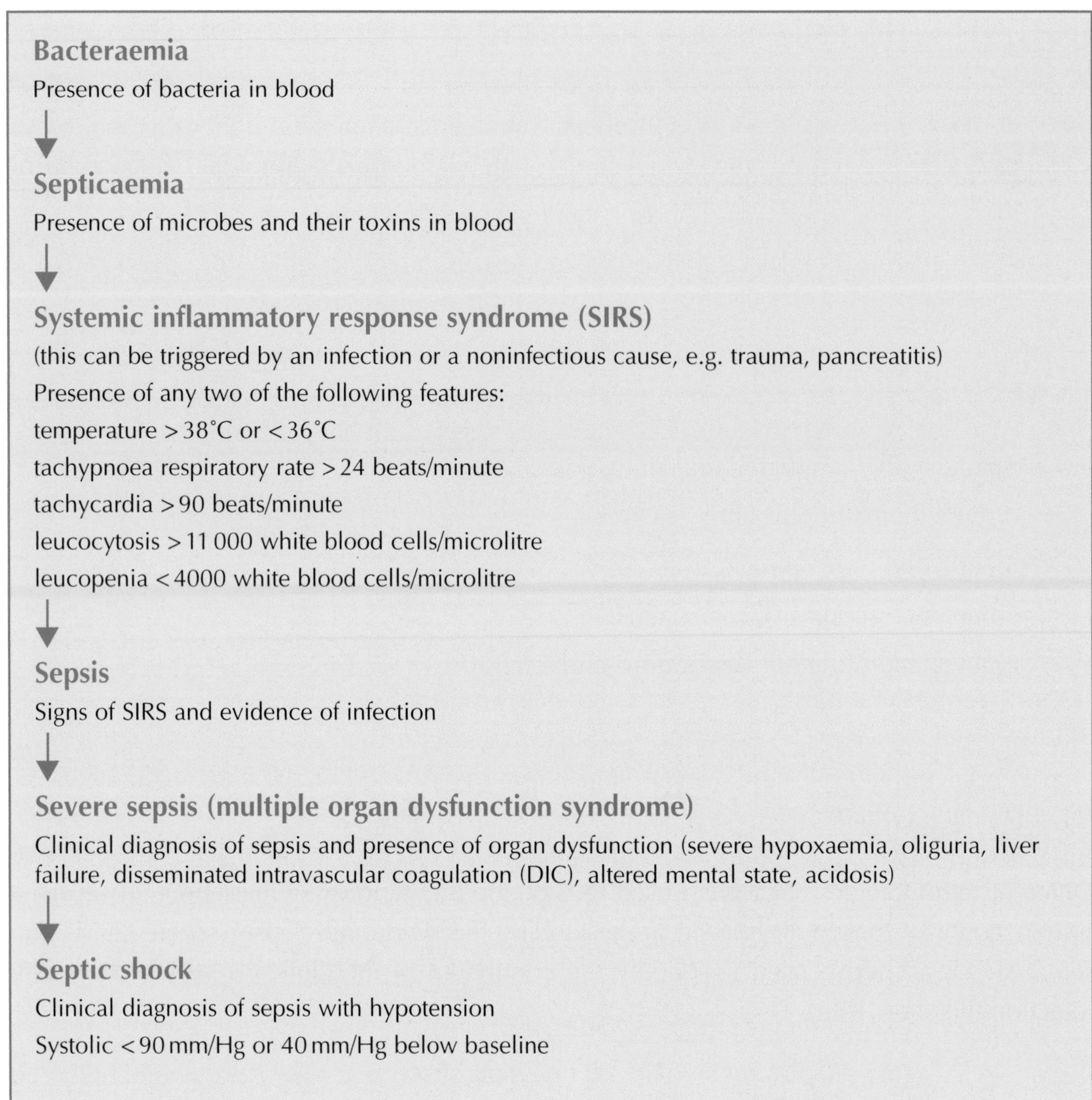

Figure 6.1 Continuum of the clinical response to severe infection

CMACE Report (2006–2008): Saving Mothers' Lives

Unlike other causes of direct deaths, the rate of maternal deaths from sepsis has risen in the latest report, and, for the first time since the inception of the report in 1952, it is now the leading cause of direct deaths. There were 29 deaths directly attributable to genital tract sepsis compared with nine in 1985–87. This has been a gradually rising trend. Substandard care was identified in 18 of 26 (69%) who died within 6 weeks of delivery. The report identified some necessary improvements to reduce deaths caused by sepsis, including education for front-line staff and encouragement to follow clear national guidelines for treatment. See Box 6.1 for causes of sepsis both within and outside the genital tract.

Box 6.1 Important causes of sepsis in obstetric patients

Pyelonephritis
Chorioamnionitis
Postpartum endometritis
Wound infection
Pneumonia, including influenza-associated respiratory infection
Acute appendicitis
Acute cholecystitis
Pancreatitis
Necrotising fasciitis
Mastitis

Microbiology

The most common microbes responsible for sepsis in the UK include *Streptococcus* Group A, B and D, followed by *Escherichia coli*. Other organisms that can cause sepsis include *Staphylococcus aureus* and the obligate anaerobic bacterium, *Fusobacterium necrophorum*.

Deaths in the latest report were most commonly due to beta-haemolytic Group A *Streptococcus*. This is not the same organism as the Group B *Streptococcus*, which is present in the vagina in many women, and may cause neonatal sepsis but is rarely a problem for the mother. Group A *Streptococcus* is a common skin or throat commensal, carried asymptomatically by up to 30% of the population. It is easily spread and is responsible for streptococcal sore throat, a very common childhood condition. Historically, puerperal fever was much more common prior to the advent of antibiotics and Group A streptococcus was responsible for the majority of infections and deaths.

Transmission in pregnant women is thought to be either through the throat as a portal of entry, or via the perineal route, even in the presence of intact membranes, as bacteria can cross this apparent barrier. Streptococcal infection has a seasonal rise in incidence between December and April. The link between pregnant women and children with Group A streptococcal sore throats is thought to be significant as a possible source of infection. In the past, there was an emphasis on the transmission of infection from caregivers to women, much reduced since the advent of strict hygiene practices in hospitals. It is thought that raising public health awareness of the risks from family members and encouraging women to follow appropriate personal hygiene practices may be helpful in reducing transmission of infection; in particular, pregnant women should be encouraged to handwash both before and after using the toilet to avoid transmitting organisms from other household members.

Other organisms seen in this latest report included: *E. coli*; *Clostridium septicum* (a compulsory anaerobe associated with gas gangrene); *Streptococcus pneumoniae*; *Morganella morganii* (Gram-negative gastrointestinal inhabitant acting as an opportunistic pathogen and resistant to beta lactam antibiotics) and one case of Panton-Valentine leucocydin (PVL) toxin producing methicillin-resistant *S. aureus* (MRSA).

Epidemiology

Groups of women over-represented in the deaths due to sepsis are women from minority ethnic groups, including asylum seekers and recent immigrants, as well as obese women. Lack of English language may have been a factor. Three women with sickle cell trait or disease died, suggesting that these women need particular care. Again, these cases were from ethnic minority groups.

The gestation at presentation and route of sepsis has been suggested as a useful method for defining cases for future comparisons, as each group may have differing methods of transmission and therefore prevention:

- unsafe abortion
- presenting with infection and ruptured membranes (genital tract sepsis)
- genital tract sepsis post delivery (including post-abortion/miscarriage)
- severe sepsis from the community, membranes intact, not in labour
- postpartum sepsis related to delivery but not involving the genital tract
- other coincidental infections, e.g. pneumonia.

Pathophysiology of sepsis

Inflammation represents the body's response to an insult, be it an infection or an injury. The initial response involves the release of primary mediators, interleukin-1 and tumour necrosis factor alpha. These are cytokines produced from activated macrophages. These primary mediators stimulate the production of secondary mediators that, in turn, activate coagulation and complement cascades. This is followed by the expression of anti-inflammatory mediators that help to contain the inflammation locally. This is the period during which there is immunoparesis. As with many other regulatory processes, there is a fine balance between the pro- and anti-inflammatory mediators.

In situations where the bacterial load is high, or there is an imbalance between pro- and anti-inflammatory mediators, inflammation becomes generalised resulting in severe sepsis. There is growing evidence that this fine balance is genetically controlled.

At a cellular level, the inducible form of nitric oxide synthase is stimulated. This causes overproduction of nitric oxide from endothelial cells, macrophages and muscle cells. Nitric oxide is the major mediator of vasodilatation and myocardial dysfunction, which result in hypotension. Superoxide radicals also react with nitric oxide to form peroxynitrate, which causes direct cellular injury.

Clinical manifestations of haemodynamic alterations

There is a decrease in arteriolar and venous tone. This causes venous pooling of blood and a drop in vascular resistance, resulting in hypotension. In the initial stages of sepsis, there is hypotension with reduced cardiac output and low filling pressures. With fluid resuscitation, cardiac output increases, resulting in a hyperdynamic circulation, but there is not much change in blood pressure owing to a reduced vascular resistance. There is an increase in pulmonary vascular resistance, resulting in raised pulmonary arterial pressures. The changes in the vascular tone differ in different vascular beds, resulting in the maldistribution of blood volume and flow. There is evidence to suggest that the ability of tissues to extract oxygen is impaired owing to mitochondrial dysfunction. This encourages anaerobic metabolism in tissues, promoting lactic acidosis.

Clinical issues and presentation

Sepsis is a complex syndrome that is difficult to define, diagnose and treat. Some of the signs and symptoms are rather vague and there is an overlap with other clinical conditions, such as placental abruption, ectopic pregnancy, influenza and gastroenteritis, resulting in an inappropriate level of clinical response.

Minimising risk from infection in the antenatal period, by avoiding unnecessary vaginal examinations and paying attention to hygiene, may reduce the incidence of sepsis. Early recognition and increased surveillance of those at risk including careful assessment of postnatal mothers, especially those with prolonged rupture of membranes, ragged membranes or possibly incomplete delivery of placenta and women with uterine tenderness or enlargement, will help to identify women developing serious infection.

A high index of suspicion and close surveillance will help in identifying women with early sepsis. There has been concern raised that maternity and community staff, who do not routinely work with sick patients, need to take much greater note of basic medical and nursing observations and care (see also Chapter 4, Recognising the seriously sick patient).

Symptoms may include:

- feeling unwell, anxiety or distress
- shivery or feverish or pyrexia
- sore throat, cough or influenza-like symptoms (pneumonia accounts for a significant number of admissions to ICU in pregnant women)
- chest pain
- vomiting and/or diarrhoea
- abdominal pain or wound tenderness
- breast tenderness, suggesting mastitis
- headache
- unexplained physical symptoms

- if pregnant, might report reduced fetal movements.

Serious clinical signs can be categorised as **Red Flag signs** as suggested by the latest CMACE report *Saving Mothers' Lives* see Box 6.2.

Box 6.2 Red flag signs

These include:

- feeling unwell including altered mental state, including unusual anxiety, agitation or reduced conscious level
- fever >38°C or hypothermia <36°C can be due to sepsis
- breathlessness: respiratory rate >20 can be related to pulmonary pathology or associated with the acidosis which accompanies severe sepsis (see below)
- tachycardia: persistently >100bpm
- prolonged capillary refill times as a measure of reduced cardiac output and effective peripheral perfusion
- hypotension with initially warm vasodilated peripheries, followed by cold extremities in advanced shock
- abdominal or chest pain – beware 'after pains' of a severity that is out of proportion to known cause and not responding to usual analgesia
- uterine or renal angle pain or tenderness
- diarrhoea and/or vomiting
- if pregnant, reduced fetal movements or an abnormal, or absent, fetal heart beat
- spontaneous rupture of membranes or offensive liquor or vaginal discharge
- persistent vaginal bleeding may be associated with uterine sepsis
- broken down perineum following birth trauma or other signs of sepsis

Monitoring and investigations

Use of a MEOWS chart may help identify early signs of deterioration. More advanced levels of observation will include hourly urine output, central venous pressure (CVP) measurement and estimates of cardiac output as practical. Regular blood gas measurements, giving serial lactate results, will help guide therapy.

Initial investigations should include:

- blood cultures – after which antibiotics can be started as appropriate (plus other swabs)
- serum lactate – ideally from an arterial sample, but a venous sample is often quicker. Any woman in whom sepsis is suspected, who has a lactate >4 mmol/l, needs to have resuscitation started immediately. Raised serum lactate is a marker for poor perfusion and tissue hypoxia from whatever cause and signifies severe illness.

- white blood cell (WBC) count which may be raised or lowered; WBC $<4 \times 10^9$ suggests severe infection
- raised C-reactive protein (CRP) can suggest early infection, which alerts staff to monitor closely
- haemoglobin level: anaemia may be present due to blood loss or haemolysis associated with sepsis
- isolated thrombocytopenia with no evidence of disseminated intravascular coagulation (DIC) is seen in more than 50% of patients
- coagulation screen, as DIC may be an accompanying feature
- renal and liver function.

Later complications include DIC, adult respiratory distress syndrome (ARDS), renal failure and hepatic failure, seen in 30–50% of patients with severe sepsis. One-third of patients who die, do so early because of refractory hypotension and the rest, who succumb late, die because of multiple organ failure.

The speed of deterioration cannot be overemphasised, so the speed of response required should not be underestimated. Puerperal sepsis can be insidious in onset and can progress rapidly to fulminating sepsis and death.

Starting treatment

DO NOT DELAY TREATMENT.

Begin resuscitation immediately in women with sepsis-induced hypotension or serum lactate >4 mmol/l. Do not wait for ICU help (although they should be informed). Every medical and nursing practitioner working with pregnant, or recently delivered, women should be aware of the cost of delay in this devastating condition. It may reach the point of being irreversible before the women can access appropriate levels of care if there is any delay on the part of the women themselves, the primary care teams or the hospital staff.

Management

Recommended by the Surviving Sepsis Campaign (www.survivingsepsis.org), which is detailed below and in its simplest terms includes:

- taking blood cultures before
- giving broad spectrum antibiotics intravenously promptly
- checking serum lactate
- fluids – crystalloid 30 ml/kg
- involving an intensivist if there is either hypotension or the lactate is >4 mmol/l (as volume support and/or vasopressors will be needed to maintain mean arterial pressure (MAP) >65 mmHg).

Much of the management will be carried out by an intensive care team, but initial recognition and early treatment can be started in the obstetric unit.

In severe sepsis, early goal-directed therapy of fluid resuscitation and aggressive haemodynamic management to predefined endpoints has been shown to reduce mortality. Two essential features of early goal-directed therapy include:

- maintaining an adequate central venous pressure to carry out other haemodynamic adjustments 8–12mmHg
- maximising mixed or central venous oxygen saturation (derived from blood gas analysis of a blood sample drawn from the central line).

The endpoints with any treatment include a normal, or above normal, cardiac output to help optimise oxygen delivery to the tissues. Despite aggressive management of septic shock, mortality is around 40%. During the course of sepsis, it is not uncommon for different organs to fail. The most common include renal, haematological, hepatic and gastrointestinal systems. Failing organs need support during this critical period; however, predicted mortality increases with increasing number of failed organs, approaching 85–100% with three or more organ failures.

Where?

Initial treatment anywhere, then will need transfer to HDU or ICU care if single or multiple organ failure.

Whom?

Involve senior staff early if sepsis suspected. Request help from anaesthetic or intensive care teams, microbiology and haematology as needed. Surgical and radiological help may be needed to identify and eradicate source of sepsis.

What?

1. Airway and breathing

Maintenance of adequate oxygenation is an important step in the resuscitation of women with sepsis. This includes a patent airway with adequate breathing and supplemental oxygen. Most patients in shock will ultimately need intubation and ventilation because of increased difficulty in breathing, development of ARDS or for primary underlying disease. Adoption of a lung-protective strategy with tidal volumes of 6 ml/kg and plateau pressures ≤30cmH_2O for mechanically ventilated patients is recommended.

Signs of respiratory insufficiency may be an indicator of onset of pulmonary oedema and need investigation and treatment urgently.

2. Circulation

(a) Fluids

Use up to 30 ml/kg crystalloid as an initial bolus of fluids over 30 minutes looking for haemodynamic improvement. Hydroxyethyl starches are **not** recommended; albumin solutions may be used as part of this volume. Early request for CVP measurements will help guide fluid therapy. Fluid requirements may be very large due to fluid maldistribution. Monitor haemodynamic measurements to ensure cardiac function and renal perfusion (may have to slow fluids if rising CVP without improvement in cardiac output or tissue perfusion).

Goals:

- MAP >65 mmHg
- CVP >8 mmHg if not ventilated, 12–15 mmHg if ventilated
- urine output > 0.5 ml/kg/h.

Fluid balance is difficult in septic shock, as there will be an inevitable tendency of fluid to leak into the lungs as a result of increased capillary permeability, myocardial dysfunction, renal impairment and a low plasma oncotic pressure. Ventilation will be required in these circumstances to counteract the effects of capillary leak and to support the myocardium.

Early expert advice is essential.

(b) Vasopressors

In patients who remain hypotensive, despite adequate fluid resuscitation, early recourse to vasopressor therapy is recommended with monitoring via an arterial catheter.

Goals:

- MAP >65 mmHg with arterial monitoring as soon as practical
- central venous oxygen saturation >70% or mixed venous >65%.

Noradrenaline administered centrally is the vasopressor of choice but can be started peripherally if urgent, preferably under guidance from the anaesthetic team. Adrenaline may be added if poorly responsive. Sensitivity to catecholamines is significantly altered in septic patients and they require much higher doses than in other clinical situations. Low-dose dopamine should not be used for renal protection.

3. Antibiotics

After obtaining blood cultures, give broad spectrum intravenous antibiotics (see Box 6.3) immediately and certainly within 1 hour of diagnosing severe sepsis or septic shock. DO NOT DELAY while awaiting results of cultures. Other swabs/fluids to be taken as clinically indicated e.g. throat, vaginal, urine, CSF. A microbiology consultation must be sought at an early stage to manage patients who are systemically ill.

Box 6.3 CEMACE advice on antibiotics (Check local protocols and doses before prescribing)

When woman not critically ill:

- co-amoxyclav 1.2 g 8 hourly plus metronidazole 500 mg 8 hourly (cephalosporin alternatives are given but not reproduced here).

If allergic to penicillin:

- clarithromycin 500 mg twice daily or clindamycin 600 mg–1.2 g three to four times daily plus gentamycin according to local protocol.

In severe sepsis or shock (seek advice):

- piperacillin–tazobactam 4.5 g 8 hourly or ciprofloxacin 600 mg 12 hourly plus gentamycin according to local protocol
- metronidazole may be added for anaerobic cover.

If Group A *streptococcus* suspected, clindamycin may be more effective than penicillin because it inhibits exotoxin production.

If there are risk factors for MRSA add teicoplanin 10 mg/kg 12 hourly for three doses, then 10 mg/kg 24 hourly or linezolid 600 mg twice daily. A full loading dose of each drug should be given, but then monitoring may be required for subsequent doses.

Treatment should be for at least 7–10 days.

4. Blood products

- Transfuse when Hb <7.0 g/dl to maintain an Hb of at least 7–9 g/dl.
- Fresh frozen plasma should be used to correct clotting abnormalities if there is active bleeding or a planned invasive procedure.
- Platelets may be needed if the count is <50×10^9/litre and surgical procedures or invasive procedures are planned. Otherwise, prophylactic platelet transfusion should be used when platelet count is <10×10^9/litre if no bleeding, or 20×10^9/litre if at high risk of bleeding.

5. Source identification and control of infection

- Identify source of infection as rapidly as possible; imaging may be required.
- Closed-space infections need surgical drainage, including evacuation of retained products of conception.
- In women with endometritis not responding to antibiotics, a septic pelvic thrombosis should be considered; these patients may require heparin together with antibiotics.
- Women not responding may have myometrial necrosis and/or abscess formation, which continue to seed into the bloodstream; in these cases, early surgical intervention, with possible recourse to hysterectomy, could save lives.

- Necrotising fasciitis is another condition that requires early surgical intervention with fasciotomy and aggressive antibiotic therapy.

Other therapies likely to be commenced in the ICU setting

6. Steroids

If hypotensive and unresponsive to fluids and vasopressors, give hydrocortisone, up to 200 mg/day. Corticosteroids should not be used in the absence of persistent shock.

Data published from a multicentre randomised trial from France has shown a better survival in patients given small-dose steroid supplementation. Preliminary data from a Cochrane meta-analysis, considering 15 randomised controlled trials of low- and high-dose corticosteroids in 2022 patients with septic shock, give further support for using hydrocortisone in septic shock.

7. Activated protein C

The inflammatory response in severe sepsis is integrally linked to procoagulant activity and endothelial activation. The inflammatory response in sepsis is procoagulant in the early stages.

However, Drotrecogin alfa (activated) – rhAPC – is no longer recommended for use in patients with sepsis.

8. Insulin

Insulin should be commenced when blood glucose is greater than 180 mg/dl and blood glucose should be maintained below this level with an insulin infusion.

9. Renal replacement

Using haemodialysis or continuous venovenous haemofiltration (CVVH). Bicarbonate should not be used to improve haemodynamic control if pH is >7.15.

Surviving Sepsis Campaign

Spearheaded by the European Society of Intensive Care Medicine (ESICM), International Sepsis Forum (ISF) and Society of Critical Care Medicine (SCCM), the Surviving Sepsis Campaign is aimed at improving the diagnosis, survival and management of patients with sepsis by addressing the challenges associated with it. The Surviving Sepsis programme aims to:

- increase awareness, understanding and knowledge
- change perceptions and behaviour
- increase the pace of change in patterns of care
- influence public policy
- define standards of care in severe sepsis

- reduce the mortality associated with sepsis by 25% over 5 years from inception.

The Surviving Sepsis Campaign, in collaboration with the Institute of Healthcare Improvement, has developed 'Sepsis change bundles' to improve the outcomes in sepsis. A 'bundle' is a group of interventions related to a disease process that, when executed together, result in better outcomes than when implemented individually. They have suggested groups of interventions to be achieved within 3 hours and then 6 hours after admission. Achievement of these standards can then be audited to spearhead further improvements in care.

Summary of sepsis management

1 High index of suspicion.
2 Act immediately.
3 Early antibiotics.
4 Monitor carefully.

Influenza A/H1N1

The recent two winter seasons have resulted in a surge of deaths due to influenza in young people. Pregnant women have been found to be seven times more likely to die from this illness than nonpregnant women in the same age group. Among this population:

- minority ethnic groups were over-represented
- clinical comorbidities contributed, e.g. asthma, paraplegia, scoliosis
- none of the women who died had been vaccinated
- presenting features were similar to any severe illness with tachycardia, tachypnoea and variable hypoxia
- CRP was unusually raised – not common with viral infections.

Treatment

There were a number of delays documented in the women who died in recognising the illness, both in making the diagnosis and in administering oseltamivir. Women died from pneumonia or ARDS and some from complications of the extracorporeal membrane oxygen (ECMO) treatment used to try to maintain oxygenation.

Recommendations:

- high index of suspicion
- good multidisciplinary team working and planning
- basic check of O_2 saturation in all women presenting with respiratory symptoms
- breathlessness as a symptom must be taken very seriously: remember it may be respiratory, cardiac or relate to a metabolic disturbance such as diabetic ketoacidosis
- viral swabs should be taken and antivirals started immediately

- antivirals can be started even if further imaging planned
- attention to infection control when admitted
- advice to pregnant women to be vaccinated with seasonal influenza vaccination.

Summary

- There is a rising mortality from sepsis in pregnancy and childbirth.
- Recognition, early aggressive therapy and early expert involvement are central to improving outcomes for those affected.
- Information on avoiding infection and reporting symptoms must be given to all women at risk.

References and further reading

1 Astiz ME, Rackow EC. Septic shock. *Lancet* 1998;351:1502–5.

2 Centre for Maternal and Child Enquiries (CMACE). Saving Mothers' Lives: reviewing maternal deaths to make motherhood safer: 2006–8. The Eighth Report on Confidential Enquiries into Maternal Deaths in the United Kingdom. *Br J Obstet Gynaecol* 2011; 118(Suppl. 1):1–203.

3 Faro S. Sepsis in obstetric and gynecology patients. *Curr Clin Top Infect Dis* 1999;19:1–82.

4 Hollenberg SM, Ahrens TS, Annane D, Astiz ME, Chalfin DB, Dasta JF, *et al.* Practice parameters for hemodynamic support of sepsis in adult patients: 2004 update. *Crit Care Med* 2004;32:1928–48.

5 Ledger WJ, Norman M, Gee C, Lewis W. Bacteremia in obstetric-gynaecologic service. *Am J Obstet Gynecol* 1975;121:205–12.

6 Parrillo JE, Parker MM, Natanson C, Suffredini AF, Danner RL, Cunnion RE, *et al.* Septic shock in humans. Advances in the understanding of pathogenesis, cardiovascular dysfunction, and therapy. *Ann Intern Med* 1990;113:227–42.

7 Rackow EC, Falk JL, Fein IA, Siegel JS, Packman MI, Haupt MT, *et al.* Fluid resuscitation in circulatory shock: a comparison of the cardiorespiratory effects of albumin, hetastarch, and saline solutions in patients with hypovolemic and septic shock. *Crit Care Med* 1983;11:839–50.

8 Task Force of American College of Critical Care Medicine. Practice parameters for haemodynamic support of sepsis in adult patients in sepsis. *Crit Care Med* 1999;27:639–56.

9 Dellinger RP, Levy MM, Rhodes A, *et al.* Surviving Sepsis Campaign: International guidelines for management of severe sepsis and septic shock. *Crit Care Med* 2013; 41:580–637.

10 Modder J. Review of Maternal Deaths in the UK related to A/H1N1 2009 Influenza (CMACE) 2010.

11 Surviving Sepsis campaign: http://www.survivingsepsis.org

ALGORITHM 7.1 Intravenous access and fluid replacement in shock (not cardiogenic collapse)

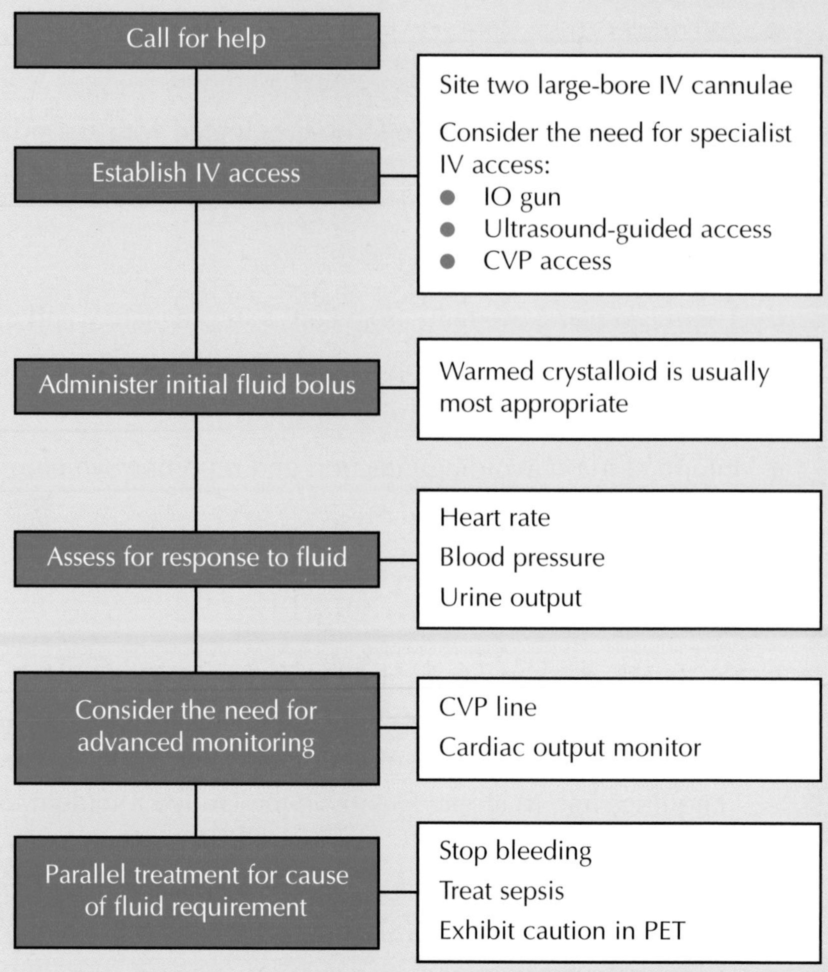

CHAPTER 7

Intravenous access and fluid replacement

Objectives

On successfully completing this topic, you will be able to:

- understand the reasons behind selection of cannula size and site
- appreciate alternatives to peripheral cannula placement
- understand fluid, blood and clotting product administration and monitoring in routine and complex clinical situations.

Intravenous access

Intravenous access is best achieved by inserting as large a cannula as possible into a large peripheral vein. Short, wide-bore cannulae deliver the fastest flow. The Hagen–Poiseuille equation describes the factors affecting the flow through a tube.

$$Q = \frac{\Delta P \pi r^4}{8 \eta l}$$

Where Q is flow, ΔP is pressure drop across the two ends of the tube, r is the radius of the tube, η is viscosity of the fluid and l is the length of the tube. The major variables we can control are ΔP, r and l.

The effect of ΔP can be demonstrated most simply by increasing the height of the infusion fluid above the patient. This will result in an observed increase in flow rate through the cannula. Simple pressure bags and more complex pneumatically controlled rapid infusion devices are available to maximise the effect on ΔP and subsequently flow rate. Great care must be taken with these devices to ensure the vein does not become damaged by the high pressure, with subsequent extravasation of fluid into the extravascular tissues, as well as the risk of delivering too much fluid too rapidly causing circulatory overload.

Because r is affected by the power 4, relatively small increases in internal diameter will have major changes on achieved flow rates. Table 7.1 demonstrates the effect on flow rates of increasing the diameter of the cannula. The length of the cannula (l) should be short to optimise rapid fluid administration.

Table 7.1 Typical flow rates under gravity through intravenous peripheral cannulae

Cannula gauge	Flow rate (ml/min)
22	36
20	61
18	96
16	196
14	343

Veins in the forearm in the obstetric patient are often large and have the benefit of not traversing a joint and therefore being easier to protect from the effects of movement. Otherwise, large veins in the antecubital fossae may be good sites for placement of peripheral intravenous cannulae for emergency fluid administration, with care taken to ensure an artery is not cannulated in error. Splinting and good fixation will be needed.

Types of large-bore cannulae

Obstetric haemorrhage can be catastrophic and extremely rapid. Intravenous devices exist (e.g. Arrow Peripheral Emergency Infusion Device [EID™] or Rapid Infusion Catheter [RIC®]) that can increase the flow rate to four times that seen through a 16-gauge cannula (Figure 7.1). The EID uses a small-gauge 'seeker' needle to permit venous puncture in patients with poor peripheral perfusion. The built-in Seldinger (guide wire) technique then allows the 6 French gauge infusion catheter to be railroaded into the vein. The RIC allows the existing peripheral access to be converted, 20 g or greater, to a 7 French gauge catheter. A Seldinger exchange wire is threaded through the existing venous access, once patency of the cannula has been established. The cannula is then removed, leaving the wire in place within the vein. The infusion catheter is then threaded over the wire to establish large bore peripheral venous access.

Rapid infusion, large gauge, short bore devices are also available for central use that make the delivery of vast amount of fluid possible in the face of torrential haemorrhage.

Alternatives to peripheral venous access

Intraosseous access

In extreme situations, the placement of intravenous cannulae may not be possible. The intraosseous (IO) technique is quick and relatively simple, particularly when assisted by a powered insertion device (Figure 7.2). This skill is taught during the face-to-face element of the MOET course.

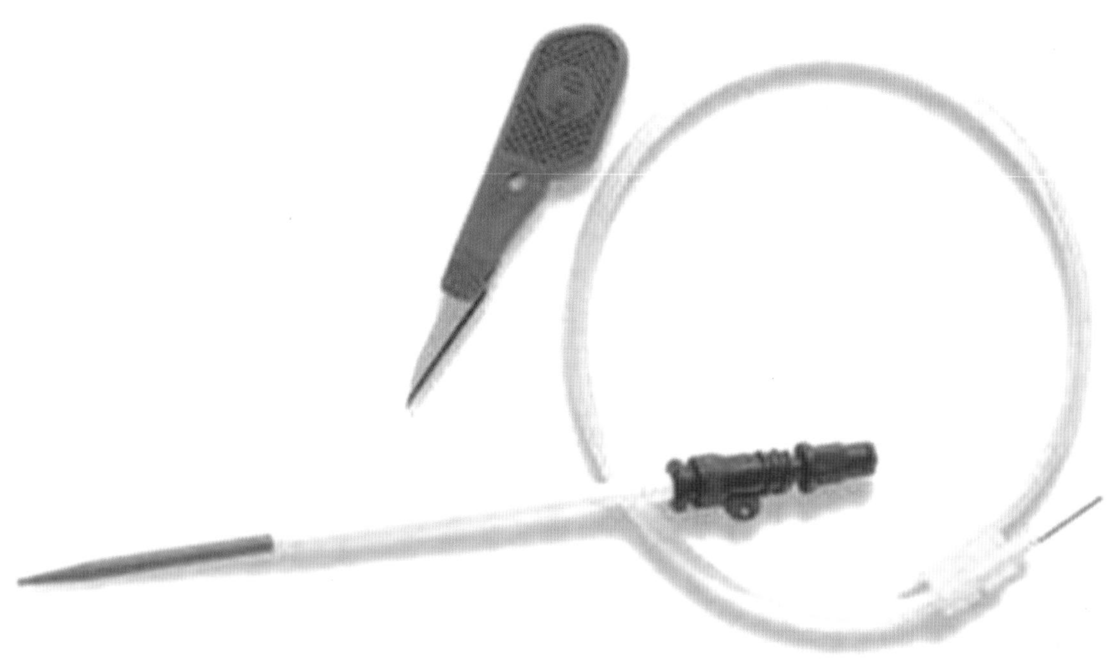

Figure 7.1 Arrow Rapid Infusion Catheter (RIC®) (with kind permission from Arrow)

TIBIAL	HUMORAL
Anterior surface, 2 cm below and slightly medial to the tibial tuberosity. 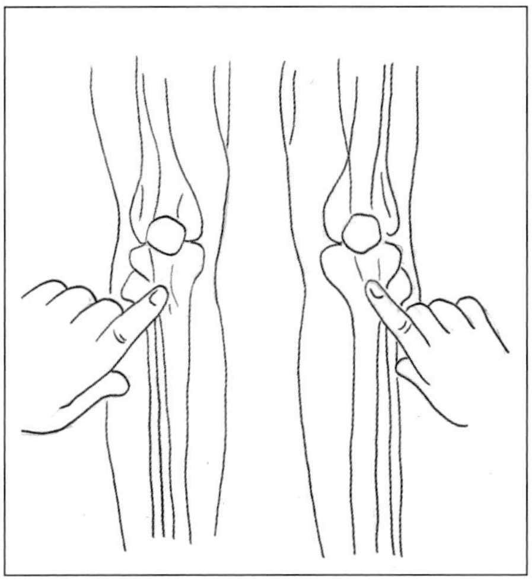	Position arm with elbow close to side, with forearm flexed so hand resting on abdomen. Anterolateral surface, 1 cm above the greater tubercle (use only in patients where landmarks can be clearly identified). 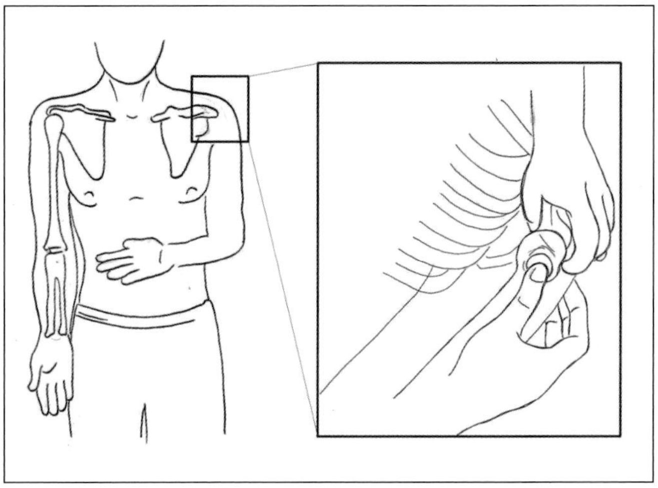

Figure 7.2 Sites for IO needle placement: tibial and humoral

Uses for IO cannulae:

- the administration of drugs
- the administration of fluid
- the aspiration of marrow, which can be used for crossmatching blood.

It must be remembered that fluid will need to be administered under pressure, as gravity alone will not be sufficient to provide adequate flow through the IO cannula.

Contraindications to use of IO cannulae:

- fracture proximal or distal to insertion site
- previous orthopaedic surgery at the site
- infection at the puncture site
- previous IO access within 24 hours at the same site should preclude the use of IO needles at that site
- the inability to palpate bony landmarks.

Figure 7.2 shows the commonly used sites for access. The humerus has advantages, in terms of flow rate and physical ease of access to the site. However, it may be covered with excessive tissue, making it impossible to establish IO access there. In this situation, it may be possible to gain access at the tibial site, where fat deposition is usually less marked. IO cannulae are available in 15, 25 and 45 mm lengths and should be chosen appropriately for the estimated amount of subcutaneous tissue to be punctured.

Complications of insertion:

- can become dislodged with subsequent high-volume infusion into the tissues
- compartment syndrome as a result of above
- sinus formation
- failure to deliver essential drugs and fluids
- infection leading to osteomyelitis.

The infection risk can be minimised by correct skin preparation, occlusive dressing and aseptic nontouch techniques when using the cannula. Modern needles can be inserted using a rapid access 'gun' with purpose-made occlusive dressings that are more secure. This will be demonstrated on the course.

While insertion of the IO cannula using the gun is relatively painless, running in the fluid can cause significant pain and local analgesia may be required. By contrast, the handheld IO needles do cause pain on insertion and, unless the patient is in extremis, local anaesthetic should be used both in the skin and above the periosteum before the needle is put in place.

CVP line access

A CVP line may help to avoid either under-transfusion or fluid overload. This requires the placement of an intravenous catheter into the central circulation. Placement is achieved most commonly by the internal jugular vein approach or from a peripheral vein in the arm using a much longer catheter. The latter is especially useful for monitoring in cases with severe DIC, as the risk of bleeding at insertion is small. However, these devices are usually single lumen and therefore only of use for monitoring. If infusion of centrally acting drugs or fluids is required, a multilumen catheter is usually placed in the internal jugular or the subclavian vein.

Femoral vein access

Access to the femoral vein is less used in the obstetric patient. Ease of access will vary hugely with the degree of obesity and the size of the uterus and may be rendered useless if obstetric manoeuvres in the lithotomy position are required. It should not be discounted in a crisis, as it can provide quick access to a central vein without requiring a head-down position or interfering with the airway. However, there is the concern of exacerbating haemorrhage from infusing fluids into the venous system that is actively bleeding.

Practical tips for use of CVP lines:

- the staff looking after them should receive training in their use
- the transducer should be zeroed at approximately the level of the heart
- the flush bag needs to be maintained at an adequate pressure, usually 300 mmHg pressure to avoid flow backtracking down the line, 300 mmHg is conventionally used and provides a steady infusion of 2–3 ml per hour via a flushing device
- heparin-containing flush bags are not usually required
- care needs to be taken to ensure all ports on the three-way taps used are capped to avoid an air embolus when the woman inhales
- care on removal of the device to maintain closed caps, a supine position and pressure over the site to avoid an air embolus
- strict asepsis when taking samples or giving drugs to avoid infected lines and subsequent bacteraemia
- removal as soon as no longer needed to reduce risk of infection or venous thrombosis.

Ultrasound-guided access

The rise in availability of portable ultrasound machines has seen huge uptake of use among anaesthetic practitioners. This technique allows direct visualisation of the vein to be cannulated. The operator can observe puncture of the vein by realtime ultrasound guidance, thus reducing the risk of inadvertent arterial cannulation or failed venous access. In the absence of adequate peripheral intravenous access, many anaesthetists would choose to use this technique to gain access to a central vein.

Ultrasound has also gained popularity in siting peripheral access cannulae in morbidly obese or oedematous women. Anatomical landmarks can be scanned to find veins, assess depth and observe direct puncture of veins that are not visible or palpable on the surface of the skin.

Venous cut down

With the advent of IO access and ultrasound-guided techniques, the need for peripheral venous cut down is greatly reduced. The technique remains useful in healthcare settings that are poorly resourced.

Intravenous fluid administration

Circulatory volumes

In everyday obstetric practice, the commonest reason for urgent fluid administration will be in the face of maternal haemorrhage. For that reason, the bulk of this section is written in the context of maternal bleeding unless otherwise commented on.

During pregnancy, we see an increase in circulating volume of approximately 40%. This means the volume increases from 70 ml/kg to 100 ml/kg, or 4900 ml to 7000 ml in a 70 kg woman. It is this expansion in circulating volume that allows the mother to compensate extremely well for blood loss; it is also the reason why we sometimes underestimate the severity of blood loss, occasionally even until the point of maternal collapse, and the signs and symptoms produced only become obvious and dramatic with life-threatening blood losses.

Maternal blood loss can be categorised into four classes of increasing severity (see Table 5.1). It is worthy of note that absolute blood loss in a smaller woman reflects a larger percentage loss of her circulating volume.

Fluid warming and pressure devices

All intravenous fluids should be warmed when their administration is rapid. The rapid administration of large volumes of cold fluid will lead to significant hypothermia. Note: it is dangerous to infuse cold fluid directly into the heart through a CVP line. There are numerous fluid warming devices available; more advanced models offer co-axial heated tubing to ensure the temperature of the fluid is maintained right up to the point of delivery in to the cannula.

Reduced maternal temperature will cause shivering in an attempt to raise body temperature resulting in an increased oxygen demand. Failure to meet this demand will increase anaerobic metabolism and metabolic acidosis. Peripheral vasoconstriction, in an attempt to reduce any further heat loss from the periphery, will also lead to decreased oxygen delivery to the tissues, which will further add to metabolic acidosis. Significant drops in temperature will also have profound effects on the efficacy of the coagulation cascade and contribute to problems with clot formation.

High-pressure infusion devices are essential. Hand-inflated pressure bags are effective but labour intensive. Hazards of any high-pressure infusion include fluid overload and air embolism.

Types of intravenous fluid

Crystalloids

Crystalloids contain small molecules therefore they exert little oncotic pressure. As a result, these fluids distribute outside the intravascular compartment with ease, making their use in volume correction transient. They are physiological solutions and remain in the circulation for about 30 minutes, before passing into the extra- and intracellular spaces. An overload may cause pulmonary and cerebral oedema (so care is needed in pre-eclampsia/eclampsia).

They are useful for the immediate replacement of lost volume in the haemorrhage situation. They are also the mainstay of fluid administration in most other circumstances, as will be discussed in the remainder of this chapter.

Hartmann's solution

Also known as Ringer's lactate or compound sodium lactate, this fluid is often the crystalloid of choice. Its ionic composition is closely matched with that of plasma.

0.9% sodium chloride ('normal' saline)

The excessive use of solutions of sodium chloride can result in hyperchloraemic metabolic acidosis and clinicians should be aware of this, and avoid their use in large volume when possible.

Dextrose solutions

Dextrose within these fluids is rapidly metabolised by the body. The remaining fluid is therefore water, which is free to rapidly distribute into intracellular tissues. This increases the risk of cerebral and pulmonary oedema. The use of dextrose solutions should therefore be reserved for the treatment of specific conditions, such as hypoglycaemia, or (in conjunction with saline) with intravenous insulin regimens to maintain glucose homeostasis in diabetic women.

Use of large volumes of hyponatraemic solutions is dangerous and can result in rapidly lowering serum and intracellular sodium levels leading to tissue oedema. Restoring sodium levels from extremes to normal is also a hazardous activity and expert advice must be sought urgently. Should a woman present with a very low serum sodium, the restoration of sodium levels must be very cautious under the guidance of an intensivist.

Synthetic colloids

Synthetic colloids are solutions containing large molecules of starch or gelatine and as a result they exert an oncotic pressure to keep fluid inside the vascular compartment. They remain in the intravascular compartment for longer than crystalloids and therefore may be useful for correcting fluid deficit associated with haemorrhage where blood products are not immediately available. Administration of synthetic colloids can be associated with different adverse effects on coagulability. This side effect is a real concern when managing severe blood loss and their use should be limited where possible. Infrequently, colloids are also associated with anaphylactic reactions. Recent concern about renal failure with use of hydroxyethyl starch solutions has led to a European suspension of use.

Crystalloid versus colloid

The debate over crystalloid or colloid as the most appropriate fluid is complex and out of the scope of this chapter. It is generally agreed that an initial infusion of crystalloid is appropriate for emergency situations requiring volume resuscitation. Colloid may have a place for volume replacement, but blood products are likely to be required for severe haemorrhage.

Blood products

Blood and blood product transfusions carry risks, so all involved must be adequately trained in patient identification and documentation, product identification and storage, as well as defrosting needs and shelf times (Table 7.2). Guidelines exist for this and there are training packages that should be undertaken and updated regularly. It is also important to be familiar with the practical transfusion requirements of blood products used, to ensure maximum benefit is gained from them.

Packed red cells

Concentrated red cells are the mainstay of treatment for volume replacement and the restoration of oxygen-carrying capacity of blood. Each pack contains approximately 220 ml of red cells and 80 ml of saline-adenine-glucose-mannitol (SAG-M) solution, giving it a shelf life of 35 days. The haematocrit varies from 55% to 70% so a plasma substitute needs to be given in an appropriate amount to provide the additional volume required.

(Fresh whole blood is not used in adult practice in the UK because release from the blood bank less than 24 hours after collection does not allow completion of a full infection screen.)

Citrate anticoagulation

In massive and rapid transfusion there may be a requirement for calcium infusion for the following reason: large volumes of citrate anticoagulants are present in stored red blood cells and FFP. Citrate binds to ionised calcium, which may result in hypocalcaemia. This in turn contributes to coagulopathy and to a negative inotropic action on the heart. Both effects can be reversed by a slow (20 minute) infusion of calcium, e.g. 10 ml 10% calcium gluconate with subsequent laboratory checks of serum calcium.

Crossmatching

Full crossmatching of blood may take up to 1 hour. In an emergency, group-specific blood may be required. A woman's blood group and presence of abnormal antibodies are usually established during pregnancy, which facilitates the provision of blood when needed. The emergency use of group-specific blood following antibody screening, as in most pregnant women in the UK, carries a risk of less than 0.1% of a haemolytic transfusion reaction, which rises to 1.0% if group-specific blood is used without antibody screening. In most circumstances, issuing of group- and rhesus-compatible blood should be possible within 5–10 minutes.

Group O Rh-negative blood should be available on the delivery suite for dire emergencies; however, its use carries a small risk of sensitisation to the 'c' antigen with possible problems for future pregnancies. It should rarely be needed.

The risk of viral transmission (e.g. hepatitis, cytomegalovirus [CMV]) is extremely low in the UK due to meticulous screening by the blood transfusion services. In order to reduce the transmission of the Creutzfeldt–Jakob (CJD) prion, the blood is further leucodepleted before being issued from the blood bank.

However, as donated blood is an expensive and limited resource with some risks attached to its use, it is agreed that in the absence of significant comorbidity the trigger for red cell transfusion, while depending most on symptomatology, is around the 7 g/dl level. The symptoms guiding transfusion include lightheadedness, shortness of breath, palpitations (due to a tachycardia) or inability to get out of bed and care for the baby, or other comorbidities such as cardiac disease.

It must be remembered that haemoglobin is currently the only readily available substance for carrying oxygen in the circulation. Even previously fit and well women can experience cardiac ischaemia, infarction and ultimately death in the face of extreme anaemia.

Fresh frozen plasma (FFP)

FFP contains clotting factors at physiological levels, which will be diluted on addition of anticoagulants. Methylene blue-treated FFP is also available. This helps to inactivate the CJD prion and is used when required for administration to neonates and children. It is extremely expensive, around 10–15 times the cost of untreated FFP.

Military and trauma experience is demonstrating increased survival when packed red cells and clotting products are administered in a ratio of 1:1 during extreme blood loss. It is not known at this stage whether this practice should be translated into the obstetric population. Present practice is variable with regard to the ratio of packed red cells to FFP. Guidance from laboratory testing is often hampered by delays in getting results, leaving clinicians to manage on clinical suspicion. If results are available and prothrombin time/activated partial thromboplastin time >1.5 times normal then 2 units of FFP will be needed as a minimum.

Table 7.2 Common blood components and their use in obstetrics

Component	Volume per unit	Dose	Number of donors	Storage	Need to defrost	Storage after defrosting	Time to transfusion	Filter required
Packed red cells	180–350 ml (mean 28 ml)	4ml/kg equivalent to 1unit will raise Hb by 1g/dl	1	Designated temperature-controlled refrigerator at 4±2°C for 35 days	No	N/A	4 hours after removal from storage	Blood transfusion set with 170–200 micron filter
Fresh frozen plasma	240–300 ml (mean 273 ml)	10–15ml/kg or 1:1 with RBC in major haemorrhage	Multiple	Designated temperature-controlled freezer at –30° for 24 months	Yes – takes 15–30min	Can be stored in blood fridge for 24 hours	4 hours after removal from storage	As above
Platelets	200–300 ml	1 adult therapeutic dose increases platelet count by $20–40x10^9$/litre	Multiple	Temperature controlled at 22±2°C with continuous agitation for 5 days	No	N/A	As soon as possible over 30–60 min – they should not be put in the fridge	As above but not through giving set which has been used for other blood products
Cryoprecipitate	100–250 ml (mean 152 ml)	2x5 donor pools (equivalent to 10 single donor units) raise plasma fibrinogen by 1g/litre	Multiple	Designated temperature-controlled freezer at –30°C for 24 months	Yes – takes 15–30min	Must be kept at ambient temperature for up to 4 hours	As soon as possible – it should not be put in the fridge	As above

Cryoprecipitate

Cryoprecipitate is another fraction of whole blood that is rich in fibrinogen and is therefore indicated in the presence of profound hypofibrinogenaemia, as may be seen in association with bleeding due to placental abruption. This means cryoprecipitate may be requested earlier in this type of haemorrhage than in a more straightforward bleed from an atonic uterus. If fibrinogen <1 g/litre give 10 units (two packs).

Platelets

Platelet packs have a limited shelf life of around 5 days. They are rarely indicated above a platelet count of 50×10^9/litre (50 000/microlitre) but may be required to raise the level to 80–100×10^9/litre if surgical intervention is planned. It is to be remembered that platelet function, not purely number, is important. This function is difficult to measure in a laboratory setting. More recently, near patient testing with devices such as platelet function analysers and thromboelastography have offered guidance on appropriate administration of clotting products.

Cell salvage

Increased cost, relative scarcity and concern over viral transmission has resulted in increased use of autologous transfusion in obstetric practice. The process involves anticoagulation, collection, filtration, washing and reinfusion of red cells at the time of surgery. Cell salvage has become a real prospect in maternal resuscitation in elective and emergency situations.

Initial concerns existed regarding the contamination of the salvaged blood with amniotic fluid, but NICE guidance has approved the use of cell salvage in obstetric haemorrhage. The quality of wash achieved by modern cell salvage machines is such that the amount of amniotic fluid reaching the circulation is minimal, akin to that experienced during a routine CS. Leucocyte depletion filters will further reduce the amount of amniotic fluid reaching the maternal circulation. Recent reports of hypotension associated with these filters have led to further ongoing discussion about the need for their use in obstetric practice.

Fetal cells can also enter the maternal circulation and women with Rh-D neg blood groups must be screened and treated appropriately with anti-D to avoid haemolytic complications in subsequent pregnancies.

Effective use of cell salvage also requires a slight change in practice for the surgeon and scrub staff. The use of suction, as opposed to swabs, will increase the yield of salvaged blood, even if the swabs are subsequently soaked in a heparin containing saline, and then aspirated into the collection jar. Blood spilt onto the drapes cannot be salvaged. The integrated suction needs to be set lower than that usually preferred by surgeons in order to minimise cell breakage. However, there has to be a realistic compromise in this to allow the surgeons to see what they are doing. It is also difficult for the assistant to retract with two hands and use the suction to provide a good field for the operating surgeon. Self-retaining retractors can be a great help.

There remains debate over the requirement to use a separate suction for the bulk of amniotic fluid at the beginning of the procedure, but current guidance from NICE does not require a double suction technique.

Cell salvage for Jehovah's witnesses

Most women who refuse blood products will accept cell salvage. However, it must be remembered and fully explained that the blood returned to the woman does not contain clotting factors: the risk of coagulation defects therefore remains as it does with homologous red cell transfusion. This is, in effect, a dilutional coagulopathy, as fluids returned gradually dilute the remaining pool of available natural clotting factors until eventually there is a catastrophic failure of the clotting mechanism. Although easily corrected in normal circumstances by administration of clotting factors, it is particularly important to emphasise this very significant limitation of cell salvage to women who refuse blood products.

Guiding fluid replacement

Clinical signs

For the vast majority of situations, fluid administration in the otherwise healthy parturient will be guided by the maintenance or restoration of easily observed clinical variables. It must be remembered that there is no place for hypotensive resuscitation in pregnant women. Raised heart rate is an early sign of absolute or relative (vasodilatatory) hypovolaemia. In general, a heart rate above 100 beats per minute should be considered sinister until proven otherwise (Table 7.3). A normal respiratory rate, normal capillary refill (less than 2 seconds) and normal pulse pressure (unless the patient is on beta-blockers) are also sensitive markers of a normal circulatory volume. It must be remembered that patients on beta-blockers have an impaired tachycardic response to hypovolaemia and also that simply abolishing systolic hypotension is not a good marker for restoration of normovolaemia.

Table 7.3 Different classes of blood loss with resulting physiological indices

	Class I	Class II	Class III	Class IV
Blood loss	15%	15–30%	30–40%	>40%
Nonpregnant (ml)	750	1000	1500	2000
Pregnant (ml)	<1000	1000–2000	2000–2700	>2700
Respiration rate (per min)	14–20	20–30	30–40	>40
Heart rate (per min)	<100	>100	>120	>140
Systolic	Normal	Normal	Decreased	Decreased
Diastolic	Normal	Increased	Decreased	Decreased
Mental state	Anxious	Anxious Confused	Confused Agitated	Lethargic
Urine (ml/h)	>30	20–30	5–15	Negligible

A normal urine output (~1ml/kg/h) is another easy to measure indicator of successful fluid homeostasis. The value of these tools as simple monitors of wellbeing is the reason why they form the basis of most early warning charts. Table 7.4 is a guide to the response to fluid resuscitation and a guide to further action.

Repeated blood gas measurements can guide fluid therapy. Metabolic acidosis may develop with severe or long-standing shock as a result of inadequate tissue perfusion and subsequent anaerobic metabolism. It is the acidosis that may be the driver for raised respiratory rate in shock. Adequate resuscitation and restoration of organ function is the best treatment. Alkalis such as bicarbonate are rarely required, and are for specialist use only.

Table 7.4 Response to resuscitation by intravenous fluids

Response type	Intervention needed
I	Signs improve and remain improved. No further fluid challenge is required.
II	An initial but unsustained improvement in vital signs followed by regression to abnormal levels. Either: • the fluid has been redistributed from the intravascular compartment to the extravascular compartments • there is continued loss (as seen in continued haemorrhage) • there is worsening of vasodilatation (sepsis/ anaphylaxis) Further fluid challenge is required. Restoration of normal variables would imply there is no further fluid loss or worsening of vasodilatation.
III	If vital signs remain abnormal then this would be considered a type III response. In the face of haemorrhage, this implies significant ongoing losses and the patient requires urgent surgery. Patients with this response in the face of sepsis will almost certainly require vasoactive drug administration to reduce the degree of peripheral vasodilatation.
IV	This group show no response to rapid fluid administration of any type. In the face of haemorrhage, this patient requires immediate surgery (to 'turn off the tap') if she is to survive. Women with sepsis are likely to require continuous vasoactive infusion to support circulation and require immediate transfer to an intensive care unit.

Advanced monitoring techniques

Our main interest when monitoring the circulation is to ensure correct filling of the left ventricle and adequate cardiac output.

Central venous monitoring

CVP is measured within the circulation via an intravenous catheter. If the entry point is from the neck veins, the tip of the catheter will sit just above the right atrium. Normal values are 0–8mmHg and act as a guide to correct volume status. Measurements from a femoral vein are more difficult to interpret.

CVP measurements are usually helpful in assessing filling of the right atrium. The assumption is made that, if the right and left sides of the heart are functioning equally effectively, the right-sided filling pressure reflects filling pressure on the left, or systemic, side of the circulation. For this to be true, we must assume that all of the interposed heart valves function normally, that the resistance in the pulmonary vasculature is normal and the elasticity (compliance) of the ventricles is normal. In many pathological states, we simply cannot rely on these assumptions being true and we may require the use of more complex cardiovascular monitoring.

There are occasions when there is left ventricular dysfunction, so that the filling pressures on either side of the heart may not be equivalent. This makes interpretation of CVP readings difficult, so that expert advice on further fluid management and appropriate cardiac support may be needed from intensive care specialists.

Conditions where CVP measurement may not be an accurate guide to fluid management:

- hypotension unresponsive to fluid therapy
- oliguria despite apparently adequate CVP measurement
- coexisting relevant disease, e.g. cardiac failure
- coexisting severe sepsis
- coexisting severe pre-eclampsia
- pulmonary oedema.

Pulmonary artery balloon tipped flotation catheters

These catheters (now rarely used) are inserted as for CVP neck lines but then traverse the right side of the heart and are positioned in the pulmonary artery. When the tip balloon is inflated to occlude the pulmonary artery, the catheter tip orifice 'sees' the pressure beyond the pulmonary vasculature i.e. left atrial pressure, thus removing some of the previously mentioned sources of error.

They are seriously invasive and can be associated with significant morbidity, including arrhythmias and rupture of the pulmonary vessels. They have been superseded in most intensive care unit settings by less invasive monitors.

Doppler probes

Transoesphageal probes can be used to employ Doppler and ultrasound evaluation of the volume status of the left ventricle. They are also able to give estimates of the cardiac output. They can only be sited in anaesthetised patients.

In the awake patient, transthoracic Doppler and peripheral arterial line traces can be interpreted by specialist machines to provide information about volume status and cardiac output.

As the monograms used by these machines are derived from nonpregnant values, the validity of these tools remains in question in the pregnant woman, but clinical research would imply that they look promising.

Clinical judgement

Often these techniques can only be performed after the woman has been transferred to an intensive care setting. This leaves the obstetrician and anaesthetist still needing good history taking, examination and monitoring skills to ensure adequate fluid replacement.

Fluid administration in special circumstances

As already discussed, fluid administration in obstetric practice is most commonly in the face of haemorrhage, where adequate prompt fluid administration is our major aim. There are, however, situations within obstetric practice where we must consider much more targeted administration of fluid.

Haemorrhage: guide to fluid therapy

- *Crystalloid:* 2 litres of warmed Ringer's or Hartmann's solution. Large volumes of crystalloid may be undesirable in view of the relatively low oncotic pressure in pregnancy and can lead to pulmonary oedema.
- *Colloid*: 1–2 litres warmed colloid until blood available. Human Albumin Solution (4% HAS) or gelatin-based solutions (see previous section).
- *FFP:* see above, or if prothrombin time/activated partial thromboplastin time >1.5 times normal. Now often issued 1:1 RBC:FFP.
- *Platelet concentrates:* if platelet count <50 x 10^9/litres. Now often issued as part of major haemorrhage pack.
- *Cryoprecipitate:* if fibrinogen <1 g/l give 10 units (two packs).

Pre-eclampsia/eclampsia (PET) (also see Chapter 24)

Fluid management prior to delivery

Matters to consider:

1. Need for preload – volume and type.
2. Fluid maintenance – volume and type.

The major concern is to avoid fluid overload. Intravenous input is limited to around 80 ml/hour in most PET protocols. If Syntocinon infusions are required, they should be given in high concentrations via a syringe driver to avoid the administration of further large volumes of fluid. The volume of this and any other infusion (magnesium, antihypertensives) should be included in the 80 ml/hour total fluids.

NOTE: Volume preload may be required either prior to the use of a vasodilator as an anti-hypertensive agent, e.g. hydrallazine or nifedipine, or prior to regional or general anaesthesia.

The degree of vasodilatation following establishment of regional anaesthesia varies and therefore the requirement for volume preload should be made on individual assessment and not be simply routine practice (see Chapter 24).

If fluid loading is required, care should be taken to ensure that the volume given is not excessive, either by using low-volume bags or administration via a volumetric pump. If hypotension does occur it can usually be controlled with low-dose vasopressor by bolus, or more commonly, by infusion.

Fluid management post delivery

In the immediate post-delivery phase, women will often have a degree of oliguria before the natural diuresis occurs. It is important not to risk fluid overload in the chase for adequate urine output. Total intravenous fluids (including drug infusions) should be limited and careful fluid balance charted. Numerous examples of fluid protocols exist around the UK; a suggested guide is shown in Chapter 24.

The correlation between CVP and volume status is poorly maintained in many pre-eclamptic patients. Previous Confidential Reports have suggested low thresholds for central venous monitoring, especially in situations where inaccuracies are likely to develop, i.e. blood loss. The use of CVP monitoring, or advanced monitoring techniques, should be a multidisciplinary decision.

Sepsis (see also Chapter 6)

Hypovolaemia is present in almost all patients with septic shock and fluid resuscitation is vital. The volumes required can be very large, as fluid is leaking rapidly into the interstitial tissues due to capillary leak caused as part of the sepsis response.

If patients do not respond to simple measures of resuscitation, CVP monitoring should be instituted to guide further fluid replacement. In severe sepsis, early goal-directed therapy of fluid resuscitation and aggressive haemodynamic management has been shown to reduce mortality. In patients who remain hypotensive despite adequate fluid resuscitation, early recourse to vasopressor therapy, with or without inotropes and ventilation, has been recommended. Evidence supports the use of noradrenaline as the vasopressor of choice. Sensitivity to catecholamines is greatly reduced in sepsis and therefore patients may require exceedingly high doses. Despite aggressive therapy, mortality from sepsis has risen in the latest CMACE report. Vigilance and early recognition remain vital if we are to improve outcome.

Cardiac disease

Response to fluid administration can be extremely unpredictable in this group of patients. Central venous monitoring, or more advanced assessment of cardiac function, may be required to guide successful and safe fluid administration. These cases require senior clinician involvement across multidisciplinary teams.

Summary

- Intravenous access should be large bore and short length.
- Haemorrhage is likely to be the commonest indication for urgent fluid administration.
- Advanced cardiovascular monitoring may be required in certain circumstances.

Further reading

1 Royal College of Obstetricians and Gynaecologists. The Management of Severe Pre-eclampsia/Eclampsia. Guideline No. 10(A). London: RCOG 2006.

2 Royal College of Obstetricians and Gynaecologists. Prevention and management of postpartum haemorrhage. Guideline No. 52. London: *RCOG* 2009 (minor revision 2011).

3 Lewis G (ed). Saving Mothers' Lives 2006–2008. Eighth Report of the Confidential Enquiries into Maternal Deaths in the United Kingdom. London: RCOG 2011.
   - Chapter 3 Pre-eclampsia and eclampsia, Neilson J (on behalf of the Centre for Maternal and Child Enquiries).
   - Chapter 4 Haemorrhage, Norman J (on behalf of the Centre for Maternal and Child Enquiries).
   - Chapter 7 Sepsis, Harper A (on behalf of the Centre for Maternal and Child Enquiries).
   - Chapter 9 Cardiac Disease, Nelson-Piercy C.

4 Sreelakshmi TR, Eldridge J. Acute hypotension associated with leucocyte depletion filters during cell salvaged blood transfusion. *Anaesthesia* 2010;65:742–4.

5 Shaz BH, Dente CJ, Harris RS, *et al.* Transfusion management of trauma patients. *Anesthesia and Analgesia* 2009;108:1760–8.

6 Chappell D, Jacob M, Hofmann-Kiefer K, *et al.* A rational approach to perioperative fluid management. *Anesthesiology* 2008;109:723–40.

7 Guideline on the Administration of Blood Components. British Committee for Standards in Haematology 2008.

8 NICE guidelines IPG 144 Intraoperative blood cell salvage in obstetrics. www.nice.org.uk/nicemedia/live/11038/30690/30690.pdf
9 Association of Anaesthetists of Great Britain and Ireland. Blood transfusion and the Anaesthetist: Intra-operative cell salvage. AAGBI Safety Guideline. London. 2009.
10 Dellinger RP, Levy MM, Rhodes A, *et al.* Surviving Sepsis Campaign: International guidelines for management of severe sepsis and septic shock. Crit Care Med 2013; 41:580–637.

SECTION 3

Resuscitation

CHAPTER 8

Airway management and ventilation

Objectives

On successfully completing this topic, you will be able to:

- understand the importance of airway patency, maintenance and protection
- identify the circumstances in which airway compromise can occur
- be able to assess and manage the airway and ventilation.

Introduction

An obstructed airway or inadequate ventilation results in tissue hypoxia within minutes and this can lead to organ failure and death. Some organs are more sensitive to hypoxia than others. For example, cerebral hypoxia, even for a short period of time, will cause agitation then a decreased level of consciousness and, eventually, irreversible or fatal brain damage.

Management of the airway is of first concern because obstruction to the airway can quickly result in hypoxia with damage or death. The next presenting threat to life results from inadequate ventilation, so attention to this is given next priority.

Supplementary oxygen must be administered to all seriously injured and ill patients through a tight-fitting facemask attached to a reservoir bag at a flow of 12–15 litres/minute (full on at the wall rotameter). The primary goal in providing supplementary oxygen is to maximise the delivery of oxygen to the cells.

As soon as monitoring in the form of pulse oximetry is available and can be reliably interpreted, oxygen delivery can be adjusted to maintain a target oxygen saturation of 94–98%. There is thought to be some evidence of potential harm in providing prolonged periods of hyperoxia. Further monitoring can be provided by the use of blood gas analysis.

Carbon dioxide is produced by cellular metabolism and carried in the blood to the lungs to be exhaled. If there is airway obstruction or inadequate ventilation, there is a build up of carbon dioxide in the blood (hypercarbia). This causes drowsiness, acidosis and a rise in intracranial pressure secondary to vasodilatation.

Airway assessment

Importance of patency, maintenance and protection of airway

The airway must be open, maintained and protected if there is risk of regurgitation and aspiration as in the heavily pregnant patient. An awake, fully conscious woman will protect her own airway. Otherwise, in an unconscious woman, the gold standard for providing a patent and protected airway is by placing a cuffed tube in the trachea, usually by endotracheal intubation. If there is a breathing problem, ventilatory support may also be necessary once you have established a patent airway.

A before B before C before D

Circumstances in which an airway problem is likely to occur

Suspect an airway problem with the following:

- the patient with a decreased level of consciousness (because there is reduced muscle tone and the tongue is likely to slip back into the pharynx)
- hypoxia
- hypotension
- eclampsia
- poisoning
- alcohol
- intracranial pathology or injury
- maxillofacial injuries
- midface fractures can move backwards and block the airway
- mandibular fractures can allow the tongue to fall backwards
- bleeding and secretions caused by these injuries can block or soil the airway
- open injuries to the neck
- direct trauma to the larynx and supporting structures
- bleeding inside the neck compressing the hypopharynx or trachea
- burns to the face and neck: swelling of the upper and lower airway due to direct burns, or inhaling hot smoke, gases or steam, will cause airway obstruction.

Airway problems may:

- be immediate (block the airway quickly) or
- be delayed (come on after a time delay – minutes or hours) or
- deteriorate with time – this is often insidious because of its slow progression and is easily overlooked (as with burns to the upper airway; consider the potential for deterioration during transfer and, if a risk, secure a definitive airway before transfer).

An airway that has been cleared may obstruct again:

- if the support for keeping the airway patent is removed (e.g. chin lift)
- if the patient's level of consciousness decreases
- if there is further bleeding into the airway
- if there is increasing swelling in or around the airway.

Assessment of airway

Talk to the patient. Failure to respond implies an obstructed airway or a breathing problem, with inability to exhale enough air to phonate, or an altered level of consciousness with the potential for airway compromise. A positive, appropriate reply in a normal voice indicates that the airway is patent, breathing normal and brain perfusion adequate.

Look to see if the patient is agitated, drowsy or cyanosed. The absence of cyanosis does not mean the patient is adequately oxygenated. Look for use of accessory muscles of respiration.

A patient who refuses to lie down quietly may be trying to sit up in an attempt to keep her airway open or her breathing adequate. The abusive patient may be hypoxic and should not be presumed to be merely aggressive or intoxicated.

Listen for abnormal sounds. Snoring, gurgling and gargling sounds are associated with partial obstruction of the pharynx. Hoarseness implies laryngeal injury. An absence of sound does not mean the airway is patent; if the airway is totally obstructed there may be total silence. Feel for air movement on expiration and check if the trachea is in the midline.

Assessment of ventilation

Establishing a patent airway is the first step, but only the first step. A patent airway allows oxygen to pass to the lungs, but this will only happen with adequate ventilation. Ventilation may be compromised by airway obstruction, altered ventilatory mechanics or by central nervous system depression. If breathing is not improved by clearing the airway, attempt to ventilate by facemask. If ventilation is possible, the airway is patent but there is a problem with spontaneous ventilation. If ventilation is not possible, this would suggest that the airway continues to be obstructed. If there is a problem with spontaneous ventilation look for a cause within the chest or an intracranial or spinal injury as a cause and assist ventilation.

Inspect: Look for chest movement and obvious injuries.

Palpate: Palpate for chest movement and palpate the back of the patient's chest for injuries.

Palpate the trachea, checking it is in the midline.

Percuss: Percussion note should be resonant and equal bilaterally.

Auscultate: Air entry should be equal bilaterally.

Airway management

- Clear the obstructed airway.
- Maintain the intact airway.
- Recognise and protect the airway at risk.

The airway is at risk from aspiration in any patient with reduced level of consciousness, but in the pregnant patient regurgitation is more likely, so the potential for aspiration is increased.

Cervical spine injury suspected

Techniques for clearing, maintaining and protecting the airway need to be modified in the trauma patient in whom cervical spine injury is suspected or present. Cervical spine immobilisation should be instituted wherever there is suspicion of injury, either by manual inline immobilisation, or by semi-rigid cervical collar, head blocks, backboard and straps.

Clearing the obstructed airway

In the patient with suspected cervical spine injury, manual inline immobilisation of the cervical spine and airway clearance manoeuvres are carried out together. In a patient with an altered level of consciousness, the tongue falls backwards and obstructs the pharynx. This can be readily corrected by head tilt/chin lift or jaw thrust manoeuvres and blood and debris cleared by suction.

Head tilt/chin lift

Tilt the head posteriorly with the intention of straightening and slightly extending the neck. At the same time, place the fingers of one hand under the chin and gently lift it upwards to bring the chin anteriorly. This will open the upper airway in 70–80% of patients. See Figure 8.1.

Do not hyperextend the neck if a cervical spine injury is suspected. Use jaw thrust rather than head tilt.

Jaw thrust

Grasp the angles of the mandible, one hand on each side, and move the mandible forward. The jaw thrust is used for the injured patient because it does not destabilise a possible cervical spine fracture and risk converting a fracture without spinal cord injury to one with spinal cord injury. This manoeuvre will open 95% of obstructed upper airways. See Figure 8.2.

Suction

Remove blood and secretions from the oropharynx with a rigid suction device (for example, a Yankauer sucker). A patient with facial or head injuries may have a cribriform plate fracture – in these circumstances suction catheters should not be inserted through the nose, as they could enter the skull and injure the brain.

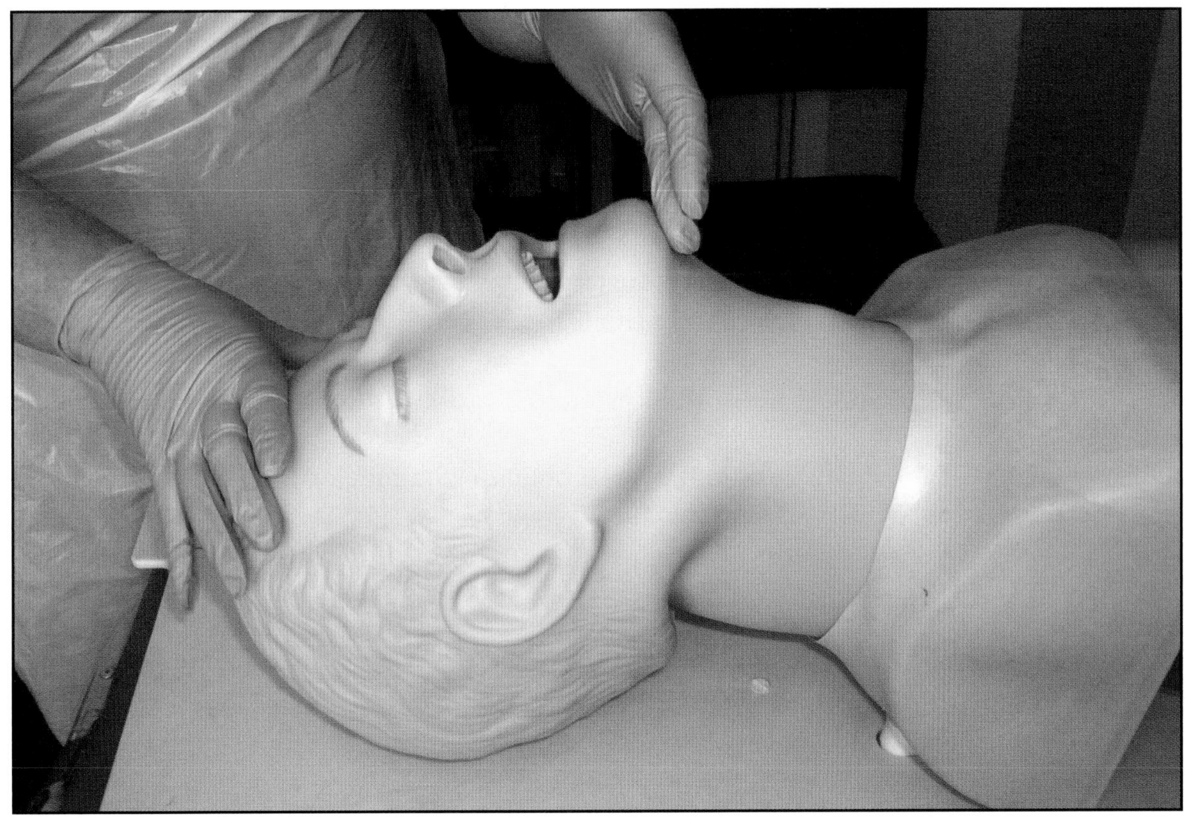

Figure 8.1 Head tilt/chin lift

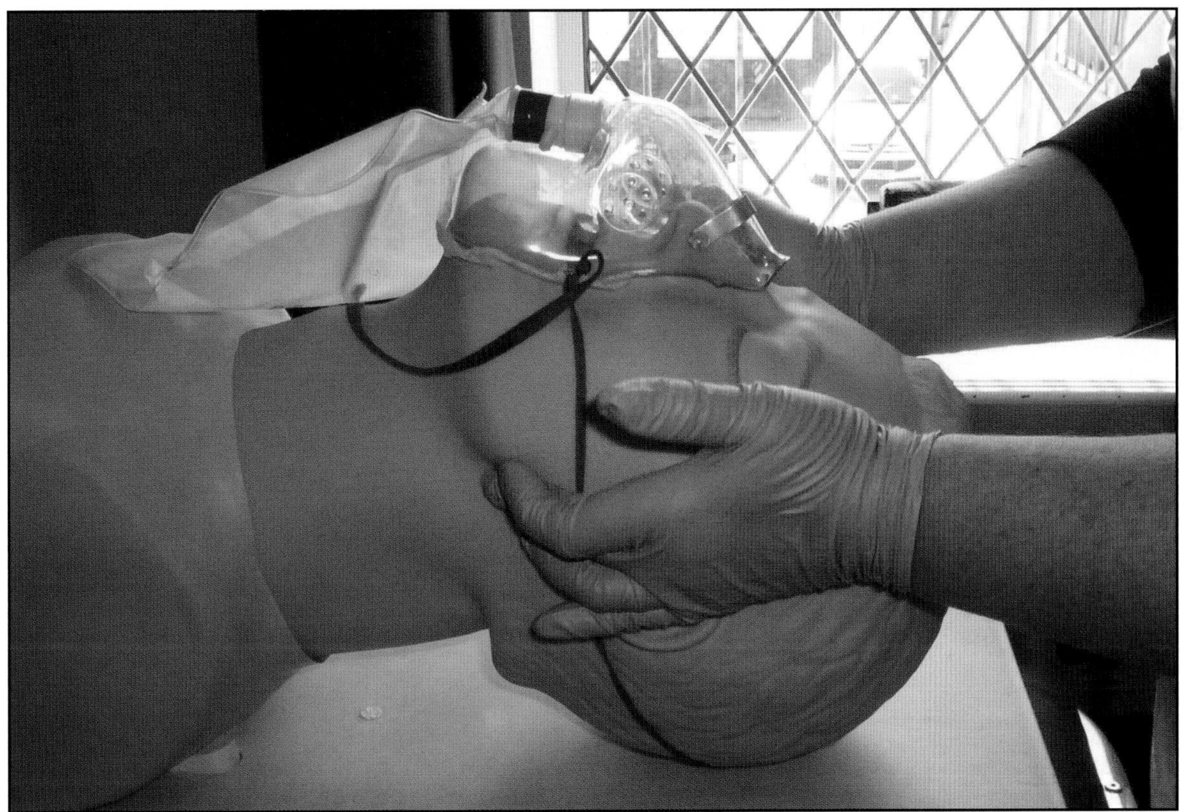

Figure 8.2 Jaw thrust

If attempts to clear the airway do not result in the restoration of spontaneous breathing, this may be because the airway is still not patent or because the airway is patent but there is no breathing. The only way to distinguish these two situations is to put either a pocket mask or facemask over the face and give breaths (either mouth-to-pocket-mask or with self-inflating bag and mask). If the chest rises, this is not an airway problem but a breathing problem. If the chest cannot be made to rise, this is an airway problem.

Clearing the airway may result in improvement in level of consciousness, which then might allow the patient to maintain her own airway.

Maintaining the airway

If the patient cannot maintain her own airway, continue with the jaw thrust or chin lift or try using an oropharyngeal airway.

Oropharyngeal airway

The oropharyngeal airway (Guedel type) is inserted into the mouth over the tongue. It stops the tongue falling back and provides a clear passage for airflow. The preferred method is to insert the airway concavity upwards, until the tip reaches the soft palate and then rotate it 180°, slipping it into place over the tongue. Make sure that the oropharyngeal airway does not push the tongue backwards as this will block, rather than open, the patient's airway. A patient with a gag reflex may not tolerate the oral airway. See Figure 8.3.

Nasopharyngeal airway

A nasopharyngeal airway is better tolerated than the oropharyngeal airway by the more responsive patient. Their use is contraindicated if there is a suspected fractured base of skull. Be aware of the potential for insertion to cause bleeding from the fragile nasal mucosa, which may soil the lungs of a patient with obtunded laryngeal or pharyngeal reflexes (the unconscious or hypotensive patient). This is especially so in pregnancy. Their use is limited to intensive care units where they might be placed by physiotherapists or anaesthetists to facilitate suctioning of pharyngeal secretions. They should only be used if there is an airway problem, an oropharyngeal airway is not being tolerated and an anaesthetist is unavailable.

Be very reluctant to use a nasal airway. They do not have a large part to play in contemporary UK anaesthetic practice because of their potential to cause bleeding, which is exacerbated in pregnancy.

Lubricate the airway and insert it gently through either nostril, straight backwards – not upwards – so that its tip enters the hypopharynx. A safety pin should be applied across the proximal end before insertion to prevent the tube disappearing into the nasal passages. Gentle insertion, good lubrication and using an airway that passes easily into the nose will decrease the incidence of bleeding.

The oropharyngeal and nasopharyngeal devices maintain the airway but do not protect it from aspiration.

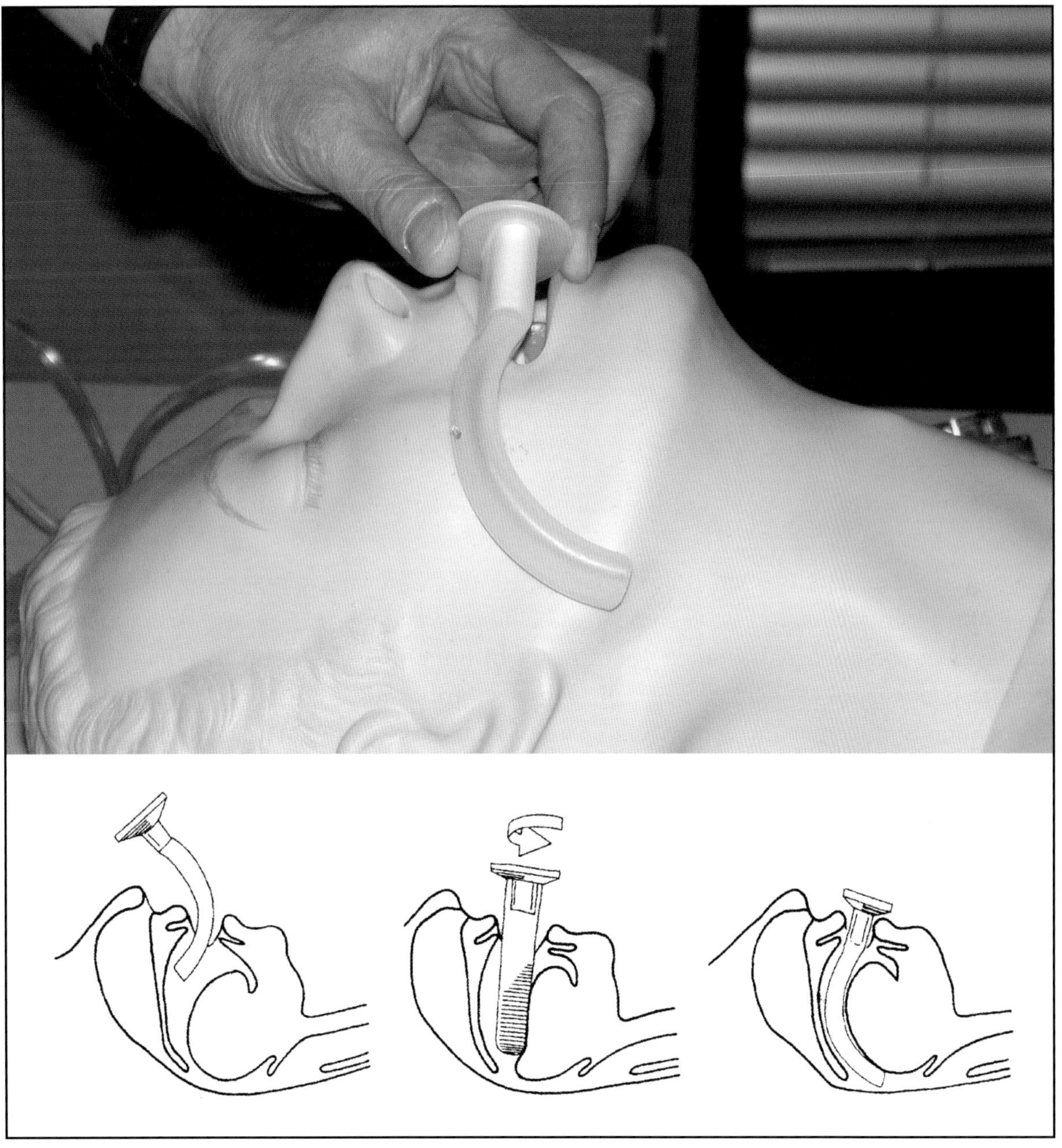

Figure 8.3 Oropharyngeal airway

Advanced airway techniques

Definitive airway is a gold standard for opening, maintaining and protecting the airway. It means that there is a cuffed tube in the trachea attached to oxygen and secured in place. Advanced airway techniques provide a definitive airway.

Advanced airway techniques may be required:

- in cases of apnoea
- when the above techniques fail

- to maintain an airway over the longer term
- to protect an airway
- to allow accurate control of oxygenation and ventilation
- when there is the potential for airway obstruction
- to control carbon dioxide levels in the unconscious patient, as a way of minimising the rise in intracranial pressure.

Advanced airway techniques are:

- endotracheal intubation
- surgical cricothyroidotomy
- surgical tracheostomy.

The circumstances and urgency determine the type of advanced airway technique to be used.

Note: The pregnant woman is at increased risk of gastric regurgitation because she has a mechanical obstruction to gastric emptying i.e. the pregnant uterus. She also has reduced tone in the lower oesophageal sphincter as a result of hormonal effects on the smooth muscle. Trauma patients are at increased risk of regurgitation because of reduced gastric emptying. Consequently, the pregnant woman (with or without trauma) without adequate pharyngeal and laryngeal reflexes (unconscious or hypotensive) is at increased risk of pulmonary aspiration. The chemical pneumonitis suffered when a pregnant woman aspirates is more severe than in a nonpregnant woman, as the gastric aspirate is more acidic in pregnancy. Consider early definitive airway, particularly in the context of a reduced conscious level.

Endotracheal intubation

In a patient with airway or respiratory compromise, the primary aim is to oxygenate the patient and this can initially be successfully achieved by positioning, use of oropharyngeal airways and use of a facemask and self-inflating bag.

If this cannot be achieved, intubation is needed. This should only be carried out without drugs where there is an urgent need for intubation, i.e. in the case of complete airway obstruction or a respiratory arrest, where the airway cannot be otherwise maintained.

It should be emphasised that heavily pregnant women are difficult to intubate and to ventilate with a bag and mask, because of weight gain during pregnancy and the potential for large breasts falling back into the working space. Consequently, for a surgeon or obstetrician, the use of a laryngeal mask airway (LMA) or a surgical airway may be the preferred option. It is usually easier to maintain an airway or ventilate by bag–valve–mask if the woman is a few degrees head up, rather than lying completely supine. This allows the weight of the breasts and abdomen to fall away from the chest. It may also make intubation easier.

Oral endotracheal intubation is most commonly used. This uses a laryngoscope to visualise the vocal cords. A cuffed endotracheal tube is placed through the vocal cords into the trachea. See Figure 8.4.

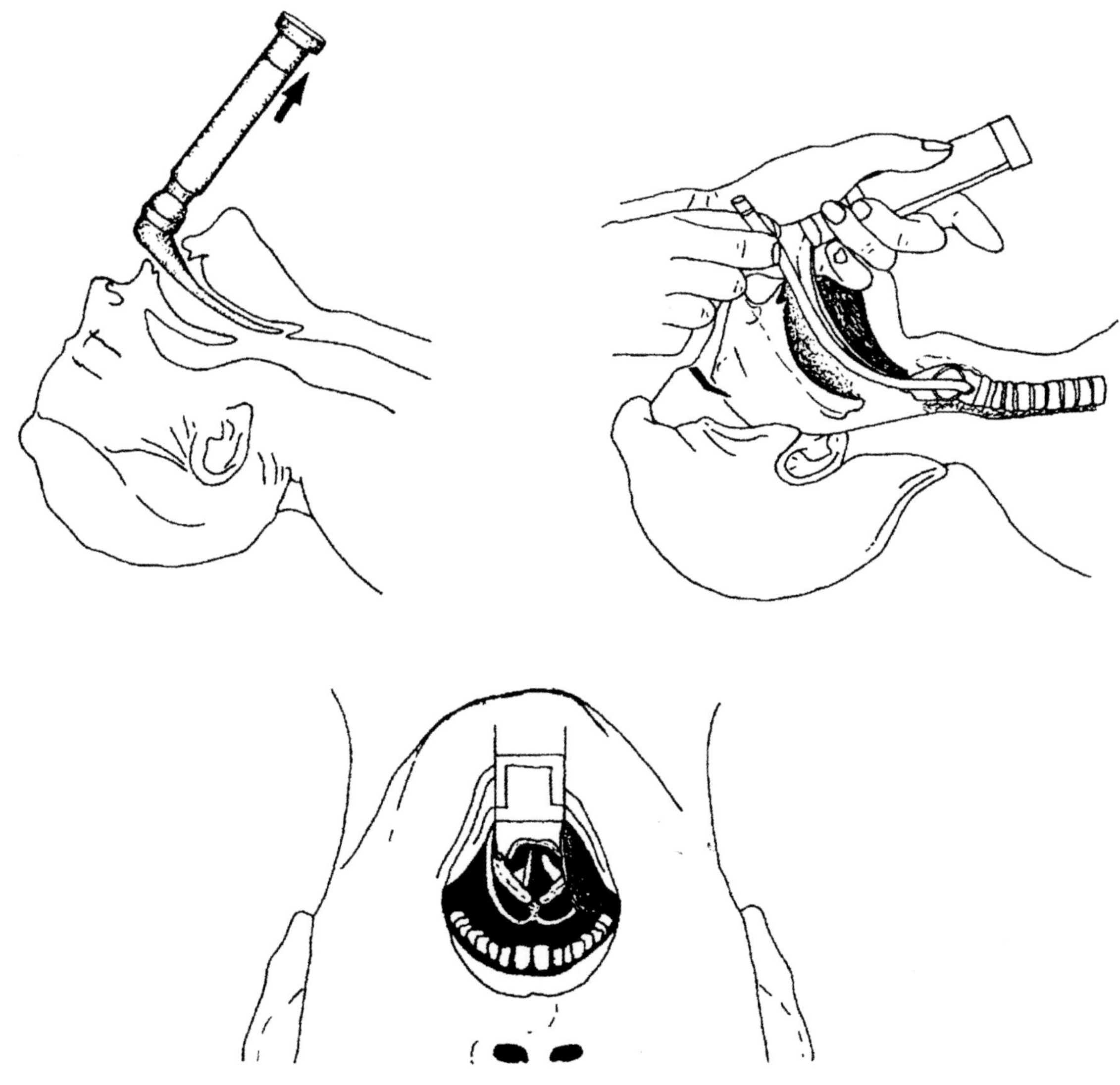

Figure 8.4 Endotracheal intubation

Tracheal intubation without using drugs is not possible unless the patient is very deeply unconscious or has sustained a cardiac arrest. If the patient is unconscious, intracranial pathology may be implied and intubation without anaesthetic and muscle-relaxation drugs will cause increases in blood pressure and intracranial pressure, which may exacerbate the intracranial condition. Intubation is therefore always a threat to patient wellbeing unless drugs are used.

Drugs should only be used to intubate by those with adequate anaesthetic training.

Where anaesthetic skills and drugs are available, endotracheal intubation is the preferred method of securing a definitive airway. This technique comprises rapid sequence induction of anaesthesia ('crash induction'):

- preoxygenation
- application of cricoid pressure

- rapid unconsciousness using drugs
- no 'bagging'
- rapid placement of endotracheal tube in trachea
- inflation of cuff before removal of cricoid pressure
- maintenance of cervical spine immobilisation when indicated.

Meticulous care must be taken to keep the cervical spine immobilised if injury to the cervical spine is suspected.

Intermittent oxygenation during difficult intubation

Inability to intubate will not kill. Inability to oxygenate will. If you can oxygenate by bag and mask, this will keep the patient alive.

Avoid prolonged efforts to intubate without intermittently oxygenating and ventilating. Practise taking a deep breath when starting an attempt at intubation. If you have to take a further breath before successfully intubating the patient, abort the attempt and re-oxygenate using the bag and mask technique.

The 2006–08 *Saving Mothers' Lives* report on maternal deaths in the UK once again identified failure to oxygenate in a patient with a difficult airway as a cause of maternal death.

Correct placement of the endotracheal tube

To check correct placement of the endotracheal tube:

- see the endotracheal tube pass between the vocal cords
- listen on both sides in the midaxillary line for equal breath sounds
- listen over the stomach for gurgling sounds during assisted ventilation for evidence of oesophageal intubation
- monitor end-tidal carbon dioxide levels; the use of capnography in the emergency intubation is increasingly recommended as a secondary method of confirming correct tube placement. Primary methods such as auscultation are still important, as in the absence of cardiac output there may be little exhaled carbon dioxide to detect. However, a capnograph may also help with ensuring continuing correct placement throughout the arrest and transfer, and presence of exhaled carbon dioxide is an indicator of restoration of cardiac output should it occur.
- if in doubt about the position of the endotracheal tube, take it out and oxygenate the patient by another method, bag and mask or surgical airway.

Other methods for maintaining the airway (not definitive airways as still unprotected)

The Laryngeal Mask Airway (LMA)

LMA (and other supraglottic airway devices) may be used to establish a patent airway and to maintain it, thereby allowing adequate ventilation to occur. In the past, LMAs have not been used in acute situations, but they are increasingly recommended as an alternative to bag mask ventilation in a cardiac arrest situation (International Liaison Committee on Resuscitation [ILCOR] guidelines). They are relatively easy to insert in nonexpert hands compared with tracheal intubation, which is important in the light of evidence from studies of intubation involving nonexperts resulting in an unacceptably high level of accidental oesophageal intubation. They may also be inserted with little, if any, interruption to cardiac compressions compared with intubation. Supraglottic airway devices do not protect the airway; consequently, there remains the potential risk of aspiration of gastric contents, which is a particular concern in pregnant women. They could be used by nonanaesthetists, in an emergency where the airway could not be maintained or ventilation reliably achieved by bag mask ventilation, in combination with an oropharyngeal (Guedel) airway. Any method of manual ventilation whether by bag-valve-mask or LMA can cause the stomach to become inflated, further predisposing to regurgitation.

Needle cricothyroidotomy

Needle cricothyroidotomy can be used to oxygenate in an emergency, but it is not a definitive airway and does not ventilate. A cannula-over-needle device is inserted through the cricothyroid membrane. This is attached to a low flow of oxygen from an insufflation device, or through oxygen tubing connected to wall oxygen at 15 litres/min, with either a Y-connector, three-way tap or side hole in the tubing at the cannula end of the tubing.

Surgical airway

A surgical airway should not be undertaken lightly and is used when:

- a hypoxic patient needing a definitive airway for resuscitation is too awake to tolerate endotracheal intubation without the use of anaesthetic drugs and there is no anaesthetist available to intubate in the time span in which the definitive airway is required
- trauma to the face and neck makes endotracheal intubation impossible
- a patient with face and neck burns requires airway protection to pre-empt delayed obstruction, but expert anaesthetic help is unavailable to carry out endotracheal intubation
- the anaesthetist cannot intubate or ventilate, e.g. at caesarean section.

Surgical cricothyroidotomy (see Figure 8.5) places a tube into the trachea via the cricothyroid membrane. A small tracheostomy tube (5–7 mm) is suitable. During the procedure, appropriate cervical spine protection must be maintained when indicated. There are also commercially available surgical cricothyroidotomy sets. A cricothyroidotomy can be replaced by a formal tracheostomy (if needed) at a later time.

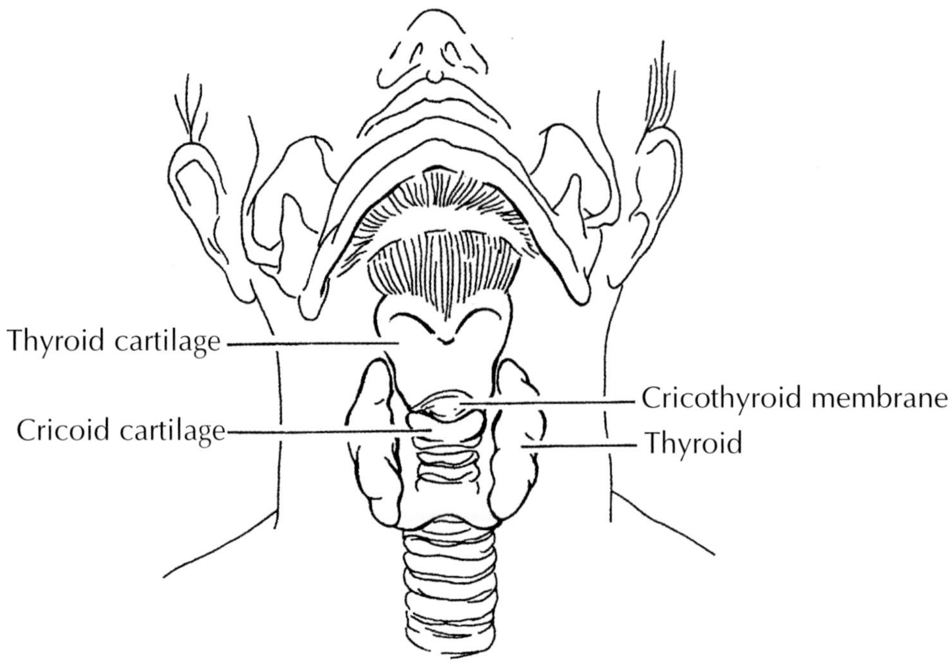

Figure 8.5 Anatomical landmarks for surgical cricothyrotomy

A formal emergency *surgical tracheostomy* takes longer and is more difficult than a surgical cricothyroidotomy. Commercial sets are available for rapid percutaneous tracheostomy using a Seldinger (guide wire) technique.

Management of ventilation

Once the airway is patent and maintained, there may be a separate requirement to assist breathing (ventilation). Spontaneous ventilation (self-ventilation) means the same as breathing. Assisted (artificial) ventilation means the patient is receiving help with breathing. The aim is to improve gaseous exchange in the lungs and to breathe for the patient if spontaneous ventilation has stopped or is inadequate. The indication for assisted ventilation is when ventilation is inadequate as in:

- chest injury
- respiratory depression due to drugs (such as opiates)
- head injury that might be causing respiratory depression and requires end-tidal carbon dioxide levels to be closely controlled to prevent cerebral vasodilatation and a consequent rise in intracranial pressure.

Assisted ventilation can be achieved by the following techniques:

- mouth-to-mouth (or nose) – unlikely in hospital
- mouth to pocket mask
- self-inflating bag to pocket mask or facemask
- self-inflating bag to endotracheal tube, LMA or tracheostomy tube
- automatic ventilation via endotracheal tube or tracheostomy tube.

Extubation

Attention to detail is also needed before extubation of any patient, even 'just' after elective surgery under general anaesthesia. The woman should be fully awake and able to protect her own airway before extubation.

Theoretically, in cases where a mother is known to have a full stomach before emergency anaesthesia, gastric contents can be reduced by gentle use of a soft, wide bore orogastric tube. However, this is rarely performed in practice as it is difficult to ensure stomach emptying. In practice, it is usual to await full awakening and utilise the left lateral or sitting position for extubation to aid the management of vomiting should it occur.

Anaesthetists should be aware of the dangers of extubation, and have a plan for rapid re-intubation should problems occur.

Summary

- Talk, look, listen, feel.
- Primary aim is to provide adequate oxygenation.
- Try simple manoeuvres, i.e. chin lift, jaw thrust, suction.
- Try simple adjuncts, namely the oropharyngeal airway.
- Tracheal intubation, endotracheal or surgical airway are gold standard because these achieve a patent airway, maintain patency and protect the airway; LMA may have a role in the absence of skilled help but does not provide a protected airway.
- Be aware of cervical spine injury during airway management.

Further reading

Centre for Maternal and Child Enquiries (CMACE). Saving Mothers' Lives: reviewing maternal deaths to make motherhood safer: 2006–8. The Eighth Report on Confidential Enquiries into Maternal Deaths in the United Kingdom. *BJOG* 2011;118 Suppl. 1:1–203.

APPENDIX 8A

Practical procedures

Oropharyngeal airway insertion

Equipment:

- a range of sizes of oropharyngeal (Guedel) airways
- tongue depressor (optional).

Procedure

The correct size of airway is selected by comparing it with the distance from the angle of the mandible to the centre of the incisors. The airway is inserted as follows:

1 Open the patient's mouth and check for debris. Debris may be inadvertently pushed into the larynx as the airway is inserted.

2 Insert the airway into the mouth either:
   - 'upside down' (concave uppermost) as far as the junction between the hard and soft palates and rotate through 180°
   - or use a tongue depressor to aid insertion of the airway 'the right way up' under direct vision.

3 Insert so that the flange lies in front of the upper and lower incisors or gums in the edentulous patient (Figure 8A.1).

4 Check the patency of the airway and ventilation by 'looking, listening, and feeling'.

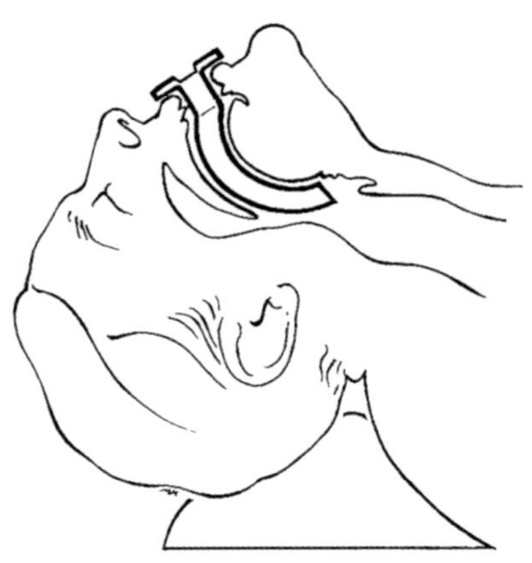

Figure 8A.1 Oropharyngeal airway in situ

Pocket mask

Equipment:

- pocket mask
- airway manikin.

Procedure

1. With the patient supine, apply the mask to the patient's face, using the thumbs and index fingers of both hands.
2. Use the remaining fingers to exert pressure behind the angles of the jaw (as for the jaw thrust), at the same time pressing the mask on to the face to make a tight seal (Figure 8A.2).
3. Blow through the inspiratory valve for 1–2 seconds, at the same time looking to ensure that the chest rises and then falls.
4. If oxygen is available, add via the oxygen inlet at 12–15 litres/min.

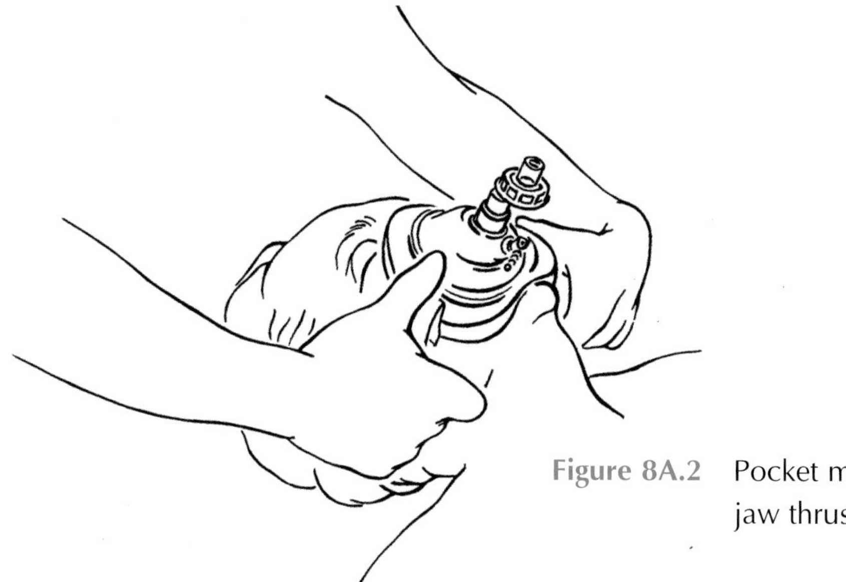

Figure 8A.2 Pocket mask in situ using a jaw thrust technique

Insertion of the LMA

Equipment:

- LMA
- lubricant
- syringe to inflate cuff
- adhesive tape to secure LMA
- suction
- ventilating device.

Procedure

Whenever possible, ventilate the patient with 100% oxygen using a bag–valve–mask device before inserting the LMA. During this time, check that all the equipment is present and working, particularly the integrity of the cuff.

1 Deflate the cuff and lightly lubricate the back and sides of the mask.

2 Tilt the patient's head (if safe to do so), open the mouth fully and insert the tip of the mask along the hard palate with the open side facing, but not touching, the tongue (Figure 8A.3a).

3 Advance the LMA, along the posterior pharyngeal wall, with your index finger initially providing support for the tube (Figure 8A.3b). Eventually, resistance is felt as the tip of the LMA lies at the upper end of the oesophagus (Figure 8A.3c). It is extremely helpful if an assistant performs a jaw thrust manoeuvre as the LMA is inserted in order to make more space for the LMA in the posterior pharynx.

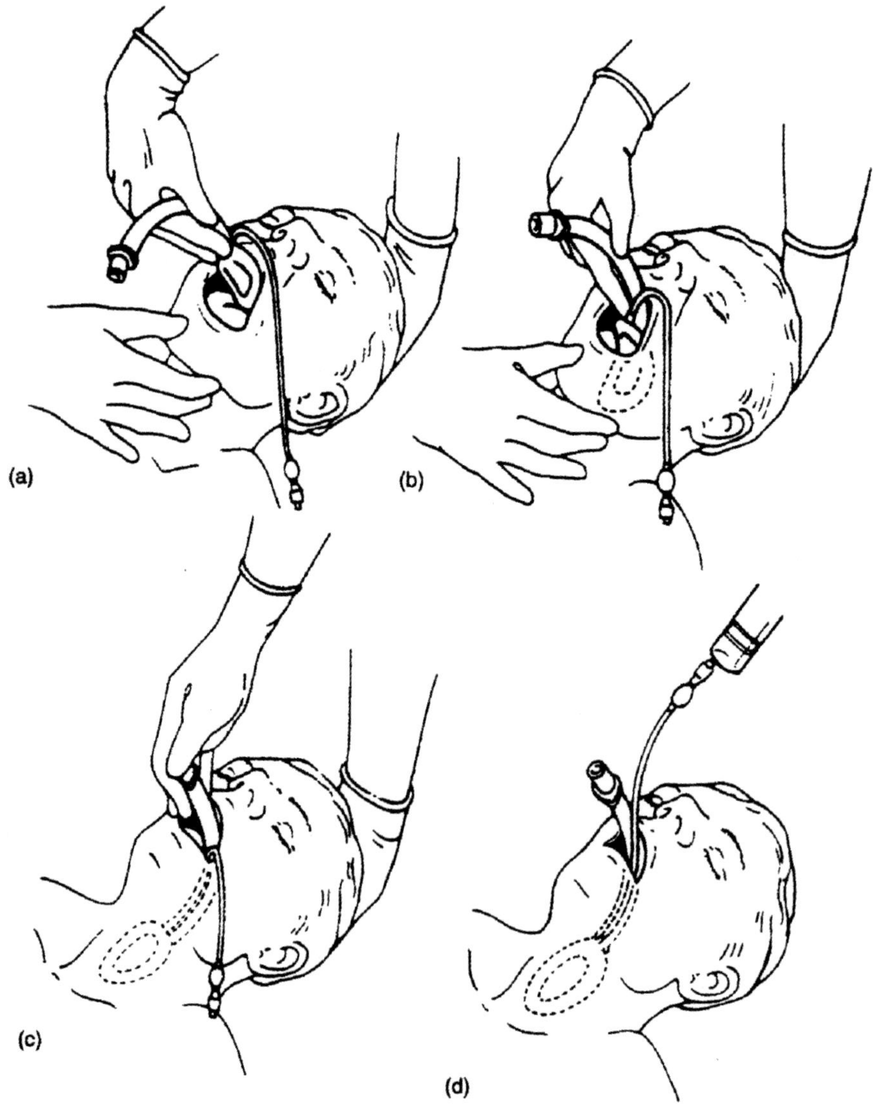

Figure 8A.3 Inserting a laryngeal mask airway

4 Fully inflate the cuff using the air-filled syringe attached to the valve at the end of the pilot tube using the volume of air shown in Table 8A.1 (Figure 8A.3d).

5 Secure the LMA with adhesive tape and check its position during ventilation as for a tracheal tube.

6 If insertion is not accomplished in less than 30 seconds, re-establish ventilation using a bag–valve–mask.

Table 8A.1 LMA sizes and inflation volumes

LMA size	Maximum inflation volume (mL)
3	20
4	30
5	40
6	50

Complications

Incorrect placement is usually due to the tip of the cuff folding over during insertion. The LMA should be withdrawn and reinserted.

Inability to ventilate the patient can be because the epiglottis has been displaced over the larynx. Withdraw the LMA and reinsert it, ensuring that it closely follows the hard palate. This may be facilitated by the operator or an assistant lifting the jaw upwards. Occasionally, rotation of the LMA may prevent its insertion. Check that the line along the tube is aligned with the patient's nasal septum; if not, reinsert.

Coughing or laryngeal spasm is usually due to attempts to insert the LMA into a patient whose laryngeal reflexes are still present.

Surgical airways

It is important to realise that these techniques are temporary measures, while preparing for a definitive airway.

Needle cricothyroidotomy

Equipment:

- cannulae 12–14 gauge
- jet insufflation equipment
- oxygen tubing with either a three-way tap or a hole cut in the side
- 20 ml syringe.

Procedure

1. Place the patient supine with the head slightly extended.
2. Identify the cricothyroid membrane as the recess between the thyroid cartilage (Adam's apple) and cricoid cartilage (approximately 2 cm below the V-shaped notch of the thyroid cartilage).
3. Puncture this membrane vertically using a large-bore (12–14 gauge) intravenous cannula attached to a syringe or use a purpose-designed curved metal cannula (Figure 8A.4).
4. Aspiration of air confirms that the tip of the cannula lies within the tracheal lumen.
5. Angle the cannula at 45° caudally and advance over the needle into the trachea.
6. Attach the cannula to an oxygen supply at 12–15 litres/minute either via a 'Y' connector or a hole cut in the side of the oxygen tubing. Oxygen is delivered to the patient by occluding the open limb of the connector or side hole for 1 second and then releasing for 4 seconds.
7. Expiration occurs passively through the larynx. Watch the chest for movement and auscultate for breath sounds, although the latter are difficult to hear.
8. If satisfactory, secure the cannula in place to prevent it being dislodged.
9. An alternative method of delivering oxygen is to use jet ventilation. This involves connecting the cannula to a high-pressure oxygen source (4 bar, 400 kPa, 60psi) via luerlock connectors or by using a Sanders injector. The same ventilatory cycle is used. This is the method designated when a metal curved needle is used with a Luer lock connector to the high pressure source.

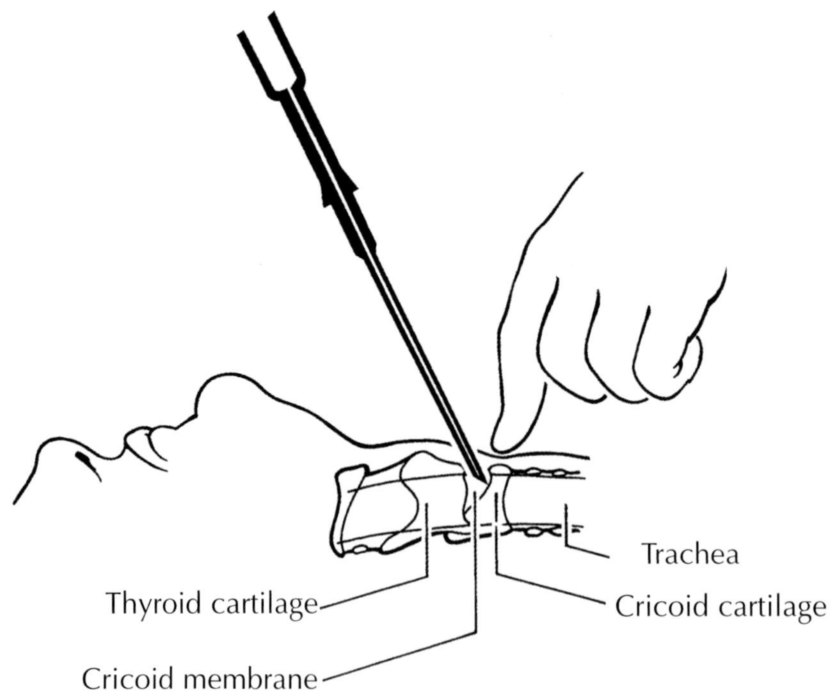

Figure 8A.4 Needle cricothyrotomy

Complications

Complications of these techniques can include:

- asphyxia
- pulmonary barotrauma
- bleeding
- oesophageal perforation
- kinking of the cannula
- subcutaneous and mediastinal emphysema
- aspiration.

Occasionally, this method of oxygenation will disimpact a foreign body from the larynx, allowing more acceptable methods of ventilation to be used.

There are two important facts to remember about transtracheal insufflation of oxygen:

1 It is not possible to deliver oxygen via a needle cricothyroidotomy using a self-inflating bag and valve. This is because these devices do not generate sufficient pressure to drive adequate volumes of gas through a narrow cannula. In comparison, the wall oxygen supply will provide a pressure of 400 kPa (4000 cm H_2O), which overcomes the resistance of the cannula.

2 Expiration cannot occur through the cannula or through a separate cannula inserted through the cricothyroid membrane. The pressure generated during expiration is generally less than 3 kPa (30 cm H_2O), which is clearly much less than the pressure required to drive gas in initially. Expiration must occur through the upper airway, even when partially obstructed. If the obstruction is complete, then the oxygen flow must be reduced to 2–4 litres/min to avoid the risk of barotrauma, in particular the creation of a tension pneumothorax.

Surgical cricothyroidotomy

Equipment:

- antiseptic solution
- swab
- syringe, needle and local anaesthetic
- scalpel
- two arterial clips
- endotracheal tube or size 5 tracheotomy tubes
- tape
- gloves.

Procedure

1. Place the patient supine if possible, with the head extended.
2. Identify the cricothyroid membrane, as described earlier.
3. Stabilise the thyroid cartilage using the thumb, index and middle fingers of the left hand.
4. If the patient is conscious, consider infiltrating with local anaesthetic containing epinephrine (adrenaline) (lignocaine 1% with epinephrine 1/200 000).
5. Make a longitudinal incision down to the membrane, pressing the lateral edges of the skin outwards to reduce bleeding.
6. Incise the membrane transversely and dilate the channel with the scalpel handle to accept a small (4–7mm) cuffed tracheostomy tube. If one of these is not immediately available, a similarly sized endotracheal tube can be used and shortened appropriately.
7. Ensure that the tube enters the tracheal lumen, rather than just running anteriorly in the soft tissues.
8. Inflate the cuff and start ventilation.
9. Check the adequacy of ventilation as described earlier and, if satisfactory, the tube can be secured.
10. Suction the upper airway via the tube to remove any inhaled blood or vomit.

An alternative technique in these circumstances is the 'Mini-Trach' (Portex). This was originally designed to facilitate the removal of secretions from the chest. The 'kit' contains everything required to create an emergency surgical airway.

1. Use a guarded scalpel to puncture the cricothyroid membrane percutaneously to the correct depth.
2. Pass the rigid, curved introducer through the puncture site into the trachea.
3. Pass the 4mm PVC flanged tracheal cannula (with a standard 15mm connector attached) over the introducer into the trachea.
4. Remove the introducer and secure the cannula via the flanges with tapes.
5. Ventilate the patient using the devices already described.

Complications

These are similar to needle cricothyroidotomy, except that bleeding is more profuse due to the larger incision. Vocal cord damage may result in hoarseness and cricoid cartilage damage may cause laryngeal stenosis.

ALGORITHM 9.1 Basic life support: pregnant woman, reproduced with the kind permission of the Resuscitation Council (UK)

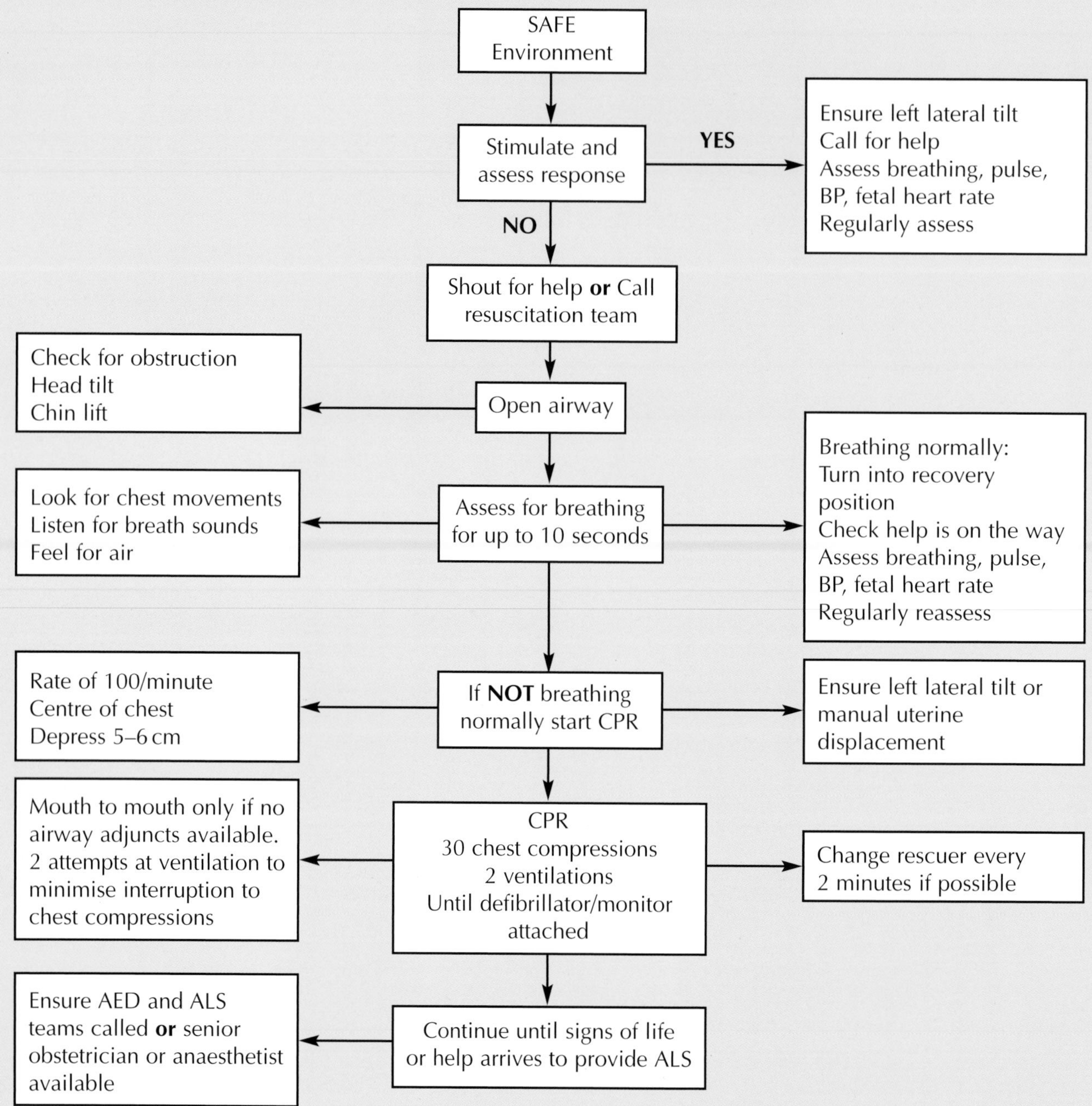

Left tilt (or uterine displacement). Empty the uterus if approx. 18–20 weeks onwards. Aim for uterine evacuation within 5 min.

ALGORITHM 9.2 Automated external defibrillator use, reproduced with the kind permission of the Resuscitation Council (UK)

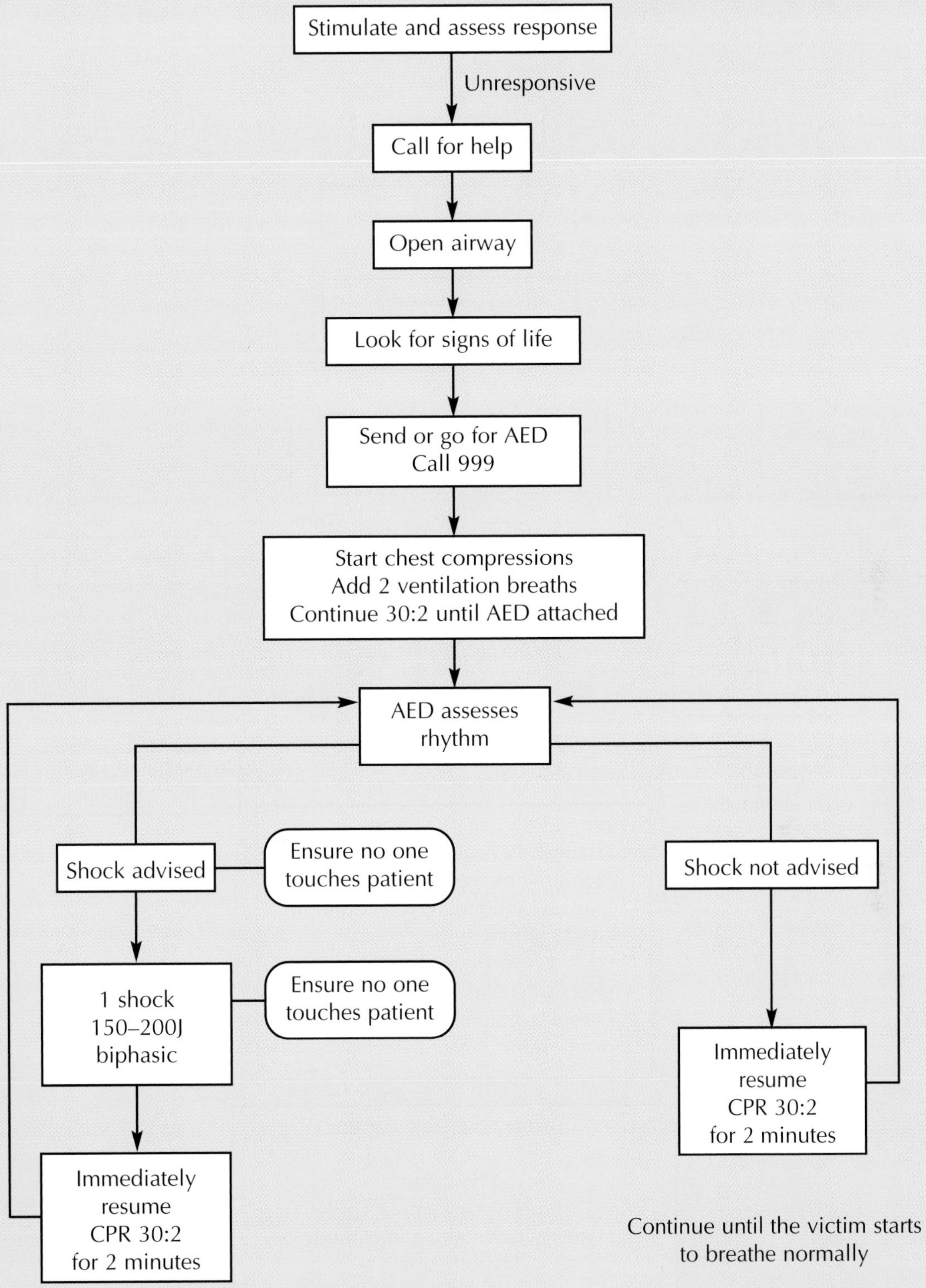

Left tilt (or uterine displacement). Empty the uterus if approx. 18–20 weeks onwards. Aim for uterine evacuation within 5 min.

ALGORITHM 9.3 Advanced life support, reproduced with the kind permission of the Resuscitation Council (UK)

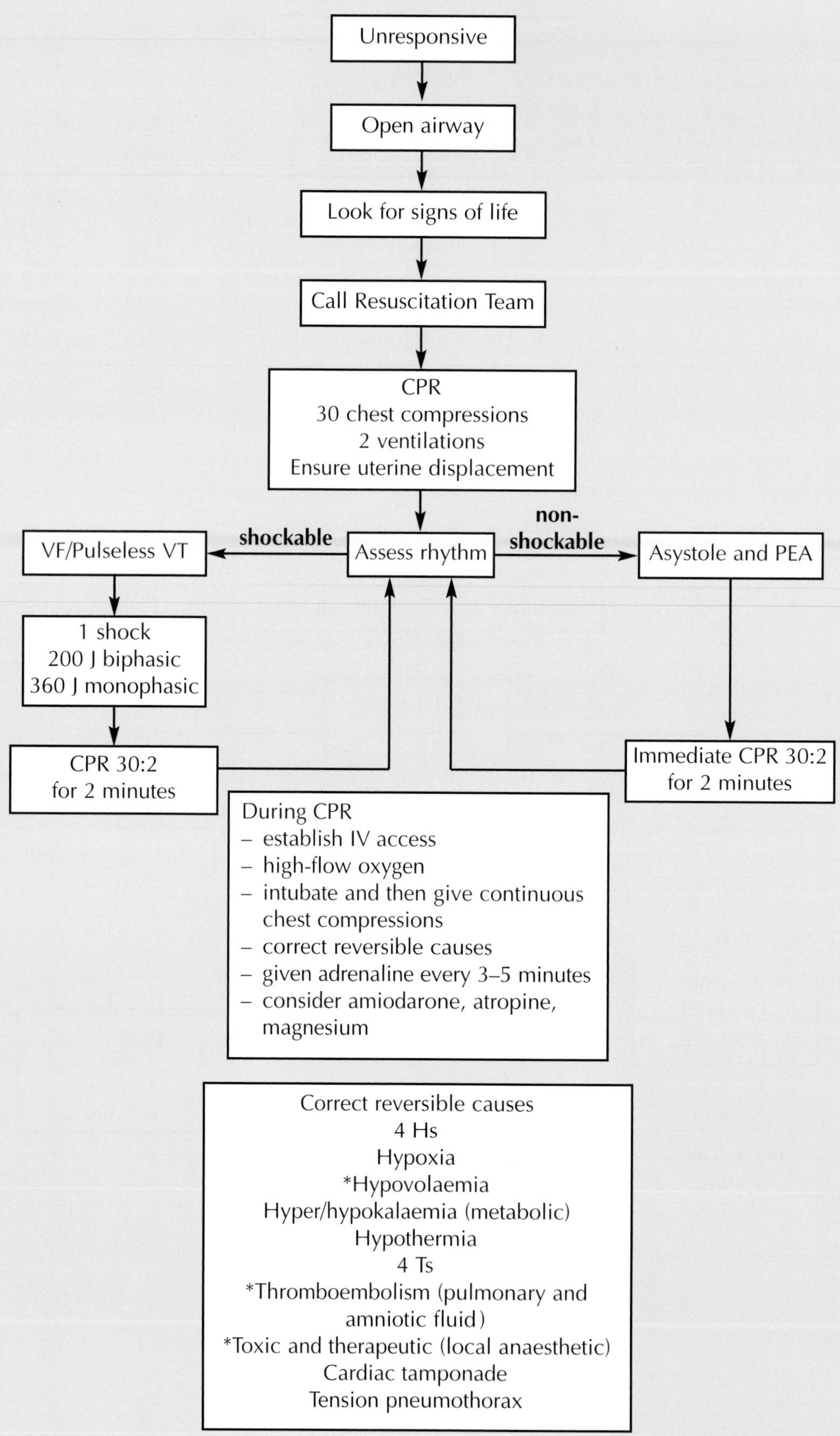

Left tilt (or uterine displacement). Empty the uterus if approx. 18–20 weeks onwards. Aim for uterine evacuation within 5 min.

*more likely in pregnancy

CHAPTER 9

Cardiopulmonary resuscitation in the nonpregnant and pregnant patient

Objectives

On successfully completing this topic, you will be able to:

- understand how to perform basic and advanced life support
- understand the importance of early defibrillation where appropriate
- understand the adaptations of CPR in the pregnant woman.

Introduction and incidence

Cardiac arrest is estimated to occur in every 30 000 deliveries. Both thromboembolism and amniotic fluid embolism are important causes of maternal death, which may present with sudden collapse. It is important that the healthcare teams know the appropriate actions to take in such an event, to improve outcome for both the mother and the child.

Basic life support

Basic life support describes the procedures that a trained *lay person* could be expected to provide. These include:

- recognising an absence of breathing or other signs of life
- knowing to ask for automated external defibrillator (AED) when summoning help
- performing chest compressions and mouth to mouth or pocket-mask breathing
- (If rescuer not happy to perform mouth to mouth breathing can continue with only chest compressions)
- minimising interruptions to chest compression while using AED.

Advanced life support

Advanced life support describes the procedures that a trained *healthcare professional* could be expected to provide. This includes all of the above, and in addition:

- the use of airway adjuncts to provide more effective ventilation
- the insertion of intravenous cannulae to give drugs
- the use of semi-automated or manual defibrillators.

It should not be necessary to perform mouth to mouth ventilation in a hospital as airway adjuncts should be close to hand.

In a hospital setting, the distinction between basic and advanced life support is arbitrary. The clinical team should be able to provide cardiopulmonary resuscitation, the fundamental components of which are:

- rapid recognition of cardiopulmonary collapse
- summoning help using a standard procedure/number
- starting cardiopulmonary resuscitation using appropriate adjuncts
- early defibrillation, when required, if possible within 3 minutes.

Recent guidelines place greater emphasis on high-quality cardiac compressions (*'push hard and fast'*) with minimal interruptions.

Management

As shown in Algorithm 9.1, the rescuer must ensure a safe environment. Try to rouse the woman by gently shaking and shouting. If no response, call for help and then return to the woman. If there is no response but there are still *'signs of life'*, then urgent medical attention should be requested and further assessment and appropriate treatment given. Signs of life include:

- normal breathing (not agonal gasps)
- movement
- coughing/gagging.

In the event of little or no signs of life, the following instructions should be carried out, simultaneously if there are multiple helpers, but of necessity are described in an appropriate order for one person.

Turn the woman onto her back with manual uterine displacement or left lateral tilt

In a noticeably pregnant woman i.e. one with a significant intra-abdominal mass (by approximately 20 weeks) it is important to minimise aortocaval compression by the uterus

(Figure 9.1). This is because aortocaval compression will significantly reduce the output that can be achieved with cardiac compressions.

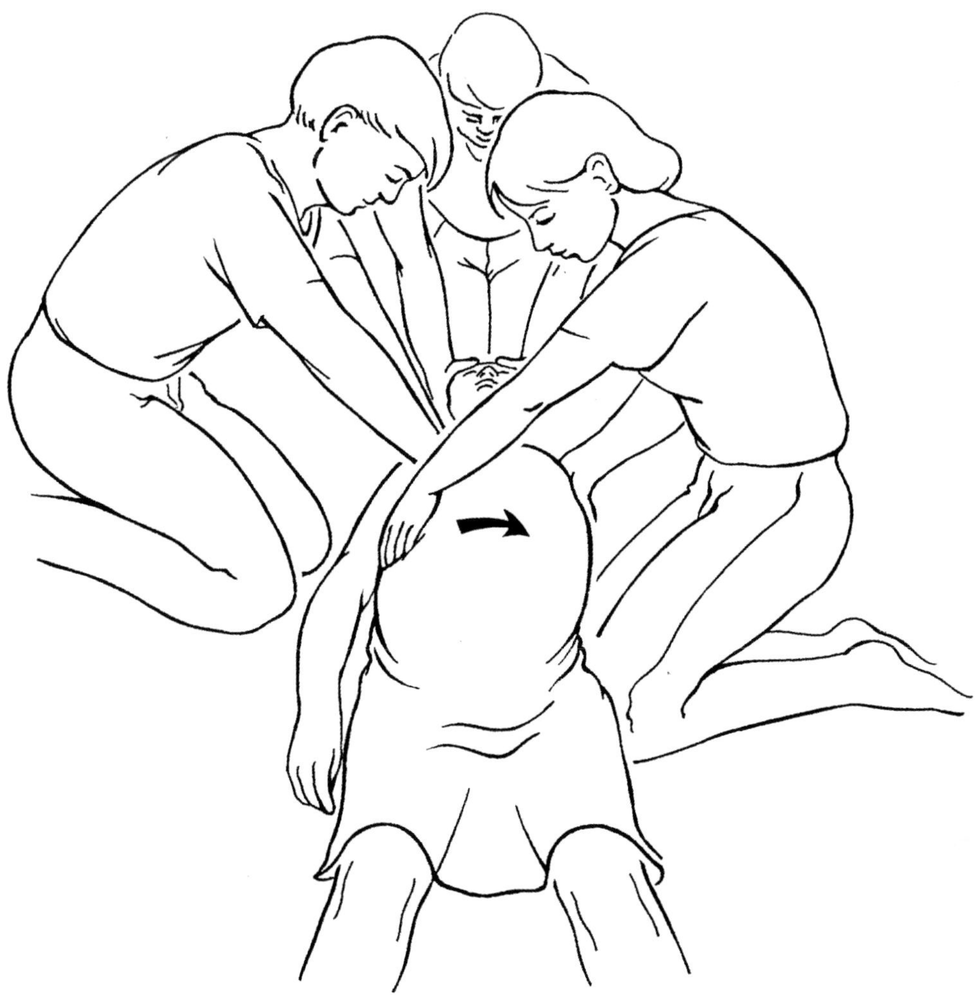

Figure 9.1 Manual displacement of the uterus to left

Open the airway

Open the mouth and briefly check for debris or foreign bodies. Use suction or forceps under direct vision to remove any obstruction, taking care not to cause trauma.

To open the airway, place your hand on the patient's forehead and gently tilt the head back. At the same time, with your fingertips under the point of the patient's chin, lift the chin to open the airway. This manoeuvre will straighten the head and neck from a slumped or flexed position, and may slightly extend the head relative to the neck. It allows more space behind the tongue in the posterior pharynx for air movement. In a conscious person, the pharyngeal muscle tone naturally maintains this space for breathing, but will be absent in the unconscious person. An oral airway may be used to provide the same space behind the tongue, with less requirement for vigorous head extension.

A jaw thrust may be required to open the airway. Do this by placing fingers *behind* both of the angles of the jaw and pushing the jaw anteriorly to displace tongue from the pharynx. If an injury to the neck is suspected, use manual inline stabilisation, avoid head tilt and use jaw thrust to open the airway.

Assess breathing (and signs of life: circulation)

Assess breathing for *no more than ten seconds* by simultaneously looking for chest movements, listening for breath sounds and feeling for the movement of air. Absence of breathing in the presence of a clear airway is now considered a marker of absence of circulation, along with absence of gagging or movement. Experienced staff may check the carotid pulse for no more than ten seconds at the same time as assessing breathing, but it is important to be aware of how difficult it is for even experienced clinicians to confirm the absence of a pulse and not to waste time before starting chest compressions. 'Unnecessary' chest compressions are almost never harmful. Gasping or agonal breathing may occur during cardiac arrest and *should not* be taken as a sign of life – it is a sign of dying and CPR should commence immediately.

If no circulation (or you are at all unsure)
give 30 chest compressions followed by two ventilations

Start CPR

(a) Chest compressions should be applied to the lower half of the sternum. Place the heel of one hand there, with the other hand on top of the first. Interlock the fingers of both hands and lift the fingers to ensure that pressure is not applied over the patient's ribs. Keep in the midline at all times. Do not apply any pressure over the top of the abdomen or lower tip of the sternum.
(b) Position yourself above the chest and with your arms straight, press down on the sternum to depress 5–6 cm at a rate of 100 to 120 beats/minute in a ratio of 30:2 compressions to ventilations. Change the person doing chest compressions about every 2 minutes to maintain efficiency, but avoid any delays in the changeover.
(c) Ventilation breaths. Keep an open airway and provide ventilation with appropriate adjuncts. This might be a pocket mask, oral airway or self-inflating bag with mask. Oxygen in high flow should be added as soon as possible.
(d) Each breath should last about 1 second and should make the chest rise as if a normal breath. Tracheal intubation should only be undertaken by experienced personnel with minimal interruption to chest compressions. The LMA may be useful as an alternative airway adjunct if intubation cannot be achieved swiftly. Once the woman is intubated, ventilation should continue at a rate of ten breaths per minute, but does not need to be synchronised with chest compressions. These should be continued without interruption.
(e) Mouth to mouth breathing is rarely necessary in the hospital setting – the important thing is to maintain a patent airway during cardiac compressions.

If it is undertaken, head tilt and chin lift should be maintained. Close the soft part of the woman's nose with your thumb and index finger. Open her mouth but maintain chin lift. Take a breath and place your lips around the mouth, making sure that you have a good seal. Blow steadily into the mouth for over 1 second, watching for the chest to rise. Maintaining head tilt and chin lift, take your mouth away and watch for the chest to fall as the air comes out. Take another breath and repeat the sequence to give another effective breath. Return to chest compressions quickly.

If circulation present but no breathing (respiratory arrest) continue rescue breathing at a rate of ten breaths/minute

Recheck the circulation every ten breaths, taking no more than 10 seconds each time. If the woman starts to breathe on her own but remains unconscious, turn her into the recovery position and apply high flow oxygen (15 litres/minute or maximum flow rate available). Check her condition and be ready to turn her back to restart rescue breathing if she stops breathing and/or compressions if necessary.

Capnography can be used in CPR. Although CO_2 levels are low, they are not nil and can be used to monitor CPR efficacy. An increase in CO_2 will indicate return of spontaneous circulation (ROSC). There is evidence that post-resuscitation hyperoxaemia is associated with a worse outcome compared with normoxaemia or hypoxaemia and so, once arterial oxygen can be monitored, aim to keep saturation between 94 and 98% by adjusting oxygen flow as needed.

Automated external defibrillation (AED)

As soon as possible, apply the defibrillator pads or paddles and pause compressions briefly to assess the rhythm. This is quicker than attaching the ECG stickers. If a shockable rhythm is identified by the AED, then continue chest compressions while the AED is charging if necessary. Follow the AED voice prompts or use manual defibrillation as appropriate (Algorithm 9.2).

The most frequent initial rhythm in the context of sudden collapse in an adult (i.e. not preceded by gradual deterioration, or illness) is ventricular fibrillation (VF). The chance of successful defibrillation diminishes over minutes. The AED enables early defibrillation by less trained personnel, as it performs rhythm analysis, gives information by voice or visual display and delivers a shock automatically (Algorithm 9.2).

Attach AED pads (or position gel pads for manual defibrillator)

Expose the chest and place one adhesive defibrillator pad on the patient's chest to the right of the sternum below the right clavicle, and one in the left midaxillary line, taking care to avoid breast tissue. Keep the axillary electrode vertical to maximise efficiency.

If defibrillation is *not* indicated CPR should be continued for 2 minutes, at which stage the AED will prompt further analysis of rhythm. If a shock is indicated, deliver it (many devices do this automatically) and immediately resume compressions for 2 minutes, after which there will be a further prompt for a rhythm analysis.

Follow the advanced life support algorithm

When trained support arrives, the rhythm should be identified as shockable or nonshockable and defibrillation instituted if indicated without delay, if not already under way. The airway should be secured and intravenous access obtained (Algorithm 9.3).

Shockable rhythms

- Shockable rhythms are treated by a single shock followed by immediate continuation of compressions without stopping for a rhythm or pulse check.
- Every 2 minutes, the rhythm should be assessed and, if necessary, a further shock delivered. The pulse is not checked *unless* there is organised electrical activity i.e. a rhythm that looks as though it might produce an output or signs of life.
- The energy used for defibrillation depends on whether a monophasic or biphasic defibrillator is used. Most modern defibrillators are biphasic as this is the most efficient way of delivering energy. The charge needed is therefore lower than on the older monophasic machines.
- The initial and subsequent shocks should be 150–200 J from a biphasic machine or 360 J from a monophasic machine
- On the shockable side of the algorithm, adrenaline, 1 mg IV, is given once chest compressions are started *after the third shock* and then after alternate shocks; i.e. approximately every 4 minutes. Amiodarone 300 mg IV is also given after the third shock.

Nonshockable rhythms

- On the nonshockable side of the algorithm (i.e. pulseless electrical activity [PEA] or asystole), adrenaline (epinephrine) 1 mg should be given as soon as intravenous access is available and thereafter, every 3–5 minutes while continuing chest compressions and ventilations at 30:2.

Reversible causes of cardiac arrest should be considered and treated as necessary. *Hypovolaemia* (from haemorrhage or sepsis) and *thromboembolism* are the most common causes of cardiac arrest/collapse in pregnancy. They are more likely to cause *nonshockable cardiac arrest.* See Chapters 5, 6, 10, 11 and 25.

Four Hs:

- Hypoxia
- Hypovolaemia (haemorrhage or sepsis)
- Hyperkalaemia and other metabolic disorders
- Hypothermia.

Four Ts:

- Thromboembolism
- Toxicity (drugs, e.g. magnesium overdose or those associated with regional or general anaesthesia)
- Tension pneumothorax
- cardiac Tamponade.

Doubt about the rhythm

If there is doubt about whether the rhythm is asystole or fine VF, CPR should be maintained and the algorithm for asystole (nonshockable rhythm) followed.

Other drugs

Sodium bicarbonate: 50 mmol IV should only be given routinely if the arrest is associated with tricyclic antidepressant overdose or hyperkalaemia. Otherwise, it should not be given routinely as it exacerbates intracellular acidosis, reduces tissue oxygen availability and has a negative inotropic effect on the myocardium. Arterial blood gases are not reliable in cardiac arrest, venous blood gases provide a better estimation of tissue pH.

Magnesium sulphate: 8 mmol (4 ml of 50% solution) may be given for refractory VF. Other indications include hypomagnesaemia, torsade de pointes (a persistent VF) or digoxin toxicity. These are unlikely in pregnancy.

Calcium: 10 ml 10% calcium chloride (6.8 mmol Ca^{2+}) IV is indicated if PEA is suspected to be due to hyperkalaemia, hypocalcaemia or overdose of calcium channel blocking drugs. Calcium maybe given as a bolus if the patient has no output, *but not in the same line as sodium bicarbonate* as this will result in precipitation. Magnesium overdose (usually in the context of treatment of pre-eclampsia) is usually reversed with calcium gluconate.

Physiological changes in pregnancy affecting resuscitation

There are a number of reasons why cardiopulmonary resuscitation is more difficult to perform and may be less effective in the pregnant than in the nonpregnant population. The presence of an increasing intra-abdominal mass compromises resuscitative efforts from about 20 weeks of gestation, but the effect will become more marked as the mother approaches term.

Vena caval occlusion

At term, the vena cava is completely occluded in 90% of healthy *supine* pregnant women and the stroke volume may be only 30% of that of a nonpregnant woman. As soon as the infant is delivered, the vena caval flow returns towards normal and adequate venous return, and consequently cardiac output is restored.

During cardiac arrest, in order to minimise the effects of the gravid uterus on venous return and cardiac output, a maternal pelvic tilt to the left of greater than 15° is recommended. The problem is that tilting the patient may delay starting compressions and itself will reduce their efficacy. The priority is to *start effective cardiac compressions as early as possible.* Therefore, preferably, aortocaval compression should be minimised through manual uterine displacement (Figure 9.1). If tilt is used, it should be between 15 and 30°.

Delivery of the fetus during cardiac arrest will increase the venous return to the heart and reduce the oxygen demands on the mother, thereby increasing the chances of successful resuscitation (see below).

Changes in lung function

Pregnant women become hypoxic faster because functional residual capacity is reduced by 20% due to the pressure by the gravid uterus on the diaphragm and the lungs – they have a smaller reservoir of oxygen to withstand apnoea. This is exacerbated by a 20% increase in the resting oxygen usage due to the demands of the fetus and uterus. These changes make it difficult to provide adequate oxygen delivery during resuscitation of a pregnant woman who is near term.

Efficacy of ventilation

In the latter half of pregnancy it is increasingly difficult to provide effective ventilation breaths during CPR, due to the increased weight of the abdominal contents and the breasts. Oesophageal sphincter tone is reduced, so the stomach is more readily inflated and the risk of passive regurgitation of stomach contents and acid aspiration into the lungs is increased. It is imperative that the airway is protected and adequate ventilation established with a cuffed endotracheal tube as early as possible, by appropriately trained staff.

Peri-arrest/perimortem caesarean section to improve chances of maternal survival

The Resuscitation Council considers that prompt caesarean delivery should be seen as part of resuscitation in cardiac arrest in advanced pregnancy. Delivery of the fetus will obviate the effects of aortocaval compression and significantly improve the chance of successful resuscitation. This will reduce maternal oxygen consumption, increase venous return, make ventilation easier and allow CPR in the supine position.

When to do it

All the evidence suggests that a caesarean delivery should begin within 4 minutes of cardiac arrest and be accomplished by 5 minutes. In practice this means preparations for surgical evacuation of the uterus should begin almost at the same time as CPR following cardiac arrest. Pregnant women develop anoxia faster than nonpregnant women and can suffer irreversible brain damage within 4–6 minutes of cardiac arrest. CPR should be continued throughout the CS and afterwards, as this increases the chances of a successful neonatal and maternal outcome.

Where to do it

The woman should *not* be transferred to an operating theatre as it will merely waste time. She should be delivered at the site of collapse, unless physically impossible. Diathermy will not be needed, as blood loss is minimal with no cardiac output. If the mother is successfully resuscitated, she can be moved to theatre to be anaesthetised and to complete the operation.

How to do it

A minimum amount of equipment is required in this situation. Sterile preparation and drapes are unlikely to improve survival. A surgical knife is sufficient.

No one surgical approach is particularly recommended and should be based on operator preference. The classical midline abdominal approach is aided by the natural diastasis of recti abdomini that occurs in late pregnancy and the relatively bloodless field in this situation. However, many obstetricians are more familiar with a lower transverse abdominal incision and can deliver a baby in less than a minute.

Open cardiac massage during surgery is a possibility when the abdomen is already open and the heart can be reached relatively easily through the diaphragm (if a midline approach has been used).

An anaesthetist should attend at the earliest opportunity to provide a protected airway, ensure continuity of effective chest compressions and adequate ventilation breaths, as well as helping to determine and treat any underlying cause (four H's and four T's).

Should resuscitation be successful and the mother regain a cardiac output, appropriate anaesthesia and pain relief will be required, and the woman should be moved to a theatre to complete the operation.

Fetal outcome

It is emphasised that CS is part of resuscitation and is carried out to improve maternal survival, and it is worthwhile once the uterus has reached the level of the umbilicus (i.e. about 20 weeks of gestation). If performed promptly, it can also improve fetal survival, although gestational age at the time of delivery also clearly influences outcome. In the 2006–08 report on maternal mortality there were no neonatal survivors among those delivered at less than 28 weeks. Of those babies delivered at >36 weeks, 47% did survive: all but one in this group involved CPR begun in hospital, illustrating the advantage of early evacuation of the uterus for the neonate as well as the mother.

Although uterine evacuation is a well-validated step in maternal resuscitation, there is still reluctance among some obstetricians to perform peri-arrest caesarean sections due to concerns about neonatal neurological damage. However, in a comprehensive review of postmortem caesarean deliveries between 1900 and 1985 by Katz *et al.*, 70% (42/61) of infants delivered within 5 minutes survived and all developed normally.[1] Only 13% (8/61) of those delivered at 10 minutes, and 12% (7/61) delivered at 15 minutes, survived. One infant in each of the groups of later survivors had neurological damage. Later series confirm the advantage of early delivery for intact fetal survival, although there are a few case reports of intact infant survival more than 20 minutes after maternal cardiac arrest. Evidence suggests that if the fetus survives the neonatal period, then the chances of normal development are good.

Make decision to abandon CPR if unsuccessful

CPR should be continued if the rhythm continues as VF/VT. A decision to abandon CPR should only be made after discussion with the consultant obstetrician and senior clinicians.

Medico-legal concerns

No doctor has been found liable for performing a postmortem CS. Theoretically, liability may concern either criminal or civil wrongdoing. Operating without consent may be argued as battery if the mother is successfully resuscitated. However, the doctrine of emergency exception would be applied because a delay in treatment could cause harm. Another criminal offence theoretically could be 'mutilation of corpse'. An operation performed to save life would not be wrongful, because there would be no criminal intent. The unanimous consensus in the literature is that a civil suit for performing perimortem caesarean is very unlikely to succeed.

Communication and teamwork

Senior input from obstetricians, anaesthetists and midwives should be obtained as early as possible. Evidence suggests that resuscitation is more likely to be successful when there is effective communication, clear leadership and good team-working. Frequently the team will be aided by a Resuscitation Training Officer. Ensure that the family is looked after and kept informed. It is vital to document timings and interventions accurately. If the mother dies, the coroner and the GP must be informed.

Logistics

- Recruit as many staff as possible. In addition to the team leader, and those performing the resuscitation, you will need an individual responsible for each of the following:
- recording events and management
- communication
- runner/porter/transport.

Summary

- Cardiopulmonary resuscitation in pregnancy follows the techniques of basic and advanced life support, combined with lateral tilt and prompt recourse to uterine evacuation.
- Rehearsing the drills and discussing perimortem caesarean sections in teaching sessions will help familiarise staff with the procedures and support them if they are unfortunate enough to face such a decision in the workplace.

Reference and further reading

1 Katz V, Balderston K, DeFreest M. Perimortem caesarean delivery: were our assumptions correct? *Am J Obstet Gynecol* 2005;192:1916–20.

2 Nolan JP. *Resuscitation Guidelines 2010 edition.* Resuscitation Council (UK), October 2010.

ALGORITHM 10.1 Amniotic fluid embolism

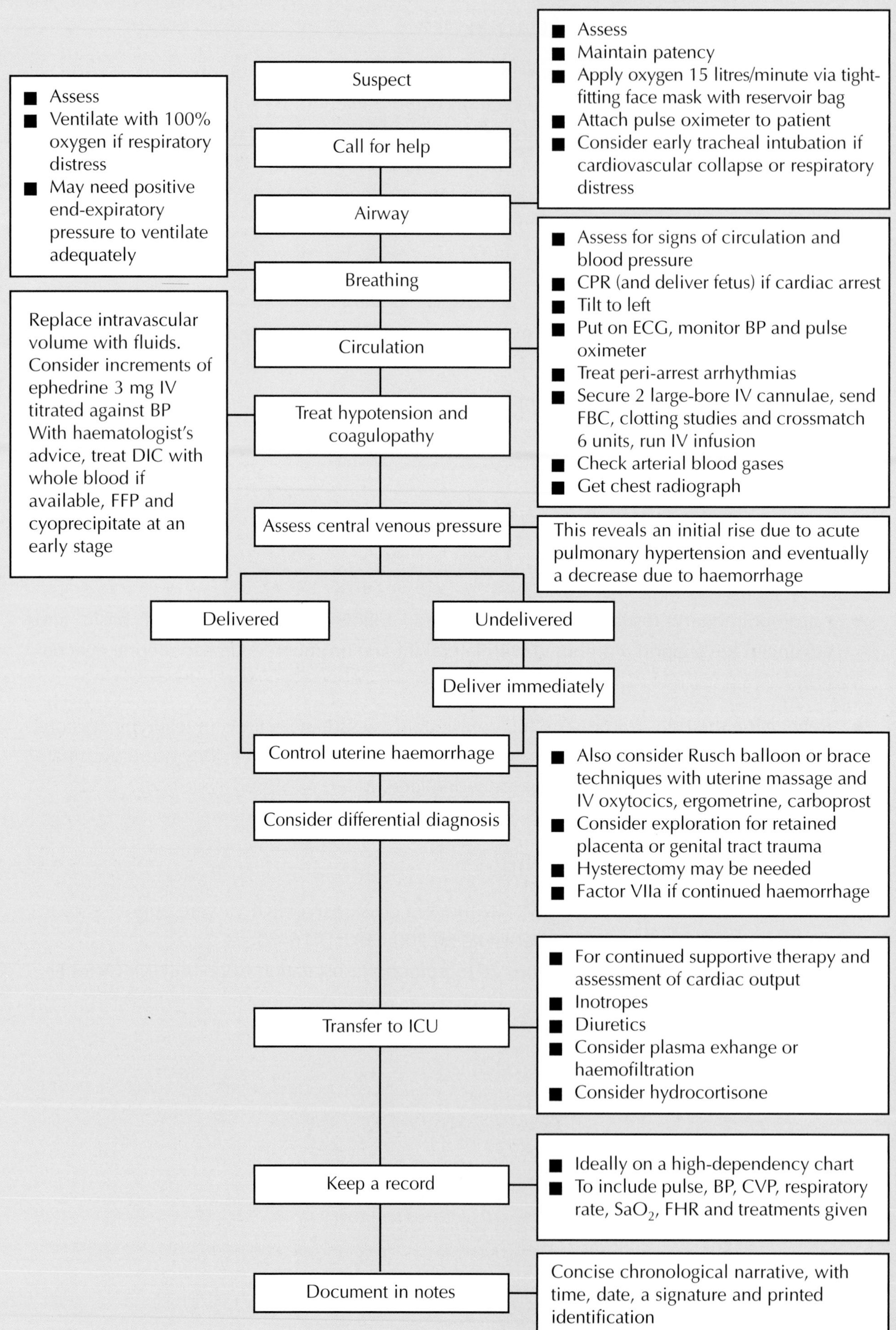

CHAPTER 10

Amniotic fluid embolism

Objectives

On successfully completing this topic, you will be able to:

- appreciate when to consider amniotic fluid embolism (AFE), facilitating early diagnosis
- manage the immediate treatment of a suspected AFE
- understand the options in treatment following initial assessment and resuscitation.

Introduction

The dramatic nature of AFE and the poor outcome with which it is associated mean that prompt and appropriate management are needed to minimise morbidity and mortality. The evidence upon which this guidance is based comes from retrospective series, including the UK Obstetric Surveillance System (UKOSS)[1] and the Confidential Enquiry into Maternal Deaths in the UK.[2] All of this evidence is observational and it is improbable that any higher quality evidence will be available. The treatments are largely reported in individual cases and so we can only establish general principles and options to be considered in any individual case.

Incidence

AFE is estimated to occur in between 1/8000 and 1/80 000 pregnancies, but because it is difficult to confirm the diagnosis there is no certainty about these figures. The latest UK figures from UKOSS suggest an incidence of one in 50 000 with a mortality rate of around 20%. The 2006–08 Confidential Enquiries into Maternal Deaths in the UK showed a death rate of 0.57 per 100 000 maternities. Over the last six triennia it has been responsible for 70 deaths, which is 9% of direct deaths.

There is wide variation in mortality from AFE worldwide, where it accounts for 13% of direct maternal deaths in France but 30% in Singapore. The percentage of direct maternal deaths caused by AFE in the US and Australia is similar to that of the UK at 7.5–10.0%.

In known AFE cases in the UK, the current mortality rate of 20% is a significant improvement on the previously gloomy outlook for women with AFE (mortality rates from the national registry in the US in 1995 suggested a mortality of 61%) and may be the result of better intensive care. However, recognition of the fact that 'milder' cases do occur may also have affected the statistics. Morbidity from this condition is also significant however, and it is particularly noteworthy that the US registry suggests that only 15% of women survived neurologically intact.

Clinical manifestations

Effects of amniotic fluid in the maternal circulation have been studied using animal models and in vitro studies. Details can be found in the further reading suggested at the end of this chapter. In summary, the effects are of:

- bronchoconstriction
- pulmonary hypertension
- left ventricular failure
- coagulopathy.

This syndrome of peripartum cardiovascular collapse with coagulopathy is similar to anaphylaxis: the response to the stimulus of fetal material in the maternal circulation is dependent upon the nature and quantity of the material and also the susceptibility of the mother. It is plausible that the effect is sometimes occlusive, sometimes a direct 'toxic' effect and sometimes a trigger to a cascade reaction. In some women, events may progress through each element. This suggests that clinical management will be aimed at supportive therapy with an understanding that the patient will pass through different phases of the clinical presentation.

The matter of amniotic fluid in the circulation is important if one is going to consider intraoperative autologous blood transfusion. This has been a concern considered in relation to the use of cell salvage for blood loss at CS; leucocyte depletion filtering seems to reduce particulate contaminants to the level equivalent to maternal venous blood. The safety of intraoperative autologous blood collection has been examined in cohort studies and no demonstrable increase in complications has been found. Cell salvage at CS has been approved by NICE and its use is recommended by RCOG in high-risk patients.

Other clinical manifestations

In order to suspect an AFE, we have to be aware of the features of the condition. The following were described by Clark in the US registry as requirements for the condition and the same features were initially used in the UK register.[3,4] To make a diagnosis, there should be:

- acute hypotension or cardiac arrest
- acute hypoxia (dyspnoea, cyanosis or respiratory arrest)
- coagulopathy (laboratory evidence of intravascular coagulation or severe haemorrhage)

- onset of all of the above during labour or within 30 minutes of delivery
- no other clinical conditions or potential explanations for the symptoms and signs.

However with knowledge of an increasing number of cases, UKOSS has refined the definition to:

Either

Acute maternal collapse with one or more of the following features:

- acute fetal compromise
- cardiac arrest
- cardiac rhythm problems
- coagulopathy
- hypotension
- maternal haemorrhage
- premonitory symptoms, e.g. restlessness, numbness, agitation, tingling
- seizure
- shortness of breath.

Excluding: women with maternal haemorrhage as the first presenting feature, in whom there was no evidence of early coagulopathy or cardiorespiratory compromise.

Or

Women in whom the diagnosis was made at postmortem examination, with the finding of fetal squames or hair in the lungs.

It is important to note that the coagulopathy may not develop if there is a rapid deterioration and the woman dies. It will be present, or develop, if the woman survives the initial collapse. It is extremely unlikely that bleeding will be the first presentation.

Symptoms and signs

The initial UK registry paper describes several initial patterns of presentation:

- maternal hypotension, shortness of breath, fetal bradycardia then delivery (14%)
- maternal loss of consciousness or seizure then delivery (35%)
- maternal collapse after delivery of baby at CS (14%)
- fetal distress and then maternal collapse (23%)
- immediately following delivery loss of consciousness or seizures (14%).

In each case it was followed by coagulation difficulties, and usually also profuse haemorrhage.

The UKOSS data describes the presentations and features shown in Table 10.1.

Table 10.1 Presentation and features of AFE

	Women exhibiting feature* $n = 60$	Women exhibiting feature as the first symptom or sign of AFE $n = 60$
Maternal haemorrhage	39 (65%)	1 (2%)
Hypotension	38 (63%)	5 (8%)
Shortness of breath	37 (62%)	12 (20%)
Coagulopathy	37 (62%)	0 (0%)
Premonitory symptoms (e.g. restlessness, agitation, numbness, tingling)	28 (47%)	18 (30%)
Acute fetal compromise	26 (43%)	12 (20%)
Cardiac arrest	24 (40%)	5 (8%)
Cardiac rhythm problems)	16 (27%)	3 (5%)
Seizures	12 (20%)	4 (7%)

Percentages are of complete data and some women had multiple features.
*Some women presented with more than one feature.

Suspecting an AFE

AFE should be part of the differential diagnosis of women who present with any of the above during labour or after delivery.

Diagnosis

The diagnosis is a clinical one. Absolute confirmation is only possible following death, with fetal squames in the maternal pulmonary circulation. However, other clinical features still need to be present to confirm the diagnosis. This is because fetal squames have been found in central venous blood in other conditions and even in the nonpregnant woman. In the living, fetal squames, or lanugo, on central venous samples cannot be taken as indicative of the diagnosis without a compatible clinical presentation.

The differential diagnosis involves considering an exhaustive list of the causes of maternal collapse in the peripartum period:

- postpartum haemorrhage (uterine atony)
- placental abruption
- uterine rupture
- eclampsia
- septic shock
- thrombotic embolus
- air embolus
- acute myocardial infarction

- peripartum cardiomyopathy
- local anaesthetic toxicity
- anaphylaxis
- transfusion reactions
- aspiration of gastric contents.

Only after exclusion of all the other causes can a diagnosis be confirmed clinically.

A clotting screen is often very abnormal, even before haemorrhage becomes apparent, and will exclude a large number of other diagnoses. When haemorrhage is already present, abnormal clotting could be secondary to the haemorrhage (but normally considerable blood loss with fluid or blood replacement needs to have occurred in the case of haemodilutional coagulopathy).

An ECG is helpful, to look for signs of myocardial damage. In AFE, often bizarre cardiac rhythms can be present thus making interpretation difficult. Arterial blood gases and a pulse oximeter may aid management but will not differentiate causes. A ventilation perfusion scan of the lungs may demonstrate defects with either pulmonary embolism or AFE.

Management

The management of AFE is supportive rather than specific. Multidisciplinary treatment with early involvement of senior, experienced staff is essential. Obstetricians, anaesthetists, intensivists and haematologists are mandatory to give the best prospect of survival.

As collapse is the predominant presentation, the initial management is basic resuscitation to maintain vital organ perfusion.

Airway/breathing

- High flow oxygen with early intubation and mechanical ventilation.

Circulation

- Cardiac arrhythmias or cardiac arrest may occur.
- Inotropic support is likely to be needed.
- Following cardiac arrest, CPR and rapid delivery, within 5minutes, aids resuscitation.
- Coagulopathy and haemorrhage are likely, requiring blood and blood products.
- Uterotonics to minimise/treat uterine atony.
- Cardiac output measurement may guide therapy.

Ensure that fluid overload does not occur, as this can lead to worsening pulmonary oedema and subsequent acute respiratory distress syndrome. This is particularly important when the coagulopathy and haemorrhage develops, in what has been described as the 'secondary' phase of the condition, when there are high filling pressures reflecting a failing left ventricle.

Vasopressors, such as phenylephrine, ephedrine or noradrenaline, are likely to be needed to restore aortic perfusion pressure.

In this secondary phase of coagulopathy and haemorrhage, prompt transfusion of fluids will be necessary to replace blood loss. This occurs at a variable point after initial presentation. The early consideration of clotting factor replacement with FFP, cryoprecipitate and platelets is important if there are signs of coagulopathy, such as haematuria or bleeding from the gums, even before massive blood loss is apparent. It is appropriate to commence this before receiving the laboratory confirmation of coagulopathy.

Cryoprecipitate may be of intrinsic value, beyond its clotting factor components, as it contains fibronectin, which aids the reticuloendothelial system in the filtration of antigenic and toxic particulate matter. The haemorrhage that occurs is usually as a result of uterine atony, which may be exacerbated by hypoxia and the coagulopathy. Hence, cryoprecipitate, by removing fibrin degradation products, may assist in the treatment of the uterine atony. Aggressive treatment of uterine atony with medical (oxytocics, ergometrine, prostaglandin) and adjunctive techniques (packing, tamponade, Rusch balloons) should be used, though early recourse to hysterectomy may be lifesaving.

The presentation of AFE can sometimes be acute fetal collapse, which is followed, a little time after, by maternal deterioration. Checking coagulation studies and monitoring pulse oximetry in women in whom there has been sudden fetal deterioration, or whose baby is unexpectedly severely acidotic, may identify abnormalities, providing the opportunity for earlier diagnosis and treatment.

The literature contains a number of case reports suggesting other specific treatments that include:

- extracorporeal membrane oxygenation (ECMO)
- prostacyclin
- nitric oxide
- plasma exchange
- haemofiltration
- cardiopulmonary bypass
- ligation of the infundibulopelvic ligament and uterine arteries
- factor VIIa.

As the condition is anaphylactoid in nature, it has also been suggested that high-dose hydrocortisone, 500 mg 6 hourly, might be appropriate, but no studies have examined this. The treatments which aim to filter or 'cleanse' the circulating blood volume may be effective in more rapidly reversing coagulation abnormalities and are similar to the use of cryoprecipitate described above.

Risk of recurrence

Further pregnancies have been reported in women with a successful outcome after AFE, all with good fetal and maternal outcome.

Neonatal outcome

In the US registry cases, 22 of 28 fetuses (79%) alive and in utero at the time of collapse survived, but only 11 (50% of survivors) were neurologically intact. In the initial UK series:

- of the 13 women who died:
  - seven babies survived: four of these were acidotic, one had hypoxic ischaemic encephalopathy and went on to develop cerebral palsy; the outcome of the other three acidotic babies seemed initially uneventful; three of the babies did well after immediate delivery
  - six babies died: one died in utero before presentation, one was a fresh still birth and the others died in the early neonatal period
- of the 18 surviving women with a fetus alive and in utero at the time of the maternal collapse:
  - four babies died
  - four had hypoxic ischaemic encephalopathy, with one developing cerebral palsy
  - two others had low cord pH
  - the other eight babies were normal.

In the later UK series 10% of babies died.

Summary

- AFE is rare and often devastating for both the woman and her baby.
- Outcomes are improving and prompt resuscitation, assessment and support may lead to a better chance of a good outcome.
- Specific therapies have not been evaluated.

References and further reading

1 Knight M, Tuffnell D, Brocklehurst P, *et al.*, on behalf of the UK Obstetric Surveillance System Incidence and Risk Factors for Amniotic-Fluid Embolism. *Obstet Gynecol* 2010;115:910–17.
2 Lewis G (ed). Saving Mothers' Lives. The Eighth Report of Confidential Enquiries into Maternal Deaths in the United Kingdom. London: *BJOG* 2011;118(Suppl. 1).
3 Clark SL, Hankins GD, Dudley DA, *et al.* Amniotic fluid embolism: analysis of the national registry. *Am J Obstet Gynecol* 1995;172:1158–67.
4 Tuffnell DJ. United Kingdom amniotic fluid embolism register. *BJOG* 2005;112:1625–9.
5 Clark SL. New concepts of amniotic fluid embolism: a review. *Obstet Gynecol Surv* 1990:45:360–8.

ALGORITHM 11.1 Pulmonary embolism

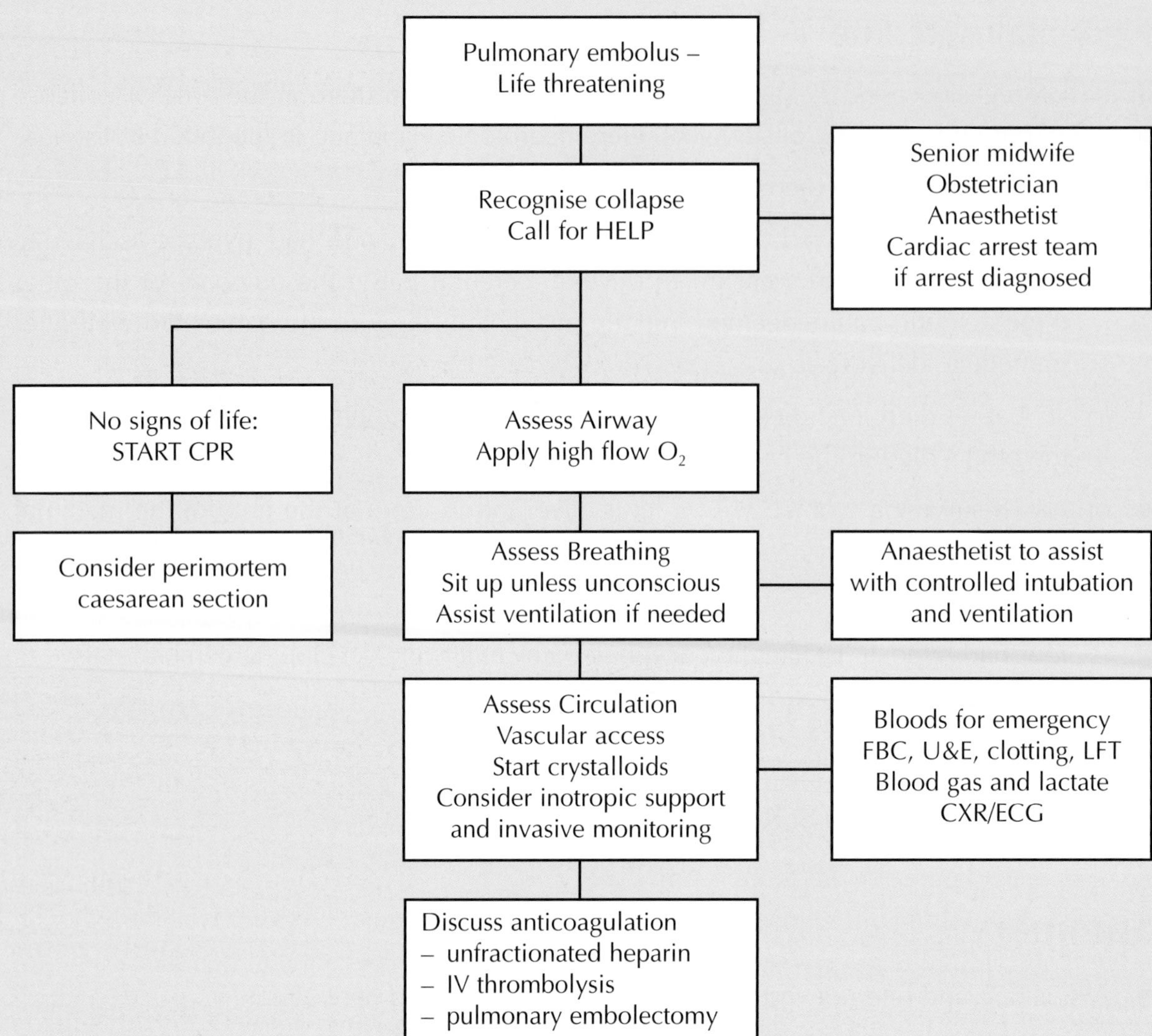

CHAPTER 11

Pulmonary thromboembolism

Objectives

On successfully completing this topic, you will be able to:

- recognise the risk factors for thromboembolism and understand the need for appropriate risk assessment and thromboprophylaxis
- recognise the features of pulmonary embolism and have an early suspicion of the diagnosis
- describe the treatment of suspected pulmonary embolism, including massive, life-threatening pulmonary embolism.

Introduction and incidence

The risk of venous thromboembolism (VTE) is significantly increased in pregnancy overall, due to a variety of important changes in the coagulation and vascular systems. There may also be a variety of other factors that can contribute to an individual's risk.

Thrombosis and thromboembolism have been the leading cause of direct maternal deaths from 1985 to 2005. By contrast, the 2006–08 Confidential Enquiry into Maternal Deaths (*Saving Mothers' Lives*[1]) reports 18 deaths from thrombosis and thromboembolism, a maternal mortality rate of 0.79/100 000 maternities, a significant decrease from the 41 deaths reported in the previous triennium and, in fact, the lowest incidence since 1985. For the first time, genital tract sepsis was the leading cause, with deaths from pre-eclampsia/eclampsia ranked second. Sixteen of the 18 deaths were attributed to pulmonary embolism and the other two to cerebral vein thrombosis. In addition, there were four late deaths attributed to pulmonary embolism.

The incidence of antenatal pulmonary embolism in the UK has recently been estimated in a prospective case–control study by UKOSS (the UK Obstetric Surveillance System) at 1.3/10 000 maternities, with a case fatality rate of 3.5% and significant severe morbidity.[2] There were 143 women with antenatal pulmonary embolisms in the study.

The period covered by the latest report is the first triennium since the publication of the RCOG guideline, '*Thromboprophylaxis during pregnancy, labour and after normal vaginal delivery,'* in 2004.[3] It is possible that the very significant fall in the rate of deaths from thromboembolism is a result of better identification of risk factors and more aggressive prophylaxis as a result of this guideline.

Of the 16 deaths from pulmonary embolism, three women died in the first trimester of pregnancy, two died after miscarriage and three after perimortem CS in the third trimester. The remaining eight died in the postpartum period, two after vaginal delivery and six after CS.

Of the 18 deaths overall, six were associated with 'major' substandard care and four with 'minor' substandard care (56% of cases). In seven women, there was inadequate thromboprophylaxis, in six there was failure to investigate chest symptoms and five cases involved a failure of appropriate referral to a consultant obstetrician.

Risk factors for VTE

Well-known additional risk factors for thromboembolism include:

- obesity
- increasing maternal age
- increasing parity
- previous VTE
- thrombophilia congenital (e.g. antithrombin 3 deficiency, protein C and S deficiency, activated protein C resistance) and acquired (lupus anticoagulant and antiphospholipid antibody)
- operative delivery
- surgical procedures in pregnancy or the puerperium.

Other recognised risk factors are: immobility; hypertensive disorders; hyperemesis; dehydration and excessive blood loss. Medical disorders such as: homocysteinuria; sickle cell disease; inflammatory bowel disease; nephritic syndrome; certain cardiac conditions and myeloproliferative disorders also increase the risk of VTE.

Risk factors were identified in only 99 of the 143 cases (70%) in the UKOSS report[2] (and 14 of the 16 deaths in *Saving Mothers' Lives*[1]), but also in 49% of controls. In the UKOSS survey, however, after adjustment, only multiparity and obesity were associated with a significantly raised odds ratio for antenatal pulmonary embolism. *Saving Mothers' Lives* also suggests that obesity is the most important risk factor, with many classic risk factors notably absent, perhaps as a result of better identification of risk factors with appropriate prophylactic treatment.

Pathophysiology

Hypercoagulability, as a result of one or more factors, results in formation of thrombus in the leg veins, on the left in up to 90% of cases and affecting the proximal ileofemoral veins in most cases. Emboli can reach the pulmonary arteries, with potentially fatal consequences. Deep vein thrombosis confined to the calf is rare in pregnancy.

Obstruction of the pulmonary arteries and release of vasoactive substances from platelets elevates pulmonary vascular resistance. The resulting increase in alveolar dead space and redistribution of blood flow impairs gas exchange. Right ventricular afterload increases, resulting in right ventricular dilatation, dysfunction and ischaemia.

Stimulation of irritant receptors causes alveolar hyperventilation. Reflex bronchoconstriction increases airway resistance and pulmonary oedema decreases pulmonary compliance.

Clinical presentation of pulmonary embolism

Pulmonary embolism can present as a massive, life-threatening event, or as a less-severe combination of symptoms with pleuritic chest pain, with or without dyspnoea, and possibly low-grade fever and haemoptysis. Clinical diagnosis of pulmonary embolism is difficult and commonly delayed because the significance of symptoms may not be appreciated by the woman or her attendants, and because there may be few signs on examination (Table 11.1).

Table 11.1 Incidence of clinical findings in pulmonary embolism

Findings	Occurrence in patients with proven pulmonary embolism (%)
Tachypnoea	89
Dyspnoea	81
Pleuritic pain	72
Apprehension	59
Cough	54
Tachycardia	43
Haemoptysis	34
Temperature >37°C	34

Although, with less severe symptoms, the differential diagnoses include chest infection, cardiac causes and pneumothorax, pulmonary embolism carries the highest risk. It should be the presumed diagnosis: treatment should be started and continued until embolism has been excluded, or a different diagnosis confirmed.

Massive pulmonary embolism may present with hypotension, severe dyspnoea, cyanosis and circulatory collapse; with central chest pain as a result of right ventricular myocardial ischaemia; or as sudden collapse, cardiac arrest or death. In this emergency situation, there may be right-sided heart failure, with increased jugular pressure, liver distension and subtle cardiac signs. As with less-severe pulmonary embolism, the presentation can be confused with that of other severe cardiopulmonary conditions, but a high index of suspicion must be maintained to avoid delay in beginning the appropriate management of a potentially life-threatening situation.

Management

The immediate management of a woman presenting with significant symptoms suggestive of pulmonary embolism, or of collapse possibly due to this condition, follows the structured approach to the severely ill patient:

1. Remember the risk factors for thromboembolism and maintain a high index of suspicion in women presenting with chest pain, dyspnoea, tachycardia or collapse.
2. Ensure a safe environment, approach the patient, 'shake and shout' if necessary.
3. Call for help: senior obstetrician, anaesthetist, on-call medical team and, in an unexplained maternal collapse or cardiac arrest, the cardiac arrest team.

   A – Assess and ensure an adequate airway, administer high flow oxygen.

   B – Assist ventilation if required, with bag and mask or intubation when appropriate personnel are present.

   C – Acquire adequate vascular access and begin fluid resuscitation. Make sure the woman is well tilted. Consider perimortem CS if in cardiac arrest with no response to CPR within minutes (see Chapter 9) and early thrombolysis if massive pulmonary embolism is confirmed, or prior to confirmation in extreme circumstances.

   D – If unresponsive and uncertain about respiration and heart rate, follow the cardiac arrest protocol.

   E – Consider exposure and environment, particularly in terms of adequate assessment of the patient, but also with regard to cooling.

Once resuscitated, move to HDU or ICU for investigation, monitoring and definitive treatment. Blood should be sent for full blood count, clotting, urea, electrolytes, liver function tests and arterial blood gases (thrombophilia screen will not affect the acute management of the situation and, if sent, should be interpreted by a haematologist). Monitoring should include non-invasive BP, pulse oximetry, ECG and hourly urine output. Chest radiograph and twelve-lead ECG should be requested. Definitive treatment may include thrombolytic therapy, pulmonary embolectomy, sedation and ventilation and invasive monitoring, as well as anticoagulation.

Investigations for patients with a possible pulmonary embolism

Chest radiograph (CXR)

CXR can exclude pneumonia, pneumothorax or lobar collapse and abnormal features associated with pulmonary embolism, such as atelectasis, effusions, focal opacities, regional oligaemia and pulmonary oedema. Radiation exposure of the fetus from a CXR is negligible. If normal, as in 50% of women with subsequently proven pulmonary embolism, bilateral leg Doppler ultrasound should be undertaken, if not yet performed, as confirmation of DVT will support the diagnosis of pulmonary embolism. The treatment is the same for both embolus and thrombus, avoiding other investigations and thereby limiting the radiation dose to the fetus.

Ventilation/perfusion (V/Q) lung scan or computed tomography pulmonary angiogram (CTPA)

If the CXR is abnormal, or if both CXR and leg Dopplers are normal, either V/Q scan or CTPA should be undertaken, depending on local availability, and after discussion with a radiologist. CTPA is recommended as the first-line investigation for non-massive pulmonary embolism, by the British Thoracic Society. There are advantages and disadvantages to both techniques and some authorities recommend V/Q scan as the initial investigation in pregnancy because of its high negative predictive value and lower radiation dose to maternal breast tissue (a risk factor for breast cancer). V/Q scan is reported as indicating a probability of the presence of a pulmonary embolism and these probabilities relate to an estimated percentage chance of an embolism being present (Table 11.2).

Table 11.2 Probability of pulmonary thromboembolism based on ventilation perfusion scan report

Scan category	Probability (%)
High probability	87
Intermediate probability	30
Low probability	14
Normal	4

Electrocardiogram (ECG)

ECG changes are nonspecific, even more so because of the electrical axis changes that occur in pregnancy. Sinus tachycardia is the most common abnormality. Right-axis deviation and right-ventricular strain may be apparent in a large pulmonary embolism, but the 'S1Q3T3' pattern is rare.

Arterial blood gases (ABG)

ABG may show a low PaO_2 and normal or low $PaCO_2$, but are nonspecific as they may be abnormal in other pathologies and may be normal with smaller emboli.

Echocardiography

Echocardiography is of limited value in pregnancy, possibly confirming a large central embolus and eliminating other causes of collapse. The latest RCOG guideline recognises that it may be of use in unstable patients as a bedside test.

Other investigations

The latest RCOG guideline[4] does not recommend the use of pulmonary angiography, otherwise the gold standard investigation for pulmonary embolism, because it carries the highest radiation exposure to mother and fetus. Spiral computed tomography (CT) and magnetic resonance imaging (MRI) have been used in the past, but both have disadvantages and neither is recommended in the RCOG guideline.

The same guideline states that D-dimer testing should not be used in the diagnosis of VTE in pregnancy. Although a negative D-dimer suggests that no VTE is present, it is not definitive. A raised D-dimer is common in pregnancy and definitive testing is still required.

Treatment

In suspected pulmonary embolism (as in DVT), the initial treatment should be with low-molecular-weight heparin (LMWH) in divided doses, twice daily, until the diagnosis is excluded. The dose depends on the particular LMWH used and there should be clear local guidelines (Table 11.3). Monitoring of anti-Xa activity (except at extremes of body weight or with other complicating factors) or platelet levels is not recommended in pregnancy.

Table 11.3 Calculation of initial doses of various LMWH by early pregnancy weight[3]

Initial dose	Early pregnancy weight (kg)			
	<50	50–69	70–89	>90
Enoxaparin	40 mg bd	60 mg bd	80 mg bd	100 mg bd
Dalteparin	5000 IU bd	6000 IU bd	8000 IU bd	10 000 IU bd
Tinzaparin	175 units/kg once daily (all weights)			

In massive, life-threatening pulmonary embolism, the recommended treatment is intravenous unfractionated heparin, because of its rapid effect and the extensive experience of its use.

The RCOG guideline suggests the following regimen for unfractionated heparin anticoagulation:

- a loading dose of 80 units/kg should be administered, followed by a continuous intravenous infusion of 18 units/kg/hour
- if a woman has received thrombolysis, the loading dose of heparin should be omitted and an infusion started at 18 units/kg/hour
- an APTT must be performed 4–6 hours after the loading dose, 6 hours after any dose change and then at least daily once in the therapeutic range; the therapeutic target APTT ratio is usually 1.5–2.5 times the average laboratory control value
- the infusion rate should, using this weight-adjusted regimen, be adjusted according to the APTT, as shown in Table 11.4.

The use of APTT monitoring of unfractionated heparin is problematic, particularly in late pregnancy, potentially leading to overdose of heparin and to bleeding problems. In these circumstances, senior haematological advice should be sought and anti-Xa activity may be useful.

Table 11.4 Infusion rates of unfractionated heparin according to APTT[3]

APTT ratio	Dose change (units/kg/hour)	Additional action	Next APTT (hours)
<1.2	+4	Re-bolus 80 units/kg	6
1.2–1.5	+2	Re-bolus 40 units/kg	6
1.5–2.5	No change		24
2.5–3.0	–2		6
>3.0	–3	Stop infusion 1 hour	6

Thromobolysis

In extreme circumstances, where there is haemodynamic compromise, thrombolytic agents such as streptokinase have been used. It is not clear whether this results in a better outcome than unfractionated heparin alone, but there are numerous case reports of its use in pregnancy, with no deaths attributed to its use.

In women in whom thrombolysis is contraindicated, thoracotomy and embolectomy might need to be considered as an urgent procedure with the advice of the cardiothoracic surgeons.

Maintenance treatment of VTE

- After the initial acute event, treatment with therapeutic doses of LMWH should be continued through the rest of the pregnancy.
- If women are receiving therapeutic doses of unfractionated heparin, they should have monitoring of their platelet count every other day until day 14 of therapy or until unfractionated heparin is discontinued, whichever is sooner.
- Women who develop heparin-induced thrombocytopenia or have heparin allergy and still require anticoagulation should be treated with danaparoid sodium or fondaparinux, with advice from a haematologist.
- Oral anticoagulants should not be used for antenatal prophylaxis of VTE, because of the side effects associated with this treatment.

Anticoagulant therapy during labour and delivery

- Once a woman on LMWH maintenance therapy thinks she is in labour, she should not inject any further heparin.
- In the case of planned delivery, LMWH maintenance therapy should be discontinued 24 hours before planned delivery.
- Regional anaesthetic techniques should not be undertaken until at least 24 hours after the last dose of therapeutic LMWH.

- A thromboprophylactic dose of LMWH should be given 3 hours after CS, or more than 4 hours after removal of an epidural catheter, if appropriate.
- The epidural catheter should not be removed within 12 hours of the most recent injection of LMWH.

Postnatal anticoagulation and review

- Therapeutic anticoagulation should be continued from the time of the thromboembolism for the duration of the pregnancy, for at least 6 weeks postnatally and also until at least 3 months of treatment has been given. Women should be offered LMWH and oral anticoagulation (although not the latter until at least 3 days postnatally), explaining the need for regular blood tests to monitor warfarin treatment. Neither LMWH, nor warfarin, is contraindicated in women who are breastfeeding. Women who have had a VTE in pregnancy should be reviewed in an obstetric medicine or a joint obstetric/haematology clinic.

References and further reading

1 Lewis G (ed.). The Confidential Enquiry into Maternal and Child Health (CEMACH). *Saving Mothers' Lives: reviewing maternal deaths to make motherhood safer – 2003–2005*. The Seventh Report on Confidential Enquiries into Maternal Deaths in the United Kingdom. London: CEMACH 2007.

2 Knight M, UKOSS. Antenatal pulmonary embolism: risk factors, management and outcomes. *BJOG* 2008;115:453–61.

3 Royal College of Obstetricians and Gynaecologists. Guideline No. 37. *Thromboprophylaxis during pregnancy, labour and after normal vaginal delivery*. London: RCOG Press 2004.

4 *Saving Mothers' Lives*: Reviewing maternal deaths to make motherhood safer: 2006–2008. *BJOG* 2011; 118:1–203.

5 Royal College of Obstetricians and Gynaecologists. Greentop Guideline No. 37b. *The acute management of thrombosis and embolism in pregnancy and the puerperium,* 2nd edn. London: RCOG Press, 2010.

6 Farquharson RG, Greaves M. Thromboembolic disease. In: James D, Steer PJ, Weiner CP, *et al.* (eds) *High risk pregnancy: management options,* 4th edn. Philadelphia: Saunders, 2011;753–61.

ALGORITHM 12.1 Newborn Life Support, reproduced with the kind permission of the Resuscitation Council (UK)

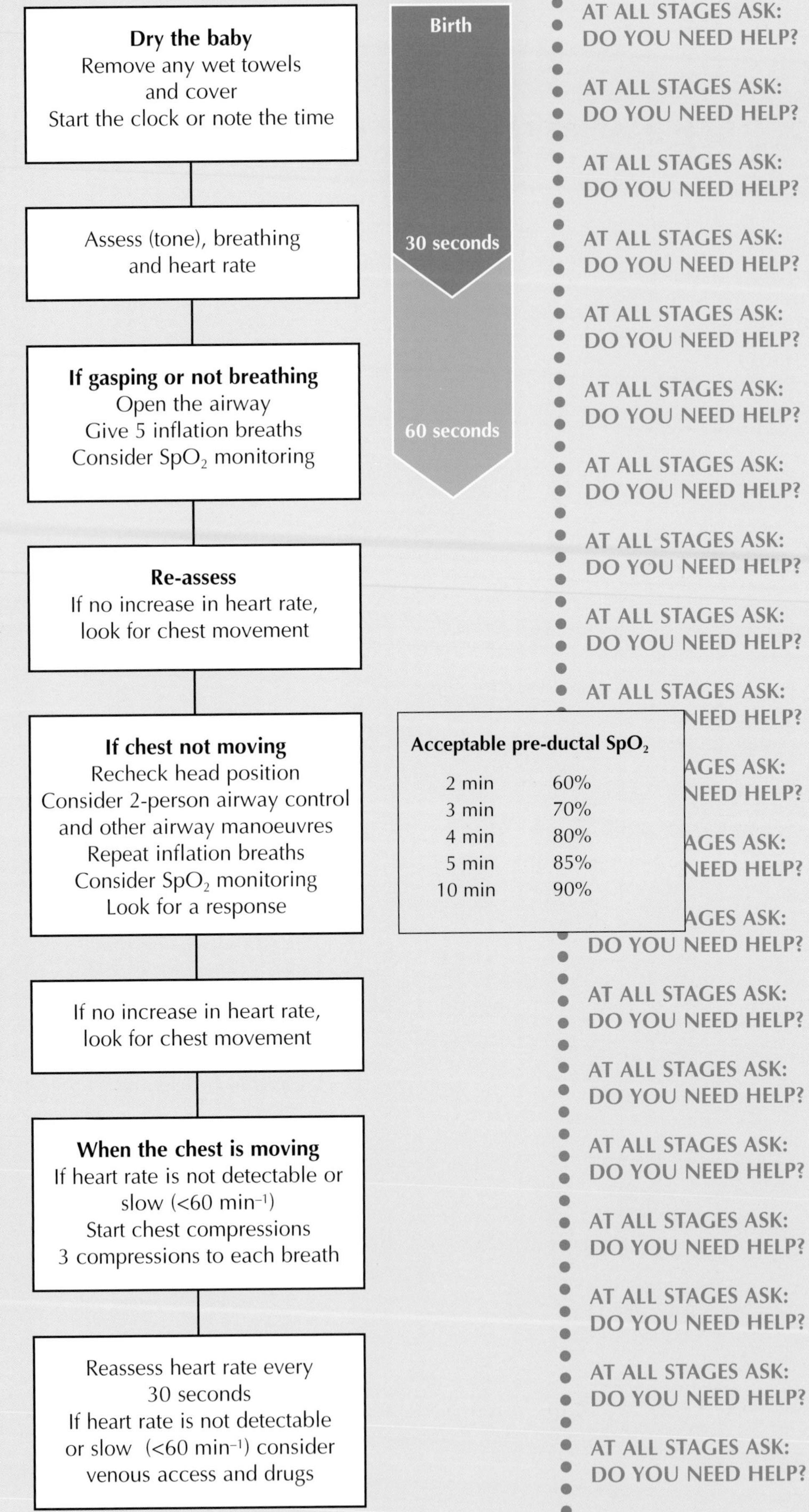

CHAPTER 12

Resuscitation of the baby at birth

Objectives

On successfully completing this topic, you will be able to:

- understand the important physiological differences in the newly born baby
- understand the equipment used for resuscitation at birth
- understand how to assess and resuscitate the baby at birth
- understand additional measures for special situations.

Introduction

The resuscitation of babies at birth is different from the resuscitation of all other age groups, and knowledge of the relevant physiology and pathophysiology is essential. However, the majority of newly born babies will establish normal respiration and circulation without help. Ideally, someone trained in newborn resuscitation should be present at all deliveries. It is advisable that those who attend deliveries attend courses such as the Newborn Life Support Course, organised by the Resuscitation Council (UK), the European Resuscitation Council or the Neonatal Resuscitation Programme, organised by the American Academy of Pediatrics. However, some babies are born in unexpected places, such as Emergency Departments. For these situations, it is important that clinicians have an understanding of the differences in resuscitating a baby at birth.

Normal physiology

At birth the baby must change from an organism with fluid-filled lungs whose respiratory function is carried out by the placenta, to a separate being whose air-filled lungs can successfully take over this function. Preparation for this begins during labour, when the fluid-producing cells within the lung cease secretion and begin re-absorption of that fluid. Delivery by CS before the onset of labour may slow the clearance of pulmonary fluid from the lungs.

During vaginal delivery, some lung fluid, perhaps 35 ml in a term baby, is expelled by passage through the birth canal. In a healthy baby, the first spontaneous breaths may generate a negative pressure of between –30 cmH_2O and –90 cmH_2O, which aerates the lungs for the first time. This pressure is 10–15 times greater than that needed for later breathing, but is necessary to overcome the viscosity of the fluid filling the airways, the surface tension of the fluid-filled lungs and the elastic recoil and resistance of the chest wall, lungs and airways. These powerful chest movements cause fluid to be displaced from the airways into the lymphatics and circulation.

After delivery, a healthy term baby usually takes its first breath within 60–90 seconds of clamping or obstructing the umbilical cord. Separation of the placenta and clamping of the cord leads to the onset of hypoxia, which is initially a major stimulant to start respiration. Physical stimuli, such as cold air or physical discomfort, may also provoke respiratory efforts.

In a 3kg baby, up to 100ml of fluid is cleared from the airways following the initial breaths, a process aided by full inflation and prolonged high pressure on expiration, i.e. crying. The effect of the first few breaths is to produce the baby's functional residual capacity. Neonatal circulatory adaptation commences with the detachment of the placenta, but lung inflation and alveolar distension releases mediators, which affect the pulmonary vasculature as well as increasing oxygenation.

Pathophysiology

Our knowledge of the pathophysiology of fetal asphyxia is based on pioneering animal work in the early 1960s. The results of these experiments, which followed the physiology of newborn animals during acute, total, prolonged asphyxia and subsequent resuscitation, are summarised in Figure 12.1.

When the placental oxygen supply is interrupted, the fetus attempts to breathe. Should these attempts fail to provide an alternative oxygen supply – as they will inevitably fail to do in utero – the baby will lose consciousness. If hypoxia continues, the respiratory centre becomes unable, through lack of sufficient oxygen, to continue initiating breathing and the breathing stops, usually within 2–3 minutes (primary apnoea, Figure 12.1).

Fetal bradycardia ensues but blood pressure is maintained, primarily by peripheral vasoconstriction and diversion of blood away from non-vital organs, and also by an increased stroke volume. After a latent period of apnoea (primary), primitive spinal centres, no longer suppressed by neural signals from the respiratory centre, exert an effect by initiating primitive gasping breaths. These deep, spontaneous gasps are easily distinguishable from normal breaths as they only occur 6–12 times per minute and involve all accessory muscles in a maximal inspiratory effort. After a while, if hypoxia continues, even this activity ceases (terminal apnoea). The time taken for such activity to cease is longer in the newly born baby than in later life, taking up to 20 minutes.

The circulation is almost always maintained until all respiratory activity ceases. This resilience is a feature of all newborn mammals at term, largely due to the reserves of glycogen in the heart. Resuscitation is therefore relatively easy if undertaken before all

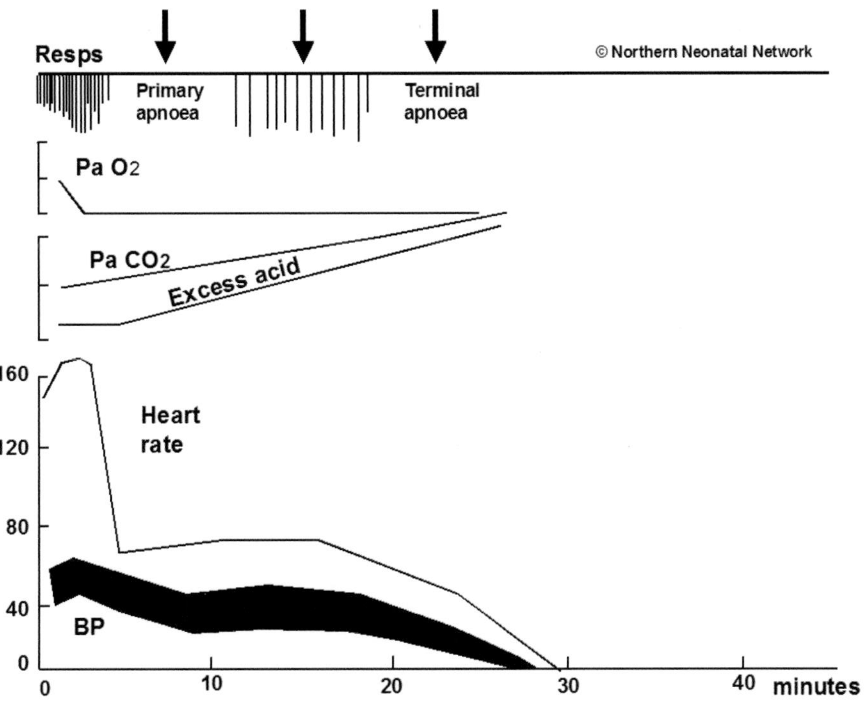

Figure 12.1 Response of a mammalian fetus to total, sustained asphyxia started at time 0 (reproduced with kind permission from the Northern Neonatal Network)

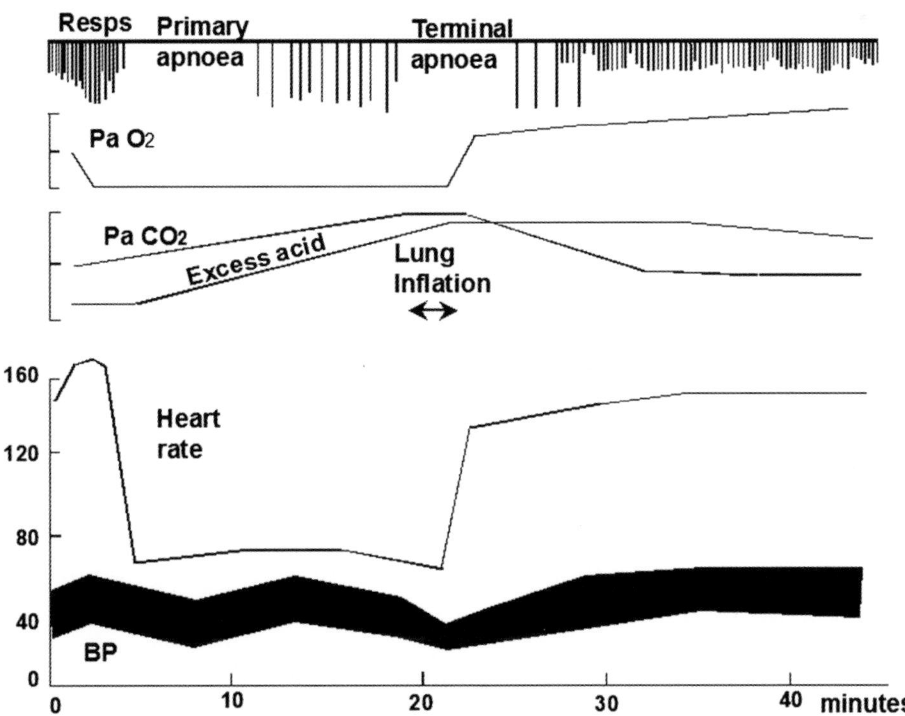

Figure 12.2 Effects of lung inflation and a brief period of ventilation on a baby born in early terminal apnoea, but before failure of the circulation (reproduced with kind permission from the Northern Neonatal Network)

respiratory activity has stopped. Once the lungs are inflated, oxygen will be carried to the heart and then to the brain provided that the circulation is still functional (Figure 12.2). Recovery will then be rapid. *Most* infants who have not progressed to terminal apnoea will resuscitate themselves if their airway is patent. Once gasping ceases, however, the circulation starts to fail and these infants are likely to need more extensive resuscitation (Figure 12.3).

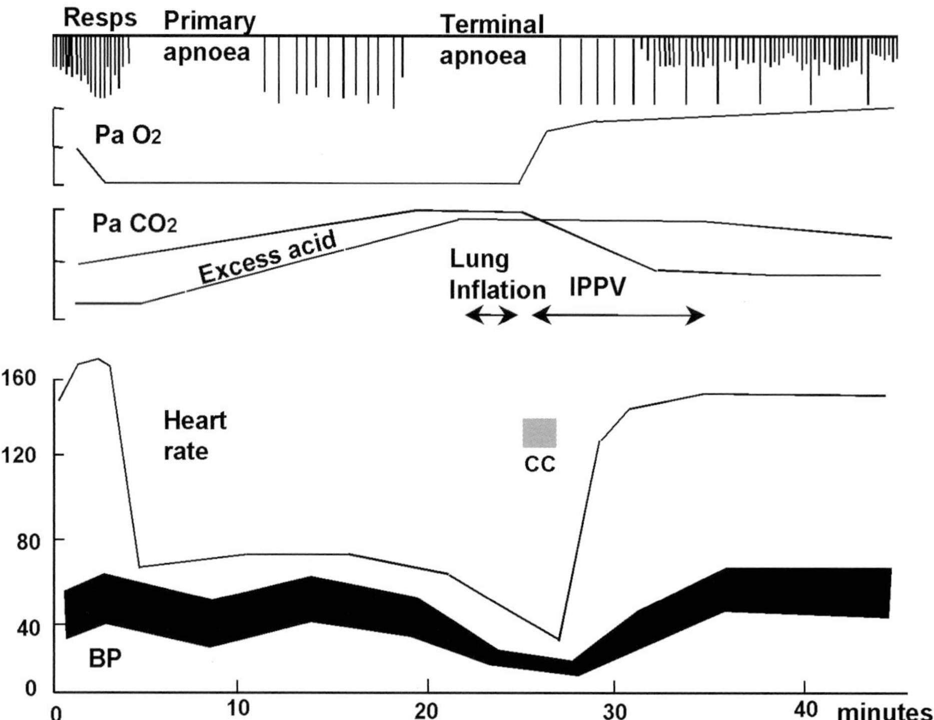

Figure 12.3 Response of babies born in terminal apnoea. In this case lung inflation is not sufficient because the circulation is already failing. However, lung inflation delivers air to the lungs and then a brief period of chest compressions (CC) delivers oxygenated blood to the heart which then responds (reproduced with kind permission from the Northern Neonatal Network)

Resuscitation

Equipment

For many newborn babies, especially those born outside the delivery room, the need for resuscitation cannot be predicted. It is therefore useful to plan for such an eventuality. Equipment that may be required to resuscitate a newborn baby is listed in Box 12.1. This will vary between departments; however, most babies can be resuscitated with a flat surface, warmth, knowledge and a way to deliver air or oxygen at a controlled pressure.

Box 12.1 Equipment for newborn resuscitation:

- a flat surface
- radiant heat source and clean dry towels (or suitable plastic bags for preterm infants used under radiant heat)
- stethoscope ± saturation monitor
- cord clamp
- scissors
- disposable gloves
- source of air and/or oxygen
- face masks
- bag-valve-mask or T piece with pressure limiting device
- oropharyngeal (Guedel) airways
- suction with catheters at least 12 Fr
- laryngoscopes with straight blades, 0 and 1
- tracheal tubes sizes 2.5 to 4.0 mm
- nasogastric tubes
- umbilical catheterisation equipment
- adhesive tape

Strategy for assessing and resuscitating a baby at birth

Resuscitation is likely to be rapidly successful if begun before the baby has become so anoxic that all potential for respiratory activity has vanished. Babies in primary apnoea can usually resuscitate themselves if they have a clear airway. As you do not know whether a newborn, apnoeic baby is in primary or terminal apnoea, you must develop a graded approach that will work in either situation. Always start by drying and covering the baby to prevent it from getting cold and then proceed as far as it is necessary down the following list:

- call for help
- start the clock or note the time
- dry and cover the baby
- assess the situation
- airway
- breathing
- chest compressions
- (drugs).

Call for help

Ask for help if you expect or encounter any difficulty, or if the delivery is outside the labour suite.

Start clock

If available, or note the time of birth.

At birth

1 There is no need to rush to clamp the cord, particularly if the baby appears well. Unless the baby is clearly in need of immediate resuscitation, wait for at least one minute from the complete delivery of the baby before clamping the cord. Keep the baby warm during this time and in the same horizontal plane as the mother.
2 Dry the baby quickly and effectively. Remove the wet towel and wrap in a fresh dry warm towel. (For very small or significantly preterm babies it is better to immediately place the wet baby in a food grade plastic bag and under a radiant heater as soon as possible).
3 During this period it is possible to assess the baby and decide whether any intervention is going to be needed.
4 Then clamp and cut the cord.

If the baby is thought to need assistance, then this becomes the priority. This may mean that the cord needs to be clamped earlier in order to deliver that assistance.

Keep the baby warm

Dry the baby off immediately and then wrap in a dry towel. A cold baby has increased oxygen consumption and cold babies are more likely to become hypoglycaemic and acidotic. They also have an increased mortality. If temperature control is not addressed at the beginning of resuscitation, it is often forgotten. Most of the heat loss is caused by the baby being wet and in a draught – hence the need to dry the baby and then to wrap the baby in a dry towel. Babies also have a large surface area to weight ratio; thus heat can be lost very quickly. Ideally, delivery should take place in a warm room, and an overhead heater should be switched on. However, drying effectively and wrapping the baby in a warm dry towel is the most important factor in avoiding hypothermia. A naked, wet baby can still become hypothermic, despite a warm room and a radiant heater, especially if there is a draught. Make sure that the head is covered as it represents a significant part of the baby's surface area (also see 'Pre-Term Babies').

Assessment of the newborn baby

While keeping the baby warm make an initial assessment by assessing:

Airway and Breathing:

- respiration – rate and quality

Circulation:

- heart rate – fast, slow, absent
- colour – pink, blue, pale
- tone – unconscious, apnoeic babies are floppy.

Unlike resuscitation at other ages, it is important to first assess the baby fully, in order to judge the success of interventions. This is most true of heart rate and breathing, which guide further resuscitative efforts. However, a baby who is white and shut down peripherally is more likely to be acidotic and a baby who is atonic is likely to be unconscious. Subsequent assessments should focus on breathing and heart rate which will guide intervention.

Respiration

Most babies will establish spontaneous regular breathing sufficient to maintain the heart rate above 100 beats/min and to improve the skin colour within 3 minutes of birth. If apnoea or gasping persists after drying, intervention is required.

Heart rate

In the first couple of minutes, auscultating at the cardiac apex is the best method to assess the heart rate. Palpating peripheral pulses is not practical and cannot be recommended. Palpation of the umbilical pulse can only be relied upon if it is $\geq$ 100 beats/min. A rate less than this should be checked by auscultation if possible or by a saturation monitor using Masimo (or similar) technology if available. A saturation monitor applied to the right hand or wrist can give an accurate reading of heart rate and saturations within 90 seconds of application (see later). An initial assessment of heart rate is vital because an increase in the heart rate will be the first sign of success during resuscitation.

Colour

Attempting to judge oxygenation by assessing skin colour is unreliable, but it is still worth noting the baby's colour at birth, as well as whether, when and how it changes. Very pale babies who remain pale and bradycardic after resuscitation may be hypovolaemic as well as acidotic.

If the baby has good tone, a good heart rate and is making respiratory effort then further help is unlikely to be needed.

Using a saturation monitor will allow a rapid assessment of heart rate and saturation within 90 seconds of application. Oxygen saturation levels in healthy babies in the first few minutes of life may be considerably lower than at other times (Box 12.2).

Box 12.2 Acceptable pre-ductal SpO_2:

2 min	60%
3 min	70%
4 min	80%
5 min	85%
10 min	90%

This assessment will categorise the baby into one of the three following groups:

1 *Regular respirations, heart rate fast (more than 100 beats/min) pink, good tone.* These are healthy babies and they should be kept warm and given to their mothers. The baby will remain warm through skin-to-skin contact with the mother under a cover and may be put to the breast at this stage.

2 *Irregular or inadequate respirations, heart rate slow (less than 100 beats/min), blue, normal or reduced tone.* If gentle stimulation (such as drying) does not induce effective breathing, the airway should be opened and, if necessary, cleared. If the baby responds, then no further resuscitation is needed. If there is no response, if necessary, progress to lung inflation.

3 *Apnoeic, or heart rate slow (less than 100 beats/min) or absent, blue or pale, floppy.* Whether an apnoeic baby is in primary or terminal apnoea (Figure 12.1), the initial management is the same. Open the airway and then inflate the lungs. A reassessment of any heart rate response then directs further resuscitation. Reassess the heart rate and respiration at regular intervals throughout.

Apnoea, low or absent heart rate, pallor and floppiness together suggest terminal apnoea. However, initial management of such babies is unchanged, although resuscitation may be prolonged.

After assessment, resuscitation follows:

- airway
- breathing
- circulation
- with the use of drugs in a few, selected, babies.

Airway

The baby should be positioned with the head in the neutral position (see Figure 12.4). The newborn baby's head has a large, often moulded, occiput, which tends to cause the neck to flex when the baby is supine on a flat surface. However, overextension may also collapse the newborn baby's pharyngeal airway, leading to obstruction. A small rolled towel placed under the neck and shoulders may help to maintain the airway in a neutral position. A jaw thrust may be needed to bring the tongue forward and open the airway, especially if the baby is floppy (Figure 12.5). Visible secretions may be removed by gentle suction with a paediatric Yankauer, or 12–14-Fr suction catheter, although secretions rarely cause airway obstruction. Blind, deep pharyngeal suction should not be performed as this may cause vagally-induced bradycardia and laryngospasm. Suction, if it is used, should not exceed 100 mmHg (9.8 kPa). The presence of thick meconium (see below) in a non-vigorous baby is the only indication for considering visualisation of the oropharynx and immediate suction.

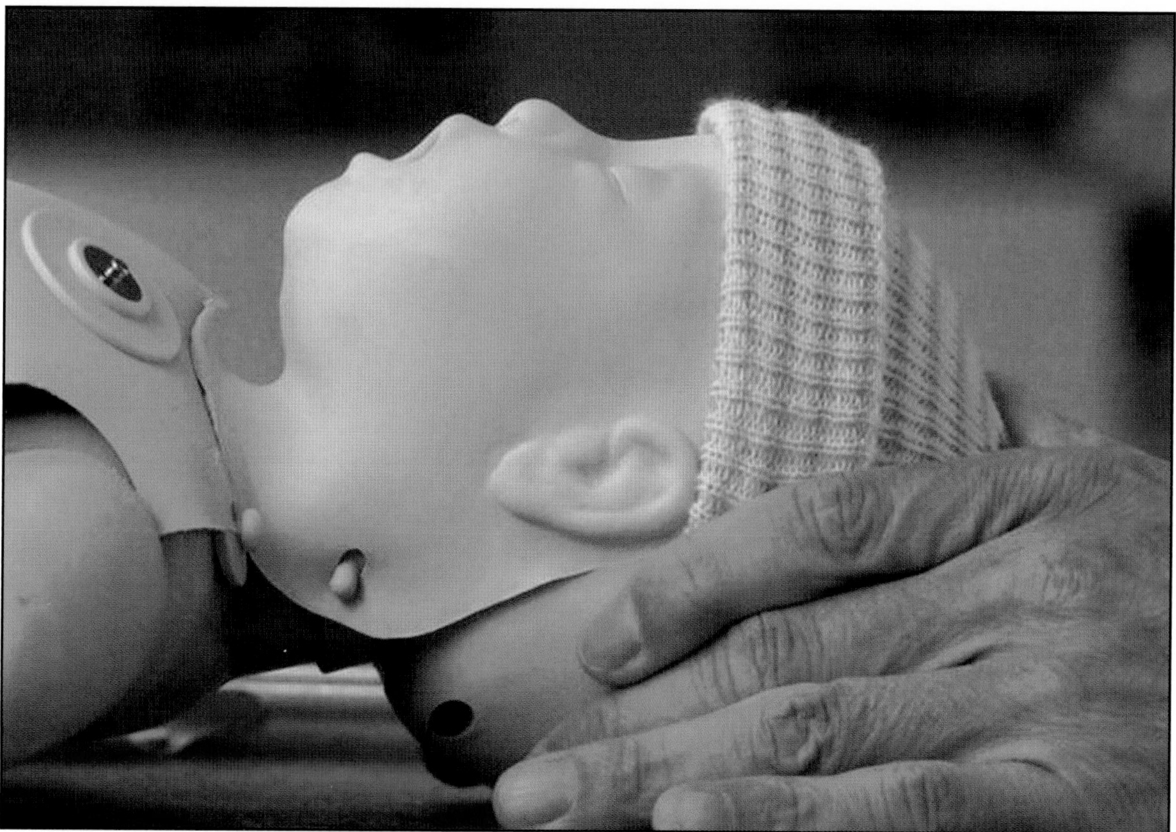

Figure 12.4 Neutral head position in newborn baby

Meconium aspiration

Meconium-stained liquor (light green tinge) is relatively common and occurs in up to 10% of births. Happily, meconium aspiration is a rare event. Meconium aspiration usually happens in term infants in utero before delivery. A large, randomised trial has shown no advantage to suctioning the airway while the head is on the perineum and this may delay resuscitation. This practice is, therefore, no longer recommended. If the baby is vigorous, a randomised trial has shown that suctioning of the trachea at any time offers no advantage either, and no specific action (other than drying and wrapping the baby) is needed.

If the baby has absent or inadequate respirations, a heart rate <100 beats/min or hypotonia, inspect the oropharynx with a laryngoscope and aspirate any particulate meconium seen using a wide-bore catheter. If intubation is possible and the baby is still unresponsive,

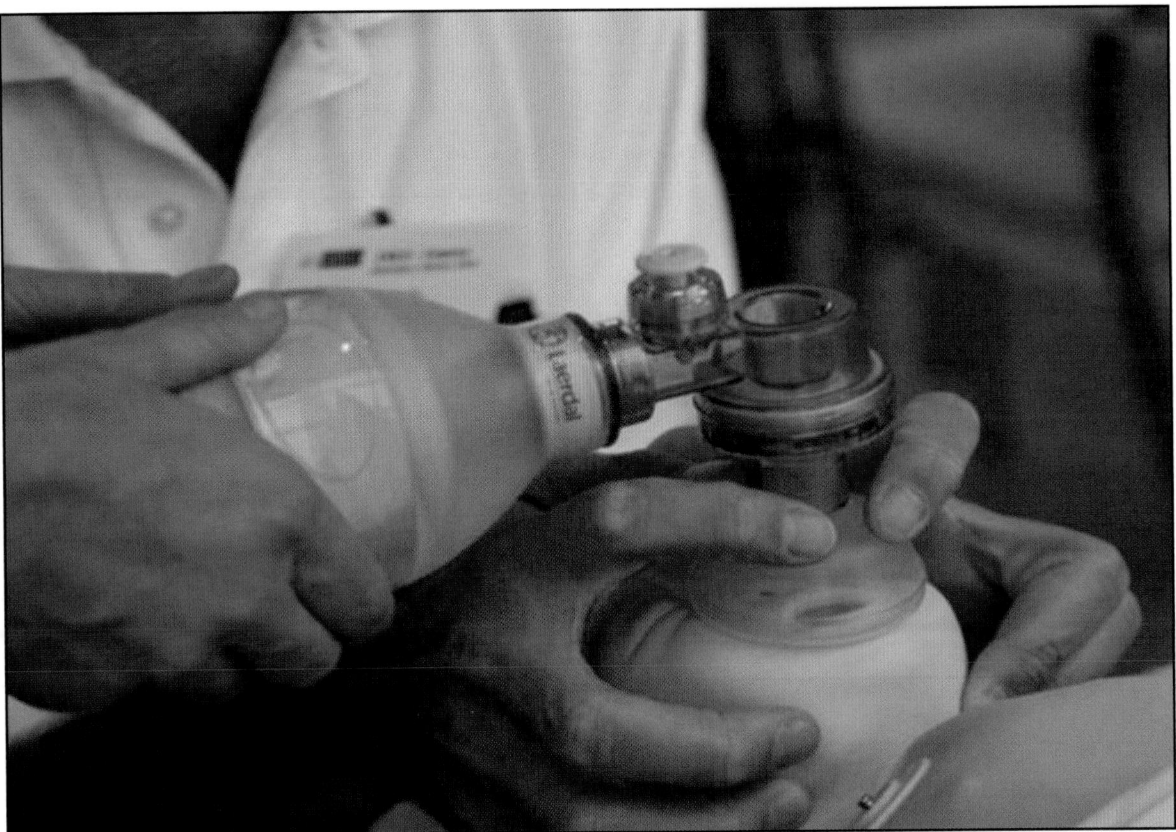

Figure 12.5 Two person jaw thrust with bag mask ventilation

aspirate the trachea using the tracheal tube as a suction catheter. However, if intubation cannot be achieved immediately, clear the oropharynx and start mask inflation. If, while attempting to clear the airway, the heart rate falls to less than 60 beats/min then stop airway clearance, give inflation breaths, start ventilating the baby and perform chest compressions (see below).

Breathing (inflation, breaths and ventilation)

The first five breaths in term babies should be 'inflation' breaths in order to replace lung fluid in the alveoli with air. These should be sustained breaths of 2–3-seconds using a continuous gas supply, a pressure limiting device and a mask. Use a transparent, circular soft mask big enough to cover the nose and mouth of the baby. If no such system is available then a 500 ml self-inflating bag and a blow-off valve set at 30–40 cmH_2O can be used to give the same 2–3-second sustained breaths (Figure 12.6). This is especially useful if compressed air or oxygen is not available.

The chest may not move during the first 1–3 breaths as fluid is displaced. Adequate ventilation is usually indicated by either a rapidly increasing heart rate, or a heart rate that is maintained at more than 100 beats per minute. Therefore, reassess the heart rate after delivery of the first 5 breaths. It is safe to assume the chest has been inflated successfully if the heart rate responds. In fluid-filled lungs, breath sounds may be heard even when the lung is not aerated.

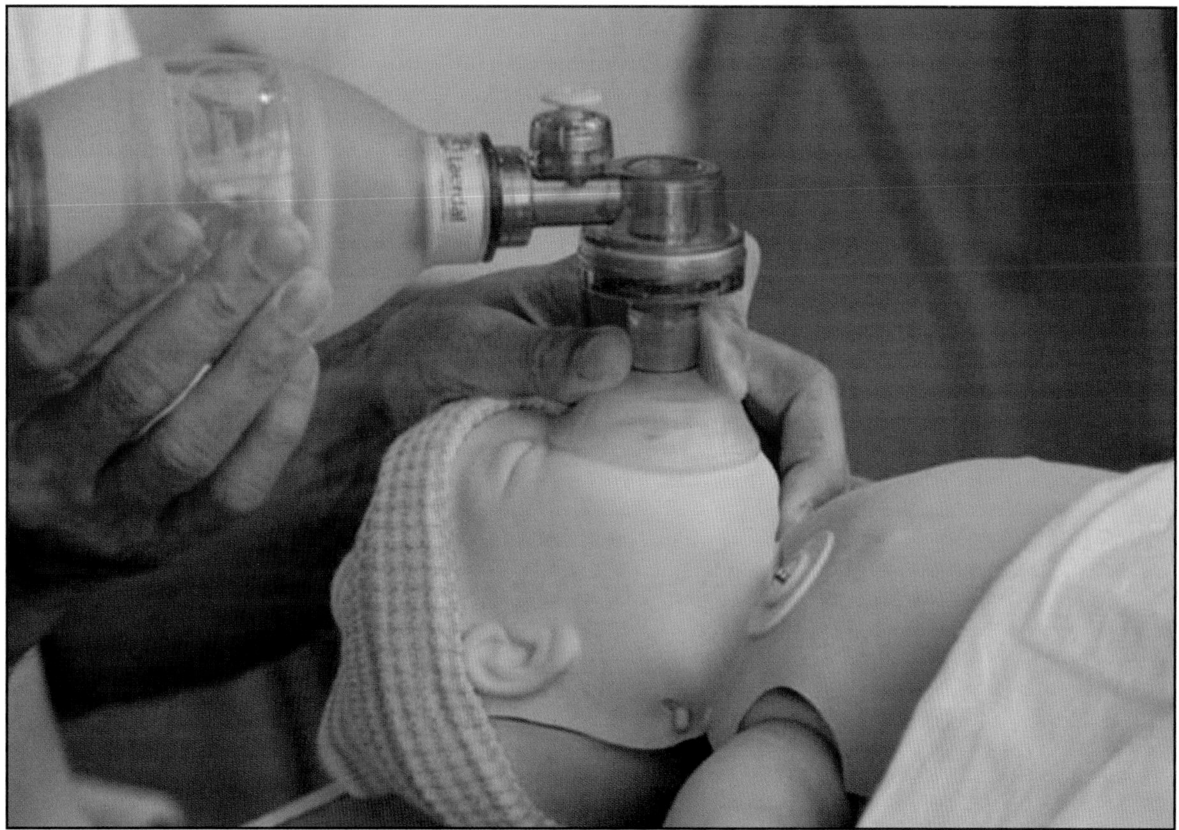

Figure 12.6 Bag mask ventilation with one-handed chin lift

Once the chest is inflated and the heart rate has increased, or the chest has been seen to move, then ventilation should be continued at a rate of 30–40 per minute. Continue ventilatory support until regular breathing is established. Where possible, start resuscitation of the baby at birth with air. There is now good evidence for this in term babies and oxygen toxicity is a real concern with premature babies. Use of the supplemental oxygen should be guided by pulse oximetry with reasonable levels listed in Box 12.2 and in Algorithm 12.1.

If the heart rate has not responded, then check for chest movement rather than auscultation as in fluid-filled lungs breath sounds may be heard without lung inflation. Go back and check airway opening manoeuvres and repeat the inflation breaths.

Circulation

If the heart rate remains slow or absent, despite adequate ventilation for 30 seconds as shown by chest movement, then chest compressions should be started. Chest compressions will help to move oxygenated blood from the lungs to the heart and coronary arteries. The blood you move can only be oxygenated if the lungs have air in them. Cardiac compromise is always the result of respiratory failure and can only be effectively treated if effective ventilation is occurring.

The most efficient way of delivering chest compressions in the neonate is to encircle the chest with both hands, so that the fingers lie behind the baby and the thumbs are apposed on the lower third of the sternum, found just below the inter-nipple line (Figure 12.7). Compress the chest briskly, *by one third of its depth.* In newborn babies, current advice is to perform three compressions for each ventilation breath (3:1 ratio).

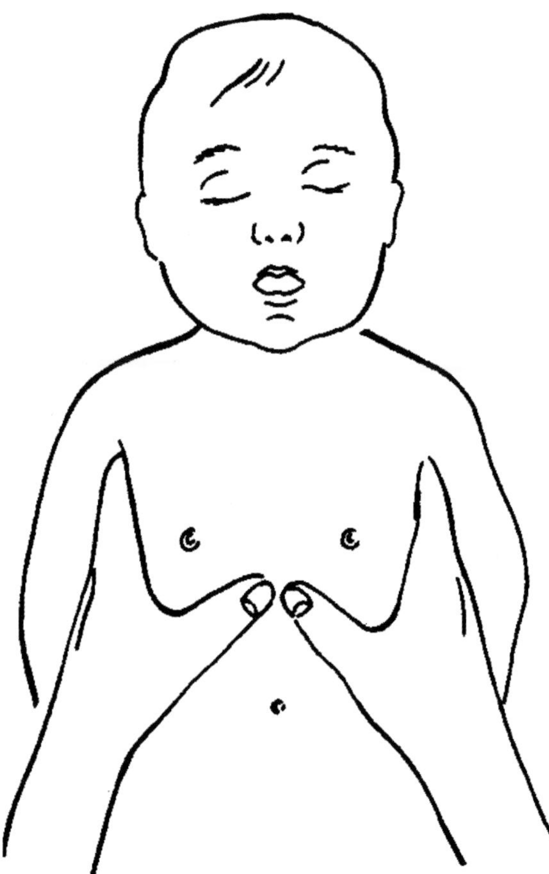

Figure 12.7 Two thumb, hand encircling chest compression in an infant

The purpose of chest compression is to move oxygenated blood or drugs to the coronary arteries in order to initiate cardiac recovery. Thus there is no point in starting chest compressions before effective lung inflation has been established. Similarly, compressions are ineffective unless interposed by ventilation breaths of good quality. Therefore, the emphasis must be upon *good-quality breaths,* followed by effective compressions. Simultaneous delivery of compressions and breaths should be avoided, as the former will reduce the effectiveness of the breaths. It is usually only necessary to continue chest compressions for about 20–30 seconds before the heart responds with an increase in heart rate. Once the heart rate is above 60 beats/minute and rising, chest compressions can be discontinued. Maintain ventilations until effective breathing or mechanical ventilation is established.

Drugs

If, after adequate lung inflation and cardiac compression, the heart rate has not responded, drug therapy should be considered. However, the most common reason for failure of the heart rate to respond is failure to achieve lung inflation, and there is *no point* in giving drugs unless the airway is open and the lungs have been inflated. Airway and breathing must be reassessed as adequate before proceeding to drug therapy. Venous access will be required via an umbilical venous line, because ideally drugs should be given centrally. The outcome is poor if drugs are required for resuscitation.

Adrenaline

The alpha-adrenergic effect of adrenaline increases coronary artery perfusion during resuscitation, enhancing oxygen delivery to the heart. In the presence of profound unresponsive bradycardia or circulatory standstill, 10 microgram/kg (0.1 ml/kg 1:10 000) adrenaline may be given intravenously. Further doses of 10–30 microgram/kg (0.1–0.3 ml/kg 1:10 000) may be tried at 3–5-minute intervals if there is no response. The tracheal route cannot be recommended, as there are insufficient data. However, if adrenaline is given via the tracheal route it is likely that doses of at least 50 microgram/kg will be required to achieve a similar effect to an intravenous dose. Such an unproven administration should not compromise airway and breathing management or obtaining umbilical access.

Bicarbonate

Any baby who is in terminal apnoea will have a significant metabolic acidosis. Acidosis depresses cardiac function. Bicarbonate 1–2 mmol/kg (2–4 ml/kg of 4.2% solution) may be used to raise the pH and enhance the effects of oxygen and adrenaline. Bicarbonate use remains controversial and it should only be used in the absence of discernible cardiac output despite all resuscitative efforts or in profound and unresponsive bradycardia.

Glucose

Hypoglycaemia is a potential problem for all stressed or asphyxiated babies. If confirmed, it is treated using a slow bolus of 2.5 ml/kg of 10% glucose intravenously, and then providing a secure intravenous glucose infusion at a rate of 100 ml/kg/day of 10% glucose. BM stix are not reliable in neonates when reading less than 5 mmol/l.

Fluid

Very occasionally, hypovolaemia may be present because of known or suspected blood loss (antepartum haemorrhage, placenta or vasa praevia, unclamped cord) or hypovolaemia may be secondary to loss of vascular tone following asphyxia (the latter is often accompanied by cardiac dysfunction). Volume expansion is initially with 10 ml/kg (if large loss suspected 20 ml/kg may be appropriate). Normal saline can be used; alternatively Gelofusine has been used safely and if blood loss is acute and severe, non-cross-matched O-negative blood should be given immediately. Albumin cannot be recommended. However, most newborn or neonatal resuscitations do not require fluid, unless there has been known blood loss or septicaemic shock.

Naloxone

This is not a drug of resuscitation. Occasionally a baby *who has been effectively resuscitated* – is pink, with a heart rate of over 100 beats/min – may not breathe spontaneously or adequately because of the possible effects of maternal opiates. If respiratory depressant effects are suspected, the baby should be given naloxone intramuscularly (200 microgram in a full term baby). Smaller doses of 10 microgram/kg will also reverse the sedation but the effect will only last a short time (20 minutes IV or a few hours IM). Intravenous naloxone has a half-life shorter than opiates, and there is no evidence to recommend intra-tracheal administration.

Response to resuscitation

The first indication of success will be an increase in heart rate. Recovery of respiratory drive may be delayed. Babies in terminal apnoea will tend to gasp first as they recover before starting normal respirations (Figure 12.3). Those who were in primary apnoea are likely to start with normal breaths, which may commence at any stage of resuscitation.

Tracheal intubation

Most babies can be resuscitated using a mask system. Swedish data suggest that if this is applied adequately, only 1:500 babies may actually need intubation. However, tracheal intubation only remains the gold standard in airway management if it is performed perfectly. It is especially useful in prolonged resuscitations, pre-term babies and meconium aspiration. It should be considered if mask ventilation has failed, although the most common reason for failure with mask inflation is poor positioning of the head with consequent failure to open the airway.

Tracheal tube placement must be assessed visually during intubation and in most cases will be confirmed by a rapid response in heart rate on ventilating via the endotracheal tube. Exhaled CO_2 detection will identify most correctly sited tubes in the presence of any cardiac output and its detection should be used to confirm tracheal tube placement.

Special cases

Pre-term babies

Unexpected deliveries outside delivery suites are more likely to be premature. Premature babies are more likely to get cold (higher surface area to mass ratio), and more likely to become hypoglycaemic (fewer glycogen stores). There are now several trials that support the use of plastic bags placed over babies of <29 weeks of gestation or <1000 g before drying in order to keep them warm. The babies should then be placed under radiant heat (see Box 12.3). The effectiveness of this technique without the radiant heater has not been tested in trial.

Box 12.3 Guidelines for use of plastic bags for pre-term babies (<29 weeks) at birth

1 Pre-term babies born below 29 completed weeks' gestation may be placed in plastic bags or wrap for temperature stability during resuscitation. They should remain in the bag until they are on the NICU and the humidity within their incubator is at the desired level. It is a way of preventing evaporative heat loss and cannot replace incubators etc. Neither should it replace all efforts to maintain a high ambient temperature around babies outside delivery suites.

2 At birth the baby should not be dried, but should be slipped straight into the prepared plastic bag or wrapping. There is no need to wrap in a towel so long as this is done immediately after birth. This gives immediate humidity. The plastic bag only prevents evaporative heat loss – once in the bag the baby should be placed under a radiant heater.

3 Suitable plastic bags are food-grade bags designed for microwaving and roasting. They should be large. The bag is prepared with a V cut in the closed end. Purpose made bags and wraps are also available.

4 The bag should cover the baby from the shoulders to the feet, with the head protruding through the V-cut. This is most easily performed if the hand is placed through the V, the head placed in the hand, and the bag drawn back down over the baby.

5 The head will stick out of the V-cut and will be dried as usual and resuscitation commenced as per standard guidelines. A hat should be placed over the head, if practical, to further reduce heat loss.

6 The standard resuscitation would be carried out without any limitations of access, but if the umbilicus is required for any access then a hole can be made above the area and the desired intervention done.

7 The bag should not be removed unless deemed necessary by the registrar or consultant.

8 After the transfer to a neonatal unit and stabilising ventilation if required, the baby's temperature should be recorded. The bag is only removed when the incubator humidity is satisfactory, and further care provided as per nursing protocols.

The more premature a baby, the less likely it is to establish adequate respirations. Preterm babies (less than 32 weeks gestation) are likely to be deficient in surfactant especially after unexpected or precipitate delivery. The surfactant, secreted by pneumocytes in the alveolar epithelium, reduces alveolar surface tension and prevents alveolar collapse on expiration. Small amounts of surfactant can be demonstrated from about 20 weeks' gestation, but a surge in production occurs at 30–34 weeks. Surfactant is released at birth due to aeration and distension of the alveoli. The half-life of the surfactant is approximately 12 hours.

Production is reduced by hypothermia (<35 C), hypoxia and acidosis (pH <7.25). In babies born before 32 weeks, one must anticipate a lack of surfactant. The effort of respiration will be increased, although the musculature will be less developed. They may require help to establish prompt aeration and ventilation, and may subsequently require exogenous surfactant therapy.

The lungs of pre-term babies are more fragile than those of term babies and thus are much more susceptible to damage from over-distension. Therefore, it is appropriate to start with a lower inflation pressure of 2.0–2.5 kPa (20–25 cmH_2O) but do not be afraid to increase this to 30 cmH_2O if there is no heart rate response.

It should be noted that very obvious chest wall movement in premature babies of less than 28 weeks' gestation may indicate excessive and potentially damaging tidal volumes.

Premature babies are more susceptible to the toxic effects of hyperoxia. Using a pulse oximeter to monitor both heart rate and oxygen saturation in these babies from birth makes stabilisation much easier. Exposing babies at birth to high concentrations of oxygen can have significant adverse longer term effects. Ranges of pre-ductal oxygen saturation found in the first few minutes of life in well preterm infants are increasingly being reported. However, normal values in well babies born before 32 weeks gestation are based upon small numbers. Therefore, at present, additional oxygen should not be given if the oxygen saturation from the right arm or wrist is above the values in Table 12.1.

Table 12.1 Saturation monitoring in premature babies

Time from birth	Acceptable (25th centile) pre-ductal saturation (%) under 32 weeks gestation above which supplemental oxygen should not be given
2 min	60
3 min	70
4 min	80
5 min	85
10 min	90

Pulse oximetry gives a quick and relatively accurate display of both heart rate and oxygen saturation which can be easily seen by all involved in the resuscitation. This is particularly useful when stabilising significantly preterm babies or when tempted to give additional oxygen to any baby. Once the oximeter is switched on, a reading can be obtained a few seconds faster if the probe is first attached to the right hand or the wrist of the baby and only then connected to the machine. Once the heart rate is displayed, it is likely that this will be more accurate than other commonly used methods of assessing heart rate.

Actions in the event of poor initial response to resuscitation

1. Check airway and breathing.
2. Check for a technical fault.
   (a) Is mask ventilation effective? Observe movement.

(b) Is the tracheal tube in the trachea? Auscultate both axillae, listen at the mouth for a large leak, and observe movement. Use an exhaled CO_2 detector to ensure tracheal tube position.

(c) Is the tracheal tube in a bronchus? Auscultate both axillae and observe movement.

(d) Is the tracheal tube blocked? If there is doubt about the position or patency of the tracheal tube, place it again. Use an exhaled CO_2 detector to check.

(e) Is a longer inflation time required?

(f) If starting in air, increase the oxygen concentration. This is least likely to be a cause, although if monitoring saturations it could be an indication for a slow increase.

3. Does the baby have a pneumothorax? This occurs spontaneously in up to 1% of newborns, but those needing action in the delivery unit are exceptionally rare. Auscultate the chest for asymmetry of breath sounds. A cold light source can be used to transilluminate the chest – a pneumothorax may show as a hyper-illuminating area. If a tension pneumothorax is thought to be present clinically, a 21-gauge butterfly needle should be inserted through the second intercostal space in the mid-clavicular line. Alternatively, a 22-gauge cannula connected to a three-way tap may be used. Remember that you may well cause a pneumothorax during this procedure.
4. Does the baby remain cyanosed despite breathing with a good heart rate? There may be a congenital heart malformation, which may be duct-dependent, or a persistent pulmonary hypertension.
5. If, after resuscitation, the baby is pink and has a good heart rate but is not breathing effectively, it may be suffering the effects of maternal opiates. Naloxone 200 micrograms IM may be considered, this should outlast the opiate effect.
6. Is there severe anaemia or hypovolaemia? In case of large blood loss, 20 ml/kg O-negative blood or a volume expander should be given. (This will usually present as a partial response to effective ventilation: the heart rate remains low at 50–100 despite good ventilation in a pale baby.)

Birth outside the delivery room

Whenever a baby is born unexpectedly, the greatest difficulty often lies in keeping the infant warm. Drying and wrapping, turning up the heating and closing windows and doors are all important in maintaining temperature. Special care must be taken to clamp and cut the cord to prevent blood loss.

Hospitals with Emergency Departments should have guidelines for resuscitation at birth, summoning help and post-resuscitation transfer of babies born within the department.

Babies born unexpectedly, outside hospital, will be at greater risk of being pre-term and of getting cold. However, the principles of resuscitation are identical to the hospital setting. Transport will need to be discussed according to local guidelines.

Discontinuation of resuscitation

The outcome for a baby with no detectable cardiac output for more than 10 minutes is likely to be very poor. Stopping resuscitation early, or not starting resuscitation at all, may be appropriate in situations of extreme prematurity (<23 weeks), birth weight of <400g, or in the presence of lethal abnormalities, such as anencephaly or confirmed trisomy 13 or 18. Resuscitation is nearly always indicated in conditions with a high survival rate and acceptable morbidity. Such decisions should be taken by a senior member of the team, ideally a consultant, in consultation with the parents and other team members and preferably before birth, if the situation has been detected at that stage.

Communication with the parents

It is important that the team caring for the newborn baby informs the parents of the progress whenever possible. This is likely to be most difficult in unexpected deliveries, so prior planning to cover the eventuality may be helpful. Decisions at the end of life must involve the parents whenever possible. All communication should be documented after the event.

Summary

- All babies need to be dried and kept warm.
- Cord clamping should follow after a minute or so from birth in most cases.
- Babies who have passed meconium who are vigorous do not need to be suctioned.
- Some babies require resuscitation involving sequentially, as needed:
  - opening the airway
  - inflation breaths
  - ventilation breaths
  - cardiac compressions.

Reference and further reading

1 Resuscitation Council. *Newborn Life Support*. London: Resuscitation Council, 2010.

SECTION 4

Trauma

ALGORITHM 13.1 Trauma

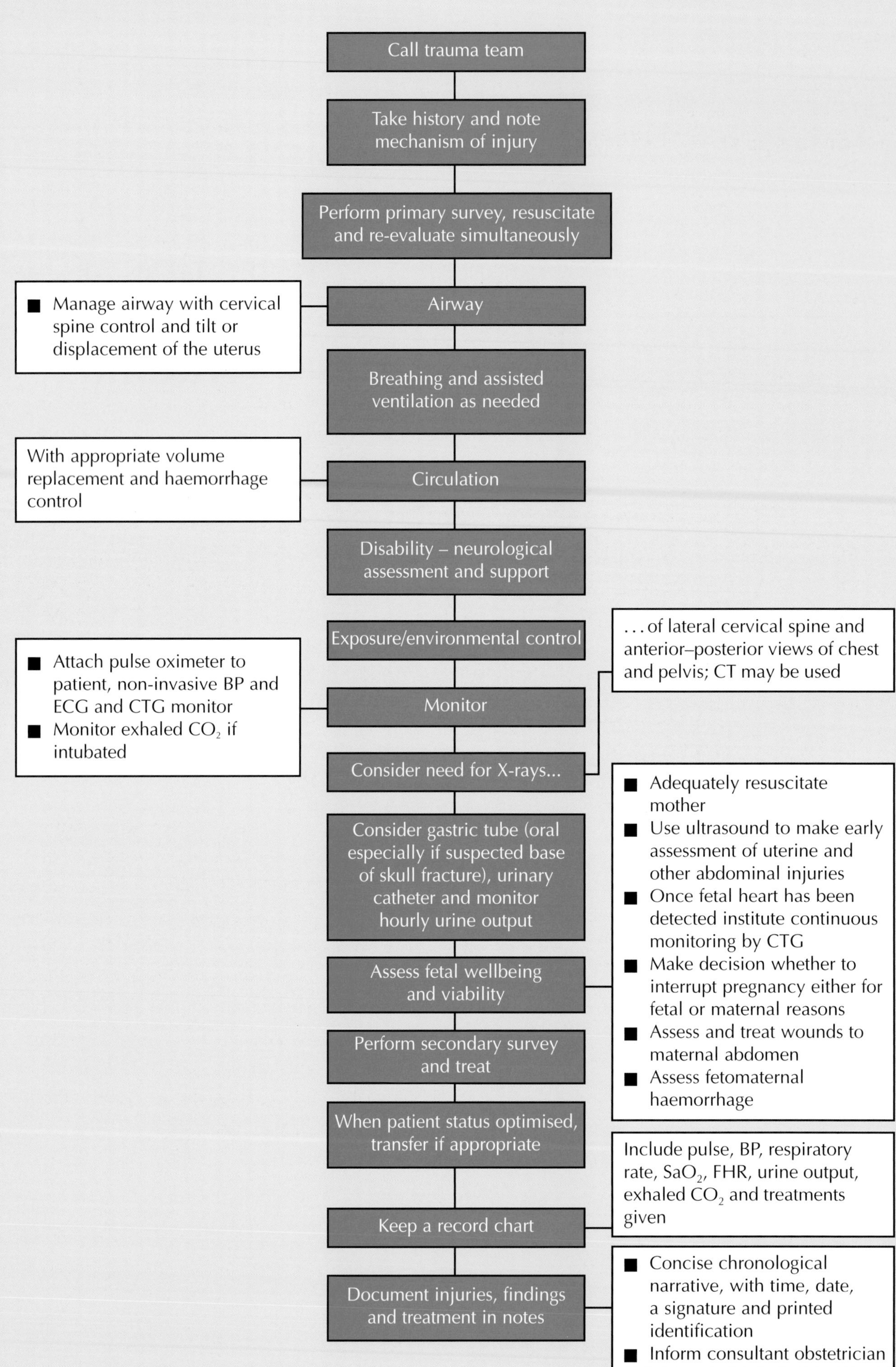

CHAPTER 13

Introduction to trauma

Trauma is an example of a multisystem, life-threatening illness. Like all life-threatening emergencies, the management of major trauma requires a systematic approach. Developing an understanding of such an approach and applying it to any life-threatening emergency will help to optimise care.

There are marked differences in the epidemiology of trauma in different countries. In the UK, there are an estimated 10 000 deaths from trauma each year – approximately 30 deaths each day, of which road traffic accidents are the most common cause.

Trauma occurs in up to 7% of pregnancies and is most commonly due to suicide (most common postnatally), road traffic accidents (equal frequency throughout pregnancy), domestic violence (more common before 18 weeks), falls (between 20 and 30 weeks) and burns.

The Confidential Enquiry into Maternal Deaths has highlighted suicide as a major cause of death recently and in the 2006–08 triennium there were 29 reported suicides. Of these deaths, 87% were by violent means, which is a less common method of suicide in the nonpregnant female. The most common methods involved hanging or jumping from a height, but self-immolation also occurred. The Enquiry reported 17 cases of road traffic accidents and 11 cases of murder, but of all the 344 deaths assessed, 34 of these women had suffered from domestic violence. The obstetrician is likely to be called to any case of trauma in the pregnant woman.

A survey of trauma deaths shows up to 33% to be preventable. These preventable deaths are largely the result of early hypoxia and hypovolaemia. Forty percent of deaths occur at the scene of the accident. Of those who survive major trauma, only 18% make a full functional recovery; many have minor disabilities, but 9% have moderate disability (usually orthopaedic, such as knee ligament injuries); and 3% have severe disability (usually neurological: spinal-cord injury, head injury). Abruption occurs in up to 70% of major trauma in pregnancy, while uterine rupture is much less likely, occurring in less than 1% of major injuries, but it is associated with a 10% maternal mortality rate. Fetal loss occurs in up to 40% of major, and 2% of minor, injuries. Fetal loss occurs in 35% traumatic abruptions and is invariable in traumatic uterine rupture. The seat belt advice, 'Above and below the bump, not over it' is regularly repeated in the confidential maternal death reports.

Analysis of trauma data shows a trimodal death distribution:

1. Instantaneous

Within seconds to minutes of the injury: deaths are due to a blocked airway, massive head injury, severe spinal-cord injury and exsanguination.

2. Early

These extend from the first few minutes to a few hours. Examples include: airway and respiratory compromise; continuing haemorrhage; and subdural and extradural haematoma. It is in this phase, often referred to as 'the golden hour' of trauma management, that properly trained individuals can save lives.

3. Late

These occur from a few hours to days or even weeks after injury. The majority are due to sepsis with associated multiorgan dysfunction. The MOET course is primarily aimed at preventing potential deaths in the 'early' phase. However, the 'late outcome' deaths (due to multiorgan dysfunction) can also be significantly influenced by vigorous and correct initial management; for example, restoration of tissue perfusion – oxygenation, antibiotics and, vitally, by recognising the need for early surgical intervention, followed by intensive medical and nursing care. The teaching is also directed at reducing and preventing disability.

The obstetrician and midwife as part of the trauma team

The pathophysiological response to trauma is altered in pregnancy and thereby the clinician's assessment of trauma may be adversely affected. The obstetrician, obstetric anaesthetist and midwife have a role in understanding anatomical and physiological changes and adapting trauma care to the pregnant woman and the fetus. While the mother takes priority and resuscitating her is helpful to the fetus, particular prompts can be helpful to the trauma team. These include: nursing the woman in left lateral tilt to enhance venous return and performing fetal monitoring to help identify the extent of the haemorrhage (as the uteroplacental circulation shuts down to preserve maternal circulation). Signs of fetal distress may aid in the diagnosis, or extent, of injury and identify the need to empty the uterus and deal with noncompressible haemorrhage. Ultrasound can be helpful in many such cases. Fetomaternal haemorrhage is also something that may need to be considered.

The sequence of care should be:

- primary survey
- assessment of the fetus
- secondary survey.

In the management of the nonpregnant trauma patient, hypotensive resuscitation is generally supported as a means of reducing severe internal bleeding before definitive haemostasis can be achieved (by surgery or embolisation); however, the permissible depth and length of hypotensive resuscitation is currently unknown. There is, however, little place for hypotensive resuscitation in pregnancy as it causes shut down of perfusion to the fetoplacental unit.

Documentation and communication

- Clear, chronological records of assessment of injuries, treatment and reassessment findings should be made and signed, timed and dated.
- Communication with the patient, with relatives and with the multidisciplinary team is essential for success.

Summary

- Major trauma is life-threatening and a systematic approach to its management can save lives.
- The obstetrician and midwife are a valued part of the trauma team as they bring expertise on pregnancy physiology to the fore.
- Maintaining oxygenation is a high priority.
- Actively restoring normovolaemia is preferable to hypotensive resuscitation when the fetus is viable, as long as this does not compromise the mother's health.

CHAPTER 14

Domestic abuse

Objectives

On successfully completing this topic, you will be able to:

- appreciate the incidence of domestic abuse
- understand the implications for the woman and fetus during pregnancy and in the postnatal period
- plan to identify cases and familiarise yourself with local support services.

Introduction

Domestic abuse is a major public health concern that threatens the health, emotional well - being and lives of women and their families.

Domestic abuse is defined, by the Department of Health,[1] as, 'Any incident of threatening behaviour or abuse (psychological, physical, sexual, financial or emotional) between adults who are, or have been, intimate partners or family members, regardless of gender or sexuality.' Women are more likely to be victims in heterosexual relationships (90%). Domestic abuse affects all social classes, all ethnic groups, occurs worldwide and affects all age groups. The broader definition allows for forced marriage, honour killings and female genital mutilation to be recognised as being part of the issue.

Scale of the problem

- One in three women experiences domestic abuse at some point in their lives.
- One in ten women will have experienced domestic abuse in the past year.
- Over one million domestic abuse incidents are recorded by the police each year.
- 30% of domestic abuse starts in pregnancy.
- 40% of women who are murdered are killed by a current or ex-partner.
- Domestic abuse is more common than violence in the street or a public house.

In the 2006–08 CMACE – *Saving Mothers' Lives* – it was reported that 11 women were murdered by their partners during, or soon after, pregnancy.[2] A total of 34 women, who died from other causes, were known to be victims of, or had self-reported, domestic abuse.

What keeps women in abusive relationships?

To outsiders it seems almost bizarre that anyone would stay within an abusive relationship, but nonetheless they do. The reasons for staying are often multiple:

Fear: If she leaves, she is afraid that she or other family members will experience more abuse or possibly be killed.

Financial: Control of her resources by her abuser.

Family: Pressures to stay with the abuser.

Father: Wanting a father figure for her children.

Faith: That she places in a religious doctrine.

Forgiveness: The abuser is often contrite.

Fatigue: From living under high and constant stress and erosion of self-esteem.

Domestic abuse and pregnancy

The incidence of domestic abuse in pregnancy is reported as being 0.9–20.1%. Domestic abuse often begins or escalates during pregnancy, or in some cases, it commences in the puerperium. The risk of moderate-to-severe abuse appears to be greatest in the postpartum period. Women suffering physical abuse are at increased risk for miscarriage, premature labour, placental abruption, low birthweight infants, fetal injury and intrauterine fetal death. Often, as a result of the abuse, women are 15 times more likely to misuse alcohol, nine times more likely to misuse drugs, three times more likely to be clinically depressed and five times more likely to attempt suicide. These all obviously have implications for both the mother and fetus.

Classically, injuries towards the pregnant abdomen, genitals and breasts are seen in pregnancy. However, the injuries can be multiple affecting any part of the woman's body. Campbell reported that 9.5% of women reported sexual abuse and 13.9% were raped by their partners.

Recognising domestic violence in pregnancy

Women who are being abused often book late and may be poor attenders. Their partners may not give them enough money to get to the hospital. Alternatively, they may attend repeatedly with trivial symptoms and appear reluctant to be discharged home. If the partner accompanies the woman, he may be constantly present not allowing for private discussion. The woman may seem reluctant to speak in front of, or contradict, her partner.

Any signs of abuse on the woman's body will be minimised. As with child abuse, the mechanism of injury often does not fit with the apparent injury. There may be untended injuries of different ages or the late presentation of injuries. A history of behavioural problems or abuse in the children may be indicative. Often the patient will give a history of psychiatric illness.

Diagnosing domestic abuse

As domestic abuse often begins or escalates during pregnancy, it is essential that we, as obstetricians and midwives, routinely ask women whether they are subject to mistreatment. Abusive pregnancies are high risk and domestic abuse is much more prevalent than most other complications of pregnancy, such as pre-eclampsia or gestational diabetes mellitus. Standard questions should therefore be included, in the same way as we would ask about medical disorders, smoking or alcohol use. Systematic multiple assessment protocols lead to increased detection and reporting of abuse during pregnancy. The mnemonic RADAR was developed, by the Massachusetts Medical Society, as a tool to guide enquiry about domestic abuse.[3]

R Routinely enquire

A Ask direct questions

D Document your findings

A Assess safety

R Review options and choices

Health professionals should be given appropriate training and education to improve awareness. Questions should be asked in a nonjudgemental, respectful, supportive manner. Obstetricians and midwives should be aware of what help is available should a woman request help. Questions, such as the following, may allow the woman to disclose the fact that she is subject to violence:

> I have noticed you have a number of bruises. Did someone hit you?
>
> You seemed frightened by your partner. Has he ever hurt you?
>
> You mention that your partner loses his temper with the children. Does he ever do so with you?
>
> How does your partner act when drinking or on drugs?

If routine questioning is to be introduced, it is important that local guidelines are developed for referral to appropriate agencies. Other strategies, such as questionnaires or information about emergency helplines in the female toilets or printed on the patient held notes, may help those women whose partners are constantly by their sides. Community midwives visiting women at home may have the privacy to discuss such sensitive matters. The provision of professional interpretation services is essential, as it is not adequate or acceptable to rely on family members to act as interpreters as this does not allow free dialogue to occur.

Documentation in the medical notes is important, even if the woman does not want to prosecute at the current time. Women often prosecute many years later and evidence of the pattern of domestic abuse helps to secure a conviction.

Medico-legal matters

Following the Domestic Violence Crime and Victims Act 2004, a case against a perpetrator can now proceed, if there is sufficient evidence, even if the victim withdraws their statement. The case proceeds in 40% of instances where the victim retracts their complaint, and health-care workers, including midwives and obstetricians, may be approached for a statement.

Communication and teamwork

Domestic abuse is an area where multiagency working is essential. No one agency is able to address all domestic abuse factors. Working collaboratively will ensure appropriate help and support is given. Unit guidelines should incorporate referral pathways for multiagency working.

Audit standard

All women should be seen on their own at least once during the antenatal period to enable the disclosure of such information.

Summary

- Domestic abuse is a major health and social problem in pregnancy.
- Domestic abuse represents a serious threat to the physical and emotional health of women and their children.
- All health professionals have an obligation to identify cases of domestic abuse and provide support and help to the victims.

Useful contacts

Women's Aid Federation of England
PO Box 391, Bristol BS99 7WS
Tel: 0117 944 4411 (office)/0808 2000 247 (helpline)
Email: helpline@womensaid.org.uk
Website: www.womensaid.org.uk

Victim Support National Office
Cranmer House, 39 Brixton Road, London, SW9 6DZ
Tel: 020 7735 9166 (enquiries)/Victim Support Line 0845 30 30 900
Email: contact@victimsupport.org.uk
Website: www.victimsupport.org.uk

Rape Crisis
PO Box 69, London, WC1X 9NJ
Tel: 020 7837 1600 (24-hour helpline)
Email: info@rapecrisis.co.uk
Website: www.rapecrisis.co.uk

Refuge
4th Floor, International House,
1 St Katharine's Way, London E1W 1UN
0808 2000 247 (24-hour national helpline)
Website: www.refuge.org.uk

Samaritans
Tel: 08457 90 90 90
Email: jo@samaritans.org
Website: www.samaritans.org

Police – Domestic Violence Group
Contact your local police station for details.

National Association of Citizens Advice Bureau
Middleton House, 115–123 Pentonville Road, London, N1 9LZ
Tele: 020 7833 2181

References and further reading

1 Centre for Maternal and Child Enquiries (CMACE). *Saving Mothers' Lives*: Reviewing maternal deaths to make motherhood safer: 2006–2008, *Br J Obstet Gynaecol* 118(Suppl. 1), 1–203.
2 Department of Health. *Responding to Domestic Abuse. A Handbook for Health Professionals*. London: Department of Health 2006.
3 Gerard M. Domestic violence: how to screen and intervene. *Registered Nurse* 2000;62:52–6.
4 Abbasi K. Obstetricians must ask about domestic violence. *BMJ* 1998;316:9.
5 Ballard TJ, Salzman LE, Gazmararian JA, *et al.* Violence during pregnancy: measurement issues. *Am J Public Health* 1998;88:274–6.
6 Bewley S, Friend J, Mezey G (editors). *Violence Against Women*. London: RCOG Press 1997.
7 Campbell JC. Nursing assessment for risk of homicide with battered women. *Adv Nurs Sci* 1986;8:36–51.
8 Covington DL, Diehl SJ, Wright BD, Piner M. Assessing for violence during pregnancy using a systematic approach. *Matern Child Health J* 1997;1(2):129.

9 Gibson E, Klein S. *Murder 1957–1968.* Home Office Research Study No 3. London: HMSO 1989.
10 Gielen AC, O'Campo PJ, Faden RR, *et al.* Interpersonal conflict and physical violence during the childbearing year. *Soc Sci Med* 1994;39:781–7.
11 Grunfeld A, MacKay K. Diagnosing domestic violence. *Canadian Journal of Diagnosis* 1997;14:61–9.
12 Heath I. Domestic violence and the general practitioner. *Matern Child Health* 1994; 19:316–20.
13 Lewis G, (ed). *Why Mothers Die 1997–1999.* The Fifth Report of the Confidential Enquiries into Maternal Deaths in the United Kingdom. London: RCOG Press 2001.
14 Lewis G (ed). *Why Mothers Die 2000–2002.* The Sixth Report of the Confidential Enquiries into Maternal Deaths in the United Kingdom. London: RCOG Press 2004.
15 Mezey GC, Bewley S. Domestic violence and pregnancy. *Br J Obstet Gynaecol* 1997; 104:528–31.
16 Royal College of Midwives. *Domestic Abuse in Pregnancy.* Position Paper No. 19. London: RCM 1997.
17 Stark E, Flitcraft A. *Women at Risk.* London: Sage 1996.
18 Widding Hedin L. Postpartum, also a risk period for domestic violence. *Eur J Obstet Gynecol Reprod Biol* 2000;89:41–5.

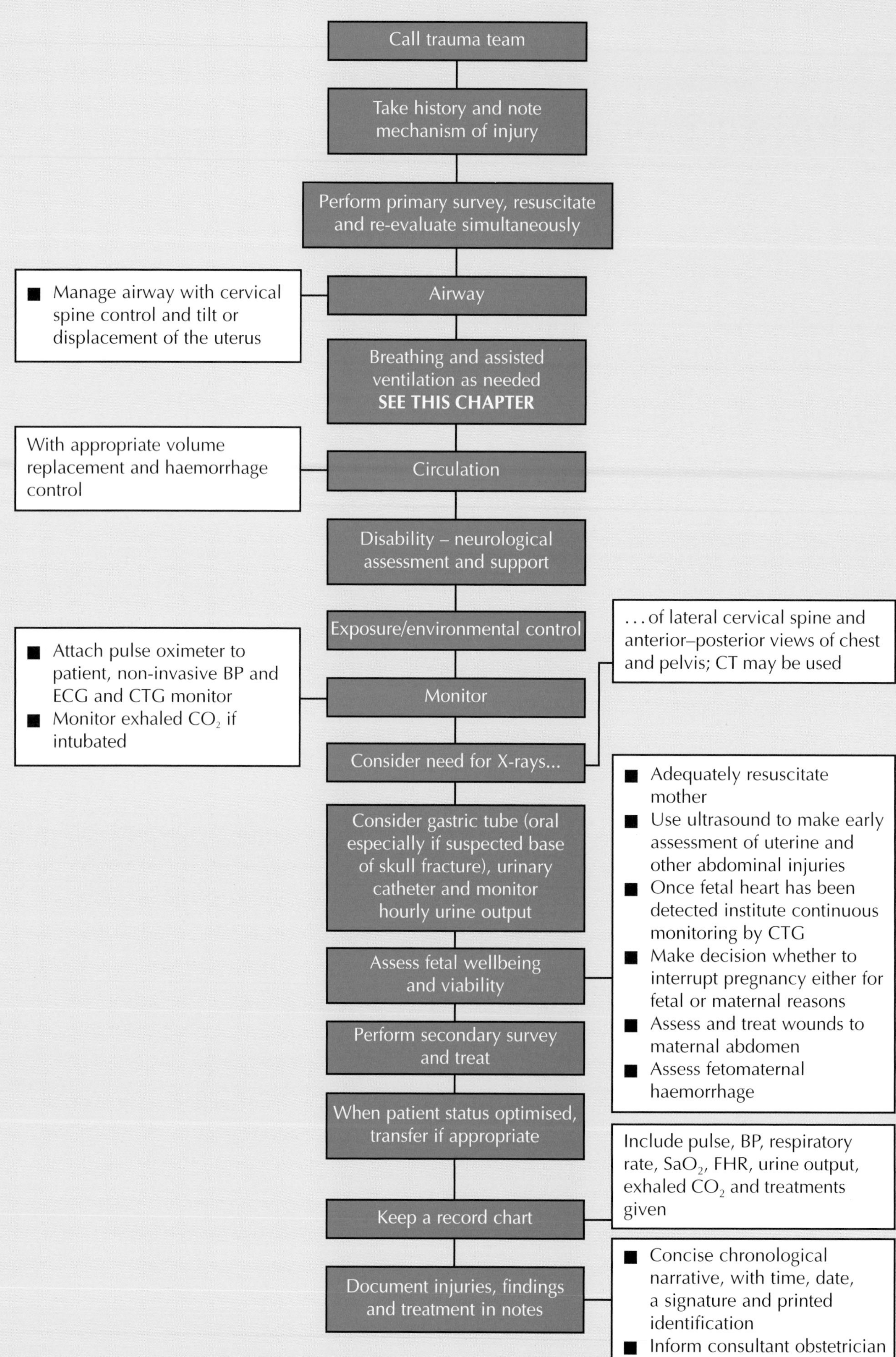
Call trauma team
Take history and note mechanism of injury
Perform primary survey, resuscitate and re-evaluate simultaneously
Airway
■ Manage airway with cervical spine control and tilt or displacement of the uterus
Breathing and assisted ventilation as needed SEE THIS CHAPTER
Circulation
With appropriate volume replacement and haemorrhage control
Disability – neurological assessment and support
Exposure/environmental control
Monitor
■ Attach pulse oximeter to patient, non-invasive BP and ECG and CTG monitor
■ Monitor exhaled CO2 if intubated
Consider need for X-rays...
...of lateral cervical spine and anterior–posterior views of chest and pelvis; CT may be used
Consider gastric tube (oral especially if suspected base of skull fracture), urinary catheter and monitor hourly urine output
Assess fetal wellbeing and viability
■ Adequately resuscitate mother
■ Use ultrasound to make early assessment of uterine and other abdominal injuries
■ Once fetal heart has been detected institute continuous monitoring by CTG
■ Make decision whether to interrupt pregnancy either for fetal or maternal reasons
■ Assess and treat wounds to maternal abdomen
■ Assess fetomaternal haemorrhage
Perform secondary survey and treat
When patient status optimised, transfer if appropriate
Keep a record chart
Include pulse, BP, respiratory rate, SaO2, FHR, urine output, exhaled CO2 and treatments given
Document injuries, findings and treatment in notes
■ Concise chronological narrative, with time, date, a signature and printed identification
■ Inform consultant obstetrician

CHAPTER 15

Thoracic emergencies

Objectives

On successfully completing this topic, you will be able to:

- identify life-threatening injuries in the chest
- identify potentially life-threatening injuries in the chest
- be aware of the skills required to manage these life-threatening injuries.

Medical emergencies, including cardiac disease, are discussed in Chapter 22. This chapter focuses on intrathoracic emergencies, mainly caused by trauma but occasionally arising spontaneously, as in the case of spontaneous pneumothorax or aortic aneurysm dissection.

Introduction

In the 2006–08 report of the Confidential Enquiries into Maternal Deaths in the UK, 29 women died from traumatic causes (17 road traffic accidents, 11 murders and one house fire).

Chest injuries are common in patients with major trauma and they are responsible for around one-quarter of trauma deaths. Many of these deaths can be prevented by the prompt recognition of life-threatening conditions and the early initiation of simple methods of treatment. Few patients will require surgery. Most are treated by the simple methods demonstrated on the MOET course of needle thoracocentesis and chest drain placement. Prompt and effective resuscitation of the mother, including the avoidance of aortocaval compression is the most effective way of ensuring good fetoplacental perfusion.

Types of injury to the chest

Chest injuries are usually classified as penetrating, blunt or both. When there are external signs of thoracic injury, intra-abdominal organs, including the gravid uterus, may also have been damaged, particularly in the later stages of pregnancy. The reverse is also true, in that obvious abdominal trauma may extend into the chest.

Initial assessment and management

An accurate history of the incident is vital. For example, the driver of a car in collision with a tree would be at risk of a traumatic brain injury, cervical spine trauma, traumatic aortic rupture, lung and myocardial contusion and abdominal trauma, in addition to many other bony and soft-tissue injuries.

The principles of management are:

- primary survey and resuscitation: life-threatening injuries discovered during the primary survey should be dealt with immediately
- assessment of fetal wellbeing and viability
- secondary survey: careful head-to-toe examination should identify any other injuries sustained
- definitive care.

Life-threatening injuries to identify and treat

Mnemonic for life-threatening injuries in the chest:

A airway obstruction

T tension pneumothorax

O open pneumothorax

M massive haemothorax

F flail chest

C cardiac tamponade

Airway obstruction

See Chapter 8.

Tension pneumothorax

The diagnosis should be considered in any trauma patient with severe respiratory distress and also, in some cases, shock. There is usually reduced air entry and reduced chest expansion but hyper-resonance on the affected side. The classic signs of tracheal deviation and distended neck veins may be very late or absent, the latter especially in those with concurrent hypovolaemic shock.

If there is any doubt, needle thoracocentesis to decompress the air, and subsequent intercostal drain placement, should be performed without delay and are very safe when performed correctly.

Open pneumothorax (sucking chest wound)

A large chest-wall defect will suck air through it with each inspiration and cause a progressive decline in pulmonary function.

The principle of management is to cover the defect in such a way as to prevent air being sucked in, but allow accumulated air to escape. An Asherman seal will be effective for small wounds or a dressing, taped securely on three sides only, for larger wounds. An intercostal drain should be placed remote to the site of injury.

Massive haemothorax

Massive haemothoraces are usually caused by damage to a systemic or pulmonary vessel. Clinical signs include evidence of hypovolaemia, decreased air entry and dullness to percussion.

The drainage of a large collection, without wide-bore intravenous access for fluid replacement, can lead to circulatory collapse when the tamponade effect is acutely lost, so intravenous access should be secured *prior to* drainage. Most haemothoraces are managed conservatively, but if after the placement of an intercostal drain the initial loss is greater than 1500 ml, or continuing losses exceed 200 ml/hour, operative intervention may be needed.

Flail chest

When a segment of the chest wall loses continuity with the rest of the thoracic cage from multiple rib fractures, that segment moves paradoxically with respiration and the segment is called a flail segment. Hypoxia is caused by trauma to the underlying lung, which can be severe. The bony injury can be extremely painful and this impairs oxygenation further. The principles of management include high concentration oxygen, insertion of an intercostal drain, careful fluid management and effective analgesia often with a thoracic epidural. A period of mechanical ventilation may be required in severe cases.

Cardiac tamponade

This occurs, infrequently, with blunt or penetrating trauma to the chest. It can be difficult to detect. It may also be seen in association with spontaneous rupture of the aorta, a well-recognised feature of women with Marfan's syndrome. In the 2006–08 maternal mortality report, seven women died from spontaneous dissection of the aorta leading to cardiac tamponade.

Signs include tachycardia, arterial hypotension, shock, distended neck veins and muffled heart sounds. It should be suspected in a hypotensive patient with a penetrating injury to the chest over the cardiac outline, either anteriorly or posteriorly. Ultrasound can quickly confirm the diagnosis. The treatment is urgent surgical exploration, but needle pericardiocentesis can be performed, under ultrasound and ECG control, if the patient is deteriorating.

Secondary survey related to the chest

A radiograph of the chest, taken in the primary survey, should be reviewed. This should be examined for bony injury, air or blood in a pleural cavity or evidence of contusion. The position of gastric and tracheal tubes, and any central venous catheters should be checked. In most cases of multiple trauma a full body CT scan will be performed. Any abnormality should be interpreted according to the mechanism of injury and the likelihood of underlying thoracic injury.

Potentially lethal chest injuries

These may not be obvious during the primary survey. They are usually described as two contusions and four disruptions:

- pulmonary contusion
- myocardial contusion
- diaphragmatic disruption
- tracheobronchial disruption
- oesophageal disruption
- aortic disruption.

Pulmonary contusion

Pulmonary contusion is usually as a result of blunt trauma to the chest and presents as hypoxia that may progress to respiratory failure. The key to successful management is to maintain a high index of suspicion, as the young pregnant population may hide the initial signs well. Any signs of respiratory impairment such as tachypnoea, low oxygen saturations, use of accessory muscles or cyanosis should prompt immediate referral to the intensive care unit. Young pregnant patients should have excellent oxygenation when breathing high-flow oxygen. If they have not, then significant contusion should be suspected.

Myocardial contusion

Myocardial contusion should be suspected whenever there is a history of blunt chest injury, although proof of significant contusion is difficult to obtain. Patients may have extra systoles, abnormal complexes or even haemodynamically significant arrhythmia.

Diaphragmatic disruption

Diaphragmatic disruption is usually associated with blunt abdominal injury and is usually found on the left side. Compression causes a radial tear in the diaphragm, allowing abdominal contents to herniate into the chest. Abdominal structures may have been damaged by the injury itself, by the placement of an intercostal drain or may become ischaemic while in the chest cavity. Oxygenation and ventilation can be severely affected.

The diagnosis should be suspected with blunt trauma to the chest or abdomen and is confirmed by chest radiograph, e.g. the presence of a gastric tube above the diaphragm. The diaphragm is usually repaired without delay.

Tracheobronchial disruption

Injuries to the larynx, trachea or bronchi need urgent attention from a senior anaesthetist. Laryngeal and tracheal injuries are rare and present with airway obstruction, subcutaneous emphysema and hoarseness. In addition, they suggest the presence of other injuries to thorax or abdominal structures. Bronchial injuries are often fatal. They may present as a pneumothorax with a continuing air leak after drain placement. Surviving patients usually require surgical repair.

Oesophageal disruption

This is usually the result of a penetrating injury, although can be caused by blunt trauma to the upper abdomen. Rupture of the oesophagus can also occur after prolonged vomiting (Boerhaave syndrome). The diagnosis is suggested by:

1. History with: pain out of proportion to other injuries; left-sided pneumothorax; particulate matter from the chest drain.
2. Mediastinal air and surgical emphysema.

Surgical repair is the treatment of choice if the diagnosis is made early, but the mediastinitis can be fatal.

Traumatic aortic disruption

The mechanism of injury here is usually a decelerating injury, such as a car crash or a fall, and those that survive to hospital have a laceration in the region of the ligamentum arteriosum and a contained haematoma. The diagnosis is made using a high index of suspicion from the history and the chest radiograph appearance of a widened mediastinum. This leads to further investigation such as CT, angiography or transoesophageal echocardiography. The treatment is surgical repair.

Summary

- Chest trauma in pregnancy involves a combination of injury to major thoracic structures with the disadvantage of a large gravid uterus that can easily impair venous return and compromise respiration.
- Most injuries can be identified by careful assessment and managed with simple measures, including the avoidance of aortocaval compression.
- Knowledge of the pathophysiology of these injuries allows the obstetrician to take part in the decision-making process and prioritise maternal, and fetal, treatment appropriately.

APPENDIX 15A

Practical procedures

Needle thoracocentesis

Equipment:

- alcohol swab
- intravenous cannula (16 gauge minimum).

Procedure

1. Identify the second intercostal space in the midclavicular line on the side of the tension pneumothorax (the side with reduced air entry, hyper-resonance and reduced chest expansion, the trachea may be deviated to the opposite side).
2. Swab the chest wall with surgical preparation or an alcohol swab.
3. Insert the cannula into the chest wall, just over the rib.
4. Remove the Luer-Lok from the catheter and listen for the escape of air as the needle enters the parietal pleura.
5. Remove the needle, leaving the plastic cannula in place.
6. Tape the cannula in place and proceed to chest drain insertion as soon as possible.

Complications

These can include:

- local haematoma
- lung laceration
- if needle thoracocentesis is attempted, and the patient does not have a tension pneumothorax, the chance of causing a pneumothorax is 10–20%; patients must have a chest radiograph and will require chest drainage if ventilated.

Chest drain insertion

(Remember intravenous access is needed before doing this.)

Equipment:

- skin preparation and surgical drapes
- local anaesthetic
- scalpel
- scissors
- artery forceps
- large clamps (two)
- chest drain tube without trocar
- suture
- underwater seal
- 10 ml syringe with orange, blue and green needles.

Procedure

1. Identify relevant landmarks. This is usually the fifth intercostal space anterior to the midaxillary line on the side with the pneumothorax (Figure 15A.1). In late pregnancy the diaphragm may be raised so the fourth intercostal space should be used. Bedside ultrasound may be helpful.
2. Swab the chest wall with surgical preparation or an alcohol swab.
3. Infiltrate with local anaesthetic.
4. Make a 2–3 cm transverse skin incision along the inferior line of the intercostal space (i.e. the superior edge of the rib below to avoid the neurovascular bundle).
5. Bluntly dissect through the subcutaneous tissues down onto the rib with artery forceps. Slip over the top of the rib and bluntly dissect through the intercostal muscles. Puncture the parietal pleura with the tip of the forceps.
6. Put a gloved finger into the incision and clear the path into the pleura.
7. Advance the chest drain tube with the aid of a clamp into the pleural space (i.e. without the trocar), directing it posteriorly.
8. Ensure that the tube is in the pleural space by listening for air movement and by looking for fogging of the tube during expiration.
9. Connect the chest drain tube to an underwater seal below the level of the patient and ensure the water level is swinging.
10. Suture the drain in place, and secure with tape (Figure 15A.2).
11. Obtain a chest radiograph.

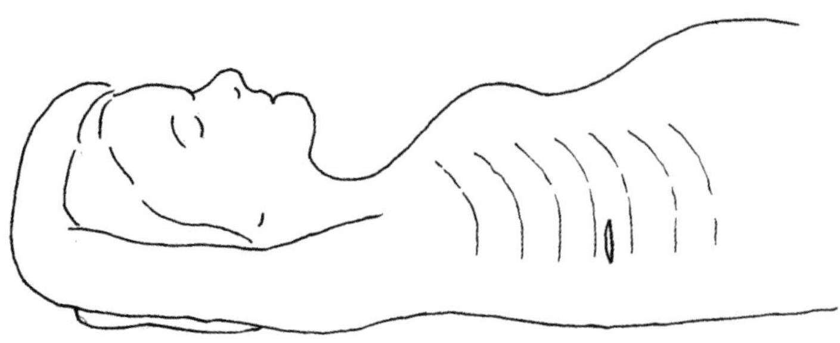

Figure 15A.1 Chest drain placement

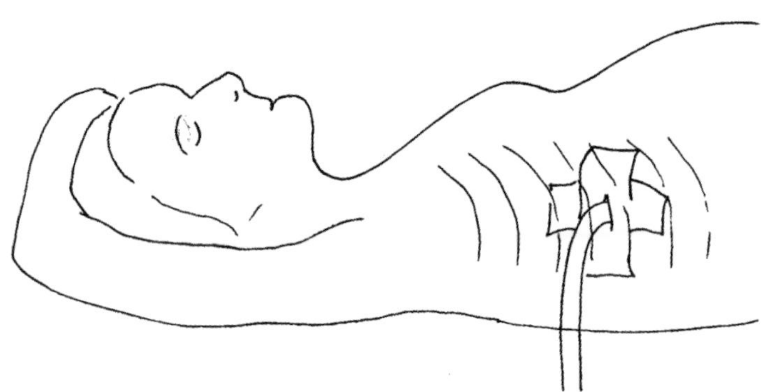

Figure 15A.2 Chest drain sutured in place and secured with tape

Prescribe appropriate antibiotics following chest drain insertion associated with trauma. Smaller bore drains may be used for drainage of air and can be inserted using a Seldinger wire, without the need for blunt dissection.

Complications

These can include:

- damage to intercostal nerve, artery or vein
- introduction of infection
- tube kinking, dislodging or blocking
- subcutaneous emphysema
- persistent pneumothorax due to faulty tube insertion, leaking around chest drain, leaking underwater seal, bronchopleural fistula
- failure of lung to expand due to blocked bronchus
- anaphylactic or allergic reaction to skin preparation.

Further reading

Laws D, Neville E, Duffy J, on behalf of the British Thoracic Society Pleural Disease Group, a subgroup of the British Thoracic Society Standards of Care Committee. BTS guidelines for the insertion of a chest drain. *Thorax* 2003;58(Suppl. 11):ii53–ii59.

CHAPTER 16

Abdominal trauma in pregnancy

Objectives

On successfully completing this topic, you will be able to:

- assess the patient who has sustained abdominal trauma, and recognise the possibility of injury
- appreciate the changes in anatomy and physiology that occur in pregnancy, and of how such changes may alter the response to trauma
- appreciate the diagnostic procedures available for the investigation of abdominal trauma, and the indications for their use
- understand the need for timely resuscitation and treatment, including surgical intervention.

Introduction

Abdominal injuries are a recurring cause of preventable deaths associated with major trauma in the pregnant and nonpregnant woman alike. Abdominal injuries in pregnancy are on the increase, from both accidental and nonaccidental causes. The prompt and accurate assessment of the presence of intra-abdominal injury, and its likely site, can be challenging and the existence of a gravid uterus makes the task more complex.

Obstetricians should become involved early in the management of victims of trauma when pregnancy is obvious or suspected. They need to be familiar with the patterns of abdominal injury in the pregnant and nonpregnant patient, and their degree of priority. They need to be aware, also, of the effects of pregnancy on the response to blood loss, affecting both mother and fetus. The mother, especially in later pregnancy, tolerates blood loss well; the fetus tolerates maternal blood loss very badly and reflects maternal hypovolaemia by demonstrating fetal distress on monitoring.

Specific challenges posed by pregnancy in assessment of the abdomen:

- the peritoneum is less sensitive
- the omentum is less able to contain local inflammation

- organ displacement occurs as the uterus enlarges; for example, the bowels are pushed upwards, which can pose diagnostic uncertainties.

The latest CMACE report (*Saving Mothers' Lives*, March 2011) records that between 2006 and 2008, 15 women died from road traffic accidents while still pregnant, and two died within 6 weeks of delivery.[1] Of the 15 pregnant women, two were pedestrians hit by motor vehicles. A perimortem caesarean section was carried out for four women in the Emergency Department. The gestations ranged from 24 to 41 weeks, and none of the babies survived.

Injuries may be blunt or penetrating. The vast majority in the UK are of blunt origin, mainly associated with motor vehicle accidents. Deceleration injuries predispose to blunt trauma, with the resulting risk of damage to viscera, including the uterus and its contents. The incidence of violent injuries is increasing, most notably domestic violence (see Chapter 14).

You must be able to identify those patients who require immediate or emergency intervention, either obstetric or surgical. A high index of suspicion is required, and early consultation with other specialties is crucial. Up to 50% of young patients with significant intra-abdominal haemorrhage will have minimal or no signs on initial assessment. Unrecognised or underestimated abdominal injury is still a cause of preventable death.

Trauma to the uterus

In the first trimester, the uterus is protected from injury by its relatively thick wall, as well as by the bony pelvis. Subsequently, it is the uterus that provides some protection to the abdominal contents, and thereby becomes increasingly vulnerable.

Abruption

As pregnancy progresses, the uterine wall becomes thinner. The uterus is elastic but the placenta is not, leading to the risk of trauma-induced abruption as the placenta shears off the uterine wall. What may seem fairly trivial trauma to the uterus may cause significant placental abruption, leading to fetal death, and also possibly leading to disseminated intravascular coagulation in the mother.

Uterine rupture

The possibility of uterine rupture should always be considered. This may be caused in a road traffic accident by blunt trauma from striking the dashboard or steering wheel, or by pressure from an injudiciously placed seat belt. The 2006–08 CMACE report restates its recommendations for the use of seat belts in pregnancy: 'Above and below the bump – not over it.' Three-point seat belts should be worn throughout pregnancy, with the lap strap placed as low as possible beneath the 'bump', lying across the thighs, with the diagonal shoulder strap above the bump, lying between the breasts. The seat belt should be adjusted to fit as snugly as comfortably possible and, if necessary, the seat should be adjusted to enable the seat belt to be worn properly. Lap belts alone are unsuitable in pregnancy.

Signs of uterine rupture include abdominal tenderness with guarding and rigidity associated with signs of hypovolaemia. The fetal lie may be transverse or oblique, with easily palpable fetal parts and inaudible fetal heart sounds. Management of suspected uterine rupture is operative exploration.

Penetrating injury

Penetrating injury, causing uterine rupture and fetal trauma, may be sustained by knife wounds, gunshot wounds or high-velocity fragments due to a blast. Other abdominal viscera, including bladder, bowel, liver and spleen, are likely to be involved in such circumstances.

Amniotic fluid embolus

Amniotic fluid embolus may occur as a result of uterine trauma. This is particularly important to recognise, in view of its high associated mortality from respiratory compromise as well as from disseminated intravascular coagulation (see Chapter 10).

Consideration of uterine rupture, amniotic fluid embolus and placental abruption may not necessarily occur to members of the trauma team without prompting from an obstetrician.

Trauma-related haemorrhage

By the third trimester, the plasma volume has expanded by 50% and this, and other physiological changes associated with pregnancy, generally increase maternal tolerance to blood loss. As an end organ, the feto-placental unit is subject to reduced blood flow, as part of the maternal response to hypovolaemia, via the release of catecholamines. Consequently, while maternal tolerance to blood loss is increased, the fetus is particularly sensitive to comparatively small reductions in maternal circulating blood volume.

As a consequence, fetal distress is evident long before the mother shows any of the classic signs of blood loss. Therefore, even modest blood loss requires careful investigation and monitoring. Significant abdominal trauma in pregnancy is associated with a high likelihood of fetal death, either early or delayed. Fluid replacement should be aggressive, in order to maintain blood volume. Hypotensive resuscitation is inappropriate in pregnancy.

Primary survey and resuscitation

A focused history takes little time, and can provide vital clues to the likelihood of abdominal injury.

It may be useful to remember the acronym 'MIST':

- Mechanism of injury
- Injuries already identified
- Symptoms and signs
- Treatment already received.

Details should also include the mechanism of restraint, if any, and details of the pregnancy. Women often carry their own obstetric notes.

An 'AMPLE' history may also be useful:

- Allergies
- Medication
- Previous medical history
- Last meal
- Events and environments related to the injury.

A Airway with cervical spine control, B breathing, Tilt

Life-threatening compromise to airway and breathing should be dealt with immediately. Cervical spine control is crucial where there is a possibility of spinal injury. It is also essential to tilt the woman as soon as possible, to avoid aortocaval compression with resulting functional hypovolaemia.

The MOET course emphasises approaching the woman with hands extended, ready to stabilise the cervical spine, while, at the same time saying 'Hello, Mrs Tilt'. High-flow facial oxygen should always be administered in the first instance.

C Circulation

Abdominal injuries may cause a 'C' problem. Blood should be taken for full blood count, group and crossmatch, and appropriate fluids should be administered (see Chapter 7). A Kleihauer test should be carried out, even if the woman is Rhesus positive, to give an indication of the extent of any fetomaternal transfusion. If a woman is known to be Rhesus negative, anti-D should be administered within 72 hours, unless the injury is remote from the uterus (e.g. isolated distal extremity injury).

It may be obvious from a brief examination during the primary survey that continuing haemorrhage is from an abdominal source, and further investigation may not be necessary. Resuscitation should continue on the way to theatre for laparotomy.

Far more frequently, intra-abdominal bleeding may only be suspected, and further investigations are required. The gravid uterus makes such investigation more difficult.

The fetal heart should be checked early in suspected abdominal injury, as placental abruption is fairly common after significant blunt trauma to the abdomen. In the hurly-burly of the emergency room, it may be difficult to hear the fetal heart with the Pinard stethoscope, and a Doppler or ultrasound machine should be obtained if possible. The mother, if conscious, is certain to be concerned about fetal wellbeing.

A fuller examination of the abdomen and pelvis, including vaginal and rectal examinations, should be performed as soon as is practicable. For further discussion of pelvic fracture see Chapter 19.

The presence of uterine contractions should be noted, as should the presence of amniotic fluid in the vagina, cervical effacement and dilatation, and the relationship of the fetal presenting part to the ischial spines. A gastric tube and a urinary catheter should be put in place.

Bleeding into the uterine muscle or into the uterine cavity is an irritant, and contractions may be the first sign of a developing abruption. Distension, tenderness, guarding and rigidity suggest injury, although a seemingly normal examination does not exclude a potentially serious injury.

Aids to diagnosis

All investigations, including radiology, should be used judiciously in the trauma patient, and must not be allowed to delay resuscitation. Remember that laparotomy may be part of the resuscitation process during the primary survey. Radiographs of the chest and pelvis should be taken and reviewed, bearing in mind the physiological widening of the symphysis pubis in the third trimester.

The most commonly used investigations to detect intra-abdominal injury are a Focused Assessment Sonography in Trauma (FAST) scan and abdominal CT scan with intravenous contrast. (See Chapter 4 Appendix: Radiology in the pregnant woman.)

FAST scan

This is a brief ultrasound examination of the left and right upper quadrant, the pelvis and the pericardium by an experienced operator, and it has become the initial investigation of choice in the presence of abdominal trauma. Good results have been achieved in pregnant trauma patients. It allows precise information to be obtained concerning the nature and extent of intra-abdominal bleeding, as well as enabling visualisation of fetal heart pulsation. The examination is noninvasive and is easily repeatable, and it may be carried out at the bedside at the same time as other diagnostic and therapeutic procedures. It may, however, fail to identify small amounts of intraperitoneal fluid, or an evolving abruption, as well as injuries to the bowel or pancreas.

A negative examination should be viewed with caution after major trauma, and may be repeated after 30 minutes. FAST scans may be more difficult to interpret in the presence of obesity, subcutaneous air and abdominal scarring.

CT

CT scanning provides a highly sensitive and specific examination in suspected abdominal trauma, and is superior to FAST scanning in detecting retroperitoneal injuries. The principle disadvantage is the risk associated with transfer to a remote radiology department, away from facilities for resuscitation and operation. Radiation risks have been considerably reduced in recent years. CT scans should be undertaken only in haemodynamically stable patients, where there is, as yet, no clear indication for emergency laparotomy.

In the patient with a viable pregnancy, abdominal delivery followed by a trauma laparotomy is likely to be the safer option for baby and mother (using a midline skin incision).

Diagnostic peritoneal lavage

Diagnostic peritoneal lavage (DPL) is seldom, if ever, undertaken in the UK these days. However, it may still have a place where FAST scanning and CT scanning are not readily available. If DPL is used in pregnancy, it should be carried out via a supra-umbilical open approach. If frank blood is found on aspiration, or where there is red or pink discolouration of the lavage fluid, intraperitoneal bleeding is confirmed.

Assessment of fetal wellbeing and viability

Outcome data in pregnant women after abdominal trauma are similar to the nonpregnant, but there is a high likelihood of fetal loss. It cannot be overemphasised that the best way of achieving a good fetal outcome is by thorough evaluation and resuscitation of the mother, thereby ensuring good placental perfusion and oxygenation.

Vasopressor drugs should be avoided where possible in the resuscitation process, as these agents may further reduce uterine blood flow, thereby worsening fetal hypoxia.

Once maternal stability has been achieved, and life-threatening injuries have been dealt with, delivery may be expedited if fetal wellbeing is in question.

Secondary survey

A resuscitative laparotomy may be required as part of the primary survey, but if not then a complete examination of the abdomen must be carried out as part of the secondary survey, regardless of whether serious injury is suspected. Pregnant patients with even apparently minor abdominal injuries should be carefully observed, as placental abruption and fetal loss may occur. Regular obstetric evaluation will be required and consideration should be given to delivering the fetus, in order to facilitate appropriate management of the mother.

Solid and hollow visceral injury

Injuries to the liver and spleen are less common in late pregnancy, due to the protection afforded by the gravid uterus, but, nevertheless, they must be taken into consideration. When such injuries are suspected, there should be a low threshold for laparotomy and CS.

Experienced staff may occasionally elect to treat selected patients conservatively, if the cardiovascular system is stable. This is particularly the case where the fetus is not viable.

Injuries to the genitourinary tract, gastrointestinal tract, the pancreas and the diaphragm may be difficult to detect, either clinically, or with FAST and CT scans. Specialised radiological investigations may be required, including urethrography, cystography, intravenous pyelography and gastrointestinal contrast studies.

Pelvic trauma

See Chapter 19.

Indications for urgent caesarean delivery in the trauma patient

These include:

- suspected uterine rupture
- suspected trauma to abdominal viscera (to allow access)
- where pelvic fixation is required to control haemorrhage
- life-threatening placental abruption
- amniotic fluid embolus
- fetal distress (bearing in mind that maternal wellbeing is the priority).

Structured laparotomy

This is required if a patient has hypovolaemic shock that cannot be explained by blood loss that is overt, in the chest or due to fractures of the pelvis or long bones. 'Blood on the floor and 4 places more' – the fourth potential site of bleeding in this *aide memoire* is the abdomen. The laparotomy should be a structured 'trauma' laparotomy, through a midline incision, with an experienced general surgeon to hand.

Summary

- Abdominal trauma in pregnancy is most commonly due to road traffic accidents in the UK, but may be due to domestic violence.
- The structured approach should be followed, bearing in mind that resuscitative laparotomy may be required as part of the primary survey.
- It must always be remembered that pregnant women tend to compensate well for blood loss. A drop in blood pressure is a late and ominous sign.
- Few clinicians in the UK have experience of dealing with major trauma in pregnancy.
- The obstetrician will tend to be involved early, and must call on skilled input from other specialties to ensure optimum outcomes for mother and baby.

References and further reading

1 Centre for Maternal and Child Enquiries *Saving Mothers' Lives* 2006–2008. *Br J Obstet Gynaecol* 2011;118(Suppl. 1).

2 American College of Surgeons. *ATLS Course Manual,* 8th edn. American College of Surgeons 2008.

ALGORITHM 17.1 The unconscious patient

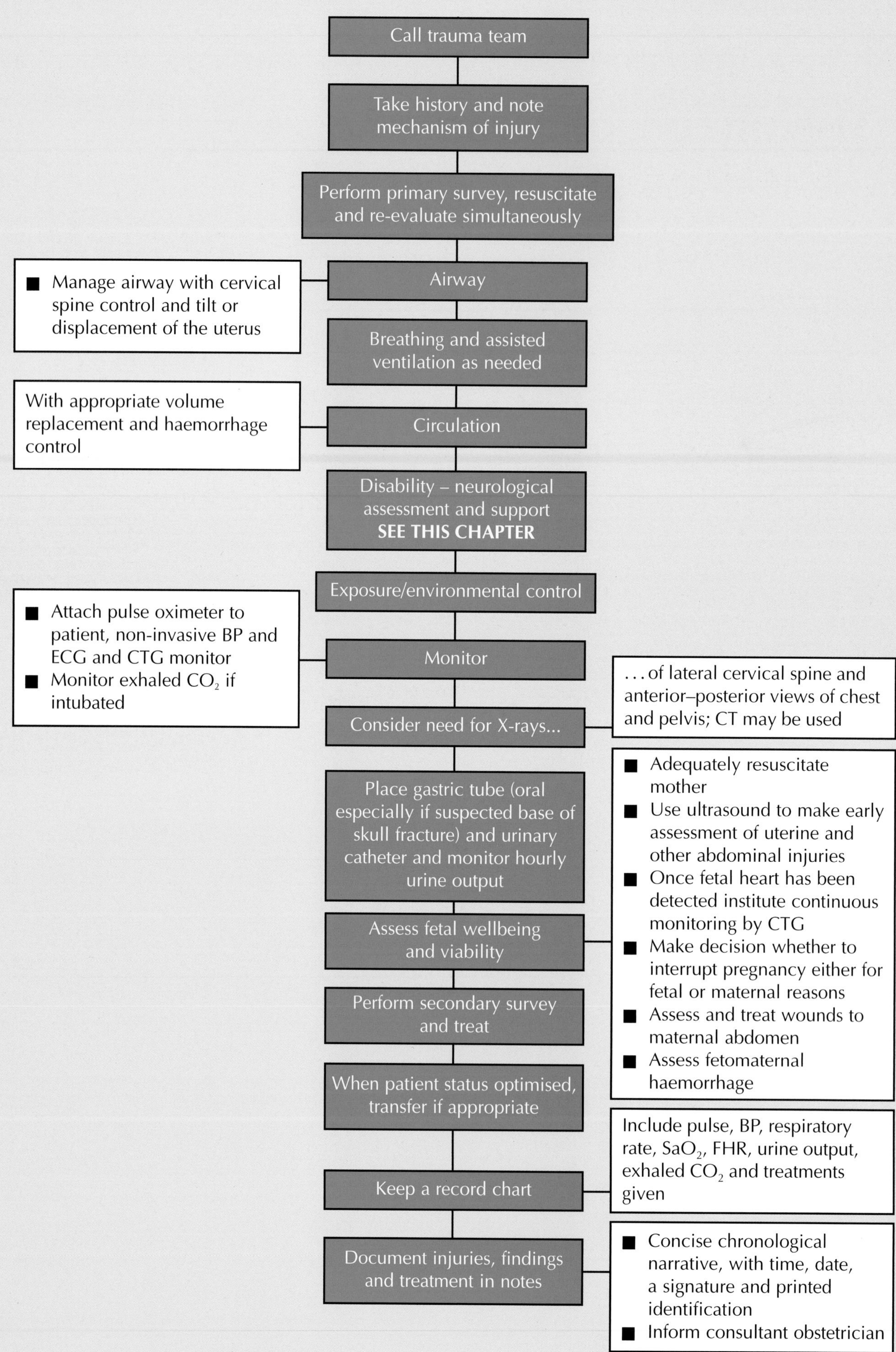

CHAPTER 17

The unconscious patient

Objectives

On successfully completing this topic, you will be able to:

- describe the principles of treatment of the unconscious patient
- understand the concept of secondary brain injury and how to prevent it
- identify types of lesion amenable to surgery (extradural and subdural haematoma).

Incidence

Each of the last three Confidential Enquiries have described approximately 40 indirect deaths in women due to disease related to the central nervous system. These include deaths from: subarachnoid haemorrhage; intracerebral haemorrhage; cerebral thrombosis and epilepsy.

The immediate management of the patient unconscious from any cause should be a basic skill of every obstetrician and midwife. The obstetric team should be aware of the potential causes of a decreased level of consciousness and treat the underlying cause, with appropriate specialist assistance where necessary.

Causes of decreased level of consciousness

A B Failure of airway or breathing: hypoxia/hypercarbia

C Failure of circulation: shock or cardiac arrest

D Failure of central nervous system:

- eclampsia or epilepsy
- intracranial haemorrhage, trauma, thrombosis, tumour or infection
- drugs, alcohol or poisoning.

Principles of treatment

Although these principles were developed in the context of trauma cases and traumatic brain injury, the same principles apply to any medical situation that threatens the supply of oxygen to the injured or uninjured brain.

Primary and secondary brain injury

Primary brain injury is the neurological damage produced by the initial event, such as a brain haemorrhage. Secondary (further) brain injury is the neurological damage caused by lack of oxygen delivery to the brain. This may be caused by:

- A B – failure of ventilation, caused by airway obstruction or inadequate breathing, resulting in poor oxygenation. In addition, both airway obstruction and inadequate breathing may lead to a rise in arterial carbon dioxide levels. This has direct consequences on intracranial pressure (ICP) (see below).
- C – failure of circulation due to shock including hypotension.
- D – intracerebral damage may cause an excessive rise in ICP, leading to reduced cerebral perfusion pressure (CPP).

Cerebral perfusion

Cerebral perfusion refers to the supply of oxygenated blood to the brain. The blood supply to the brain is more complex than other organs, because the brain is enclosed inside a rigid box. The volume of this box is fixed, so one component can only increase in volume at the expense of another, or at the expense of an increase in ICP. The main components inside the box are:

- brain substance or space-occupying lesions
- cerebrospinal fluid
- cerebral blood vessels and the blood contained within these vessels
- extracellular fluid.

CPP is the mean arterial pressure (MAP) of blood in the brain minus the resistance to flow from the mean ICP:

CPP = MAP–ICP

- any factors affecting MAP or ICP will affect CPP and potentially contribute to further neuronal damage
- adequate blood pressure (MAP) must be maintained to maintain CPP
- any rise in volume of intracranial contents may need to be controlled if the normal mechanism of cerebral autoregulation of ICP has failed:
  - brain tissue can increase in volume as a result of tumour growth or there may be increased volume caused by blood clot; both conditions may require surgery

- cerebrospinal fluid can increase in volume if there is an obstruction to free drainage of the fluid, e.g. by blood clots leading to hydrocephalus and can be drained by temporary or permanent surgical shunts
- cerebral blood volume can increase if the arterial carbon dioxide levels are allowed to rise resulting in cerebral vasodilatation; carbon dioxide levels can be reduced by maintaining a clear airway and controlling ventilation to restore a normal level of $PaCO_2$
- extracellular fluid levels can increase as a result of response to injury, such as around tumours or following cell damage caused by a major head injury; this is difficult to treat but careful fluid management avoiding excess intravenous fluids will be part of the care
- raised ICP may also be due to obstruction of venous drainage from the head from pressure on the neck veins, head down position or excess intrathoracic pressure.

Normal MAP = 70–90 mmHg
Normal ICP = 10 mmHg
If CPP is less than 50 mmHg, cerebral hypoxia may follow

There are limits beyond which the MAP itself will contribute to a rise in ICP: systolic BP >160 mmHg. This rise may be caused by known factors such as pre-eclampsia and may lead to a disastrous intracranial haemorrhage. Some women may have unknown risk factors, such as an intracranial aneurysm, and will be particularly vulnerable to surges in MAP.

Priorities in management to prevent secondary brain injury

1. Primary survey and resuscitation
2. Assessment of fetal wellbeing and viability
3. Secondary survey.

It follows that preventing a rise in ICP or a fall in cerebral perfusion is vital for the overall management and prevention of brain injury.

1. Primary survey and resuscitation

A Airway

Clear the airway. A patient with a reduced level of consciousness is more likely to have a compromised airway as the tongue falls back into the posterior pharynx. Further, she is at risk of aspiration as she has obtunded laryngeal reflexes.

B Breathing

Adequate ventilation ensures that the brain receives blood containing enough oxygen, thereby preventing further brain injury. Adequate ventilation prevents the accumulation of carbon dioxide. Ventilation may be impaired by a reduced level of consciousness. Raised intrathoracic pressure (as happens in tension pneumothorax) will compromise venous drainage from the head and raise ICP.

C Circulation

An adequate BP is required to maintain CPP. Use fluids and vasopressors appropriately. In a trauma situation, hypotension resulting from other injuries must be swiftly recognised and managed to prevent secondary brain injury. It is equally important to remember that excessive fluids are rarely needed in an isolated head injury and may contribute to worsening cerebral oedema.

In trauma, never assume that an isolated head injury is the cause of hypotension. Scalp lacerations may bleed profusely but not sufficiently to cause shock. Always presume that hypotension is due to lesions outside the brain, not brain injury, and look for a source of blood loss elsewhere or other cause of hypotension such as tension pneumothorax or spinal lesion.

Cushing's response (progressive hypertension, bradycardia and slowing of respiratory rate) is an acute response to rapidly rising ICP and is a premorbid sign. This needs urgent attention, which may include establishing controlled ventilation, use of mannitol and/or urgent surgery.

D Disability

A decrease in level of consciousness is the marker of brain injury. Generally, the more deeply unconscious a patient becomes and the longer this persists, the more serious is the injury.

AVPU: a rapid assessment of conscious level is made in the primary survey. Is the patient **A**lert, responding to **V**oice, only responding to **P**ain, or **U**nresponsive?

Pupillary responses may help to identify the degree of intracranial compromise and the possibility of a unilateral space-occupying lesion. Additional measures:

- avoid head-down position, head up if possible
- avoid ties around the neck, e.g. for an endotracheal tube
- ensure that any cervical collar in place is not compressing neck veins
- control fluid therapy carefully
- avoid rises in intrathoracic pressure
- rapid access to surgery may be required to evacuate blood clot if present
- high-dose steroids may reduce swelling associated with brain tumours
- control convulsions.

2. Assessment of fetal wellbeing and viability

When the mother is adequately resuscitated, the further wellbeing of the fetus must be considered. Timing of delivery should be considered in the patient about to undergo neurosurgical treatment, or a prolonged period of intensive care, or who is unlikely to recover consciousness. Delivery of the term fetus may be appropriate if a prolonged period of intensive care is anticipated. Physiological complications that develop in the long-term intensive care patient (coagulopathy, sepsis, etc.) may complicate a continuing pregnancy.

3. Secondary survey

The head and neurological examination assesses:

- pupillary function
- lateralising signs, e.g. limb weakness
- level of consciousness by the Glasgow Coma Scale (GCS)
- evidence of a base of skull fracture
- evidence of a depressed fracture.

The mini-neurological examination serves to determine the severity of the brain injury and the likelihood of a surgically treatable lesion. When applied repeatedly, it can be used to determine objectively any neurological deterioration. It is supplemented by CT scanning.

Pupillary function

Evaluate the pupils for their equality and response to bright light. A difference in diameter of the pupils of more than 1mm is abnormal but a local injury to the eye may be responsible for this abnormality. Normal reaction to a bright light is brisk constriction of the pupil; a more sluggish response may indicate brain injury. Pressure on the third cranial nerve (oculomotor) will result in a dilated pupil on the same side ('ipsilateral') as the injury.

Lateralising signs, such as limb weakness

Observe spontaneous limb movements, tone and reflexes for equality. If movement is negligible then assess the response to a painful stimulus. Any delay in onset of movement or lateralisation of movement following a painful stimulus is significant. Obvious limb weakness localised to one side suggests an intracranial injury causing brain compression on the opposite side. Damage to the motor or sensory cortex (or tracts leading from them) will result in a motor or sensory deficit on the opposite side to the injury.

Level of consciousness

The GCS provides a quantitative assessment of the level of consciousness. It is the sum of scores awarded (Table 17.1) for three types of response.

Table 17.1 GCS scoring

Response	Score
Eye opening response	
Spontaneous (open with normal blinking)	4
Eye opening to speech	3
Eye opening only to painful stimulus	2
No eye opening despite painful stimulus	1
Verbal response	
Orientated, spontaneous speech	5
Confused conversation but answers questions	4
Inappropriate words i.e. recognisable words without sense	3
Incomprehensible sounds	2
No verbal response	1
Motor response	
Obeys commands	6
Localises purposive response to painful stimulus	5
Withdraws from painful stimulus	4
Abnormal flexion to painful stimulus (decorticate response)	3
Abnormal extension to painful stimulus (decerebrate response)	2
No response to painful stimulus	1

Eye opening (E)

The scoring of eye opening is not possible if the eyes are so swollen as to be permanently shut. This fact must be documented.

Verbal response (V)

The scoring of verbal response is not possible if the patient cannot speak because of endo - tracheal intubation. This fact must be documented.

Motor response (M)

The best response obtained for either of the upper extremities is recorded even though worse responses may be present in other extremities.

Subsequent reassessment of the GCS can be used to detect any deterioration. For example, if the GCS has decreased by two points or more, deterioration has occurred. A decrease of three points or more is a bad prognostic indicator and demands immediate treatment.

Box 17.1 Severity of head injuries is classified as follows:

Score 8 or less = severe

Score 9 to 12 = moderate

Score 13 to 15 = minor

Changes in vital signs

Changes in the GCS may be accompanied by changes in vital signs indicating deterioration. Rising ICP due to brain swelling or expanding haematomas inside the head can cause pressure on the respiratory and cardiovascular centres in the brain stem. This produces respiratory or cardiovascular abnormalities such as changes in heart rate (slows down) and blood pressure (rises), change in breathing pattern and rate (slows down).

Types of head injury

Severity of head injury is classified based on the GCS (Box 17.1). Primary brain injury may be diffuse or focal.

Diffuse primary brain injury

Blunt injury to the brain may cause diffuse brain injury, particularly when rapid head motion (acceleration or deceleration) leads to widespread damage within the brain substance. Such injuries form a spectrum, extending from mild concussion to severe injury known as diffuse axonal injury.

Concussion is a brain injury accompanied by a brief loss of consciousness and, in its mildest form, may cause only temporary confusion or amnesia. With mild forms of concussion, most patients will be only slightly confused and may be able to describe how the injury occurred. They are likely to complain of mild headache, dizziness or nausea. The mini-neurological examination will not show lateralising signs. With more severe concussion there is a longer period of unconsciousness, longer amnesia (for time both before and after the injury) and there may be focal signs. The duration of amnesia needs to be recorded.

Diffuse axonal injury is so severe as to cause a characteristically long coma in 44% of cases. The overall mortality rate is over 30%, rising to 50% in its most severe form. The treatment of such injury involves prolonged, controlled ventilation in an intensive care unit.

Focal primary brain injury

Contusions are caused by blunt injury producing acceleration and deceleration forces on the brain tissue, resulting in tearing of the small blood vessels inside the brain. Contusions can occur immediately beneath the area of impact, when they are known as coup injuries, or at a point distant from the area of impact in the direction of the applied force, when they are known as contrecoup injuries. If the contusion occurs near the sensory or motor areas of the brain, these patients will present with a neurological deficit. Precise diagnosis requires appropriate imaging (CT scanning).

Haematomata within the skull may arise either from meningeal vessels or from vessels within the brain substance. They are defined anatomically; such a classification is useful as it has implications in terms of remedial surgery, urgency and prognosis.

Intracranial, extracerebral bleeding

Extradural haemorrhage

Extradural haemorrhage is caused by a tear in a dural artery, most commonly the middle meningeal artery. This can be torn by a linear fracture crossing the temporal or parietal bone and injuring the artery lying in a groove on the deep aspect of the bone.

Isolated extradural haemorrhage is unusual, accounting for only 0.5% of all head injuries and less than 1.0% of injuries causing coma. The importance of early recognition of this injury lies in the fact that, when treated appropriately, the prognosis is good because of the lack of underlying serious injury to brain tissue. If unrecognised, the rapidly expanding haematoma causes the ICP to rise, reducing cerebral perfusion and leading to cerebral hypoxia, coma and death.

The typical symptoms and signs of extradural haemorrhage are:

- loss of consciousness followed by a lucid interval (which may not be a complete return to full consciousness)
- secondary depression of consciousness
- dilated pupil on the side of injury
- weakness of the arm and leg on the contralateral side to the injury.

Subdural haemorrhage

Subdural haemorrhage is more common than extradural haemorrhage and is found in 30% of all severe head injuries. The mortality rate is up to 60% because, in addition to the compression caused by the subdural blood clot, there is often major injury to the underlying brain tissue. The haematoma can arise from tears in the bridging veins between the cortex and the dura or from laceration of the brain substance and the cortical arteries.

The typical symptoms and signs of subdural haemorrhage are:

- varying levels of consciousness, depending on the underlying brain damage and rate of haematoma formation

- dilated pupil on the side of the injury
- weakness of the arm and leg on the contralateral side to the injury.

Initial treatment:

- prevent secondary brain injury
- urgent evacuation of the haematoma where surgically amenable.

Delay in the treatment of extradural haemorrhage beyond 2 hours, and delay in the treatment of subdural haemorrhage beyond 4 hours, worsens the prognosis.

Subarachnoid haemorrhage

Where haemorrhaging has occurred into the subarachnoid space, the irritant effect of the bloody cerebrospinal fluid causes headache, photophobia and neck stiffness. On its own, this is not serious, but prognosis is poor if it is associated with a more severe head injury.

Intracerebral laceration

Through-and-through injuries, side-to-side injuries and injuries in the lower region of the brain stem all have a poor outcome.

All foreign bodies found protruding from the skull must be left in place. These should only be removed at a neurosurgical unit. Skull radiographs will show the angle and depth of penetration. Care must be taken during transfer to ensure that there is no further penetration.

Open brain injury in a conscious patient carries a good prognosis if surgery is not delayed. Scalp haemorrhage should be stopped, entrance and exit wounds covered with sterile dressings, and the patient transferred to a neurosurgical unit.

Other injuries

Scalp wounds

The scalp is arranged in layers. It is highly vascular and a laceration will often result in profuse haemorrhage. The bleeding point should be located and the haemorrhage arrested. This may include the use of haemostatic surgical clips and ligatures, particularly where the laceration is deep. Direct pressure may not be sufficient. The wound should be inspected carefully for signs of skull fracture and irrigated to remove debris and dirt.

Gentle palpation of the scalp wound, wearing a sterile glove, may enable the clinician to diagnose the presence of a skull fracture. If an open or depressed fracture is detected, close the wound with sutures, apply a dressing, consider antibiotics and transfer the patient to a neurosurgical unit. Do not remove any bone fragments at this stage.

Skull fractures

Although skull fractures are common, many major brain injuries will occur without the skull being fractured, and many skull fractures are not associated with severe brain injury. The current primary investigation of choice for the detection of acute, clinically important brain injuries is CT imaging of the head rather than a plain skull radiograph.

Linear skull fractures

These are particularly important when the fracture crosses the line of intracranial vessels, indicating an increased risk of intracranial haemorrhage.

Depressed skull fractures

All depressed skull fractures should be referred for neurosurgical assessment. They may be associated with underlying brain injury and may require operative elevation to reduce the risk of infection in more serious cases.

Open skull fractures

By definition, there is direct communication between the outside of the head and brain tissue, because the dura covering the surface of the brain is torn. This can be diagnosed if brain tissue is visible on examination of the scalp wound or if cerebrospinal fluid is seen to be leaking from the wound. These fractures all require operative intervention and the risk of infection is high. Discuss the use of prophylactic antibiotics with the neurosurgical team.

Basal skull fractures

The base of the skull does not run horizontally backwards but diagonally. Basal skull fractures will produce signs along this diagonal line. They can be diagnosed clinically in the presence of cerebrospinal fluid leaking from the ear (otorrhoea) or the nose (rhinorrhoea). When cerebrospinal fluid is mixed with blood it may be difficult to detect. Bruising in the mastoid region (Battle's sign) also indicates basal skull fracture, but the bruising usually takes 12–36 hours to develop. Blood seen behind the tympanic membrane (haemotympanum) may also indicate a basal skull fracture. Fractures through the cribriform plate are frequently associated with bilateral periorbital haematomas. Subconjunctival haematoma may occur from direct orbital roof fracture, in which case there is no posterior limit to the haematoma.

All these signs may take several hours to develop and may not be present in a patient seen immediately after injury. Basal skull fractures are difficult to diagnose from plain radiographs but are detectable on a CT scan of the head. Discuss with the neurosurgical team.

Summary

- Remember the A B C D E routine.
- Prevent secondary injury by preventing hypoxia, hypercarbia and hypovolaemia.
- Establish a working diagnosis.
- Constantly repeat the mini-neurological examination.
- Consider the best management of the fetus.

Further reading

1 NICE. CG56 Head Injury Guideline: National Institute for Health and Clinical Excellence 2007 (http://guidance.nice.org.uk/CG56/Guidance).

ALGORITHM 18.1 Spine and spinal cord injuries

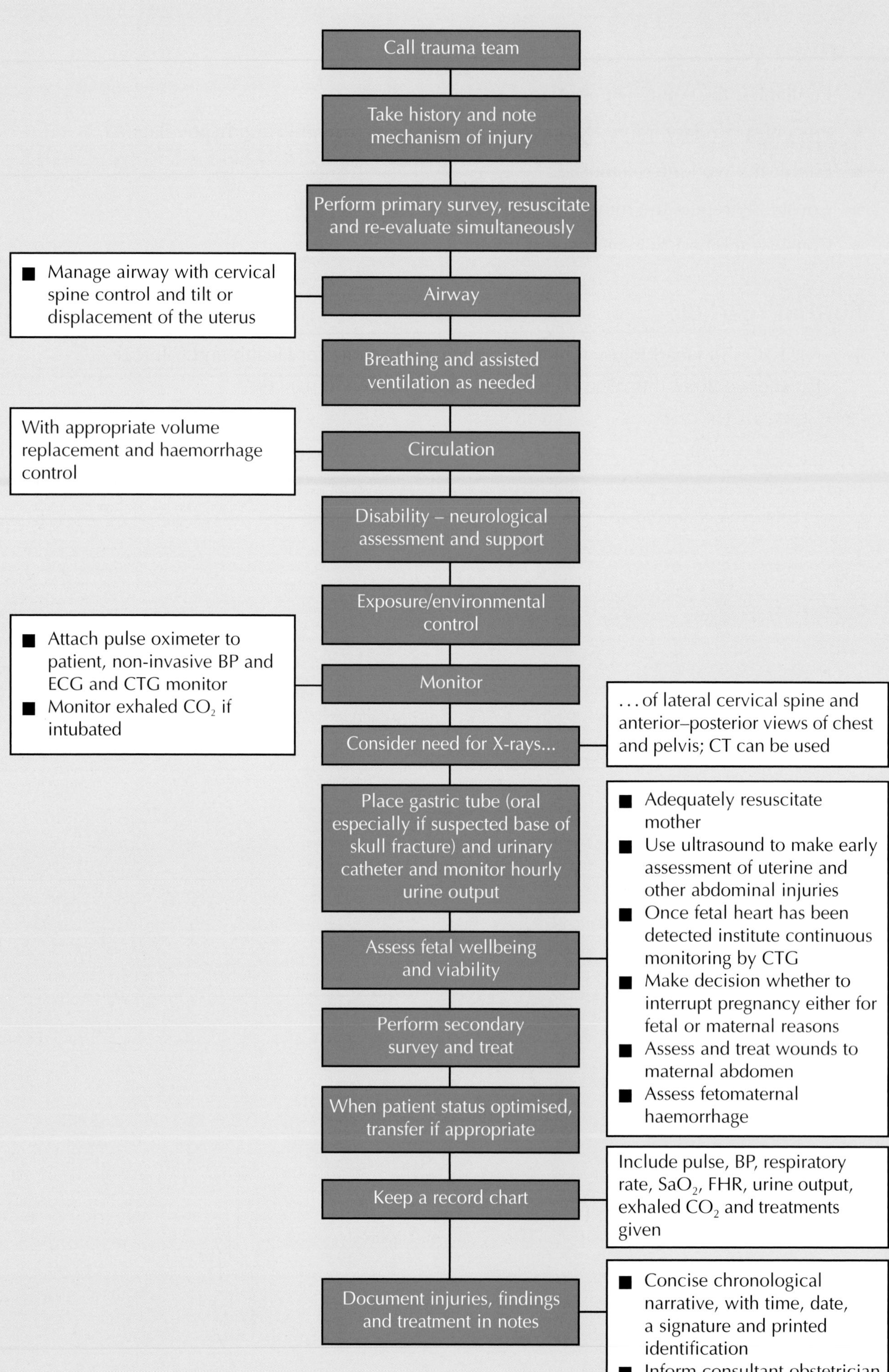

CHAPTER 18

Spine and spinal cord injuries

Objectives

On successfully completing this topic, you will be able to:

- recognise circumstances in which spinal trauma is likely to occur
- understand the importance and techniques of spinal immobilisation
- identify and evaluate spinal trauma.

Introduction

In the context of this chapter, spinal injuries refer to injuries to the bony spinal column, the spinal cord or both. There can be an injury to the bony spine without injury to the spinal cord, but there is significant risk of cord injury in these circumstances.

Failure to immobilise a patient with a spinal injury can cause or exacerbate neurological damage. Failure to immobilise a patient with an injury to the bony spine (without cord injury at that stage) can cause avoidable injury to the spinal cord. Evaluation of the spine and exclusion of spinal injuries can be safely deferred, as long as the patient's spine is protected.

A spinal injury should always be suspected:

- in falls from a height (however it is possible to injure the spine in a fall from a standing position, e.g. fall due to a convulsion)
- in vehicle collisions, even at low speed
- when pedestrians have been hit by a vehicle
- where persons have been thrown
- in sports field injuries, e.g. rugby
- in a person with multiple injuries
- in a person with injury above the clavicle (including the unconscious patient – 15% of unconscious patients have some form of neck injury)
- in the conscious patient complaining of neck pain and sensory and/or motor symptoms
- in drowning victims.

Persons who are awake, sober, neurologically normal and have no neck pain are extremely unlikely to have a cervical spine fracture. However, neurosurgical or orthopaedic opinion should always be sought if an injury is suspected or detected.

The cervical spine is more vulnerable to injury than the thoracic or lumbar spine.

Approximately 10% of patients with a cervical spine fracture have a second associated noncontiguous fracture of the vertebral column. Hence, if a cervical spine fracture is diagnosed, other spinal fractures should be suspected.

Immobilisation techniques

If injury to the spine is suspected, the whole spine should be immobilised until examination, radiography and supplementary radiological investigations have excluded spinal injury. Injury can only be excluded by an orthopaedic, neurosurgical or a suitably skilled Emergency Medicine doctor. Immobilisation should be carried out by maintaining the spine in the neutral position.

Cervical spine

Immobilisation of the cervical spine is achieved by:

- manual inline immobilisation of the head or
- semi-rigid cervical collar plus blocks on a backboard (which may be a headboard or full spine board and straps, see Figure 18.1); collars are correctly sized by following the manufacturer's instructions.

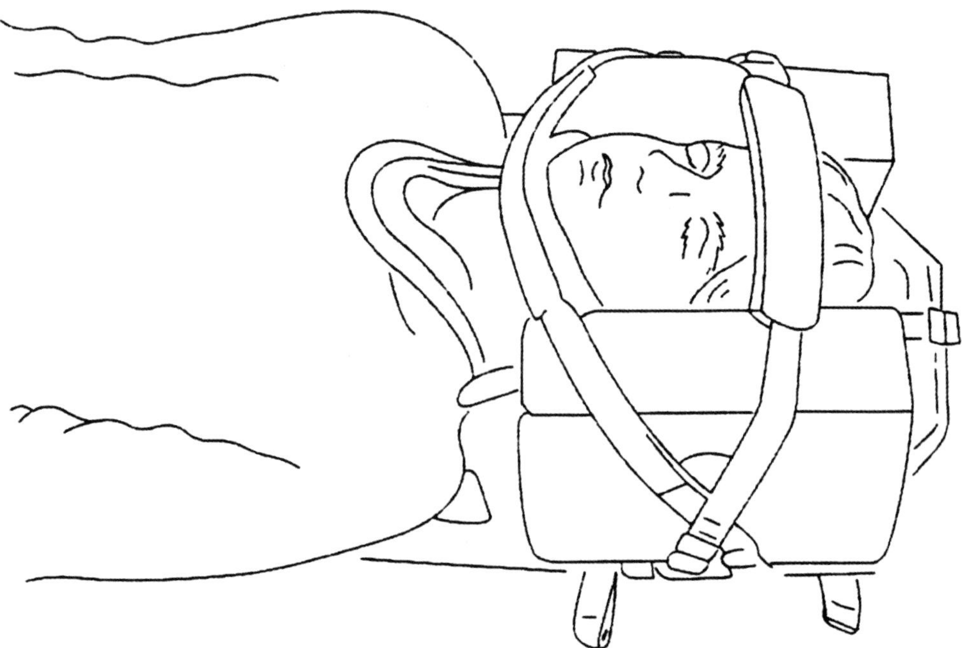

Figure 18.1 Immobilisation of the cervical spine using collar, blocks, tape and headboard

Thoracic and lumbar spine

The thoracic and lumbar spine should be immobilised by a long spine board. Inadequate, or even prolonged, immobilisation with a spine board has its own complications, with the possibility of worsening any injury and the risk of pressure sores if prolonged immobilisation is undertaken. Hence, the long backboard is usually a transportation device. Early assessment by neurosurgeon or orthopaedic surgeon is undertaken to allow removal from the device. If this is not feasible the injured patient should be log-rolled every 2 hours while maintaining spinal integrity.

To avoid supine hypotension in the heavily pregnant patient, the right hip should be elevated to 10 to 15 cm with a wedge (Figure 18.2) and the uterus displaced manually. If a pelvic fracture is suspected, manual displacement of the uterus is recommended, rather than elevation of the hip. Alternatively, the whole patient can be tilted to the left, if on a long spine board, by putting a wedge under the board.

Evaluation of a patient with a suspected spinal injury

Spinal injuries may cause problems that are identified in the primary survey, affecting airway, breathing or circulation, or the injury may itself be identified during the secondary survey.

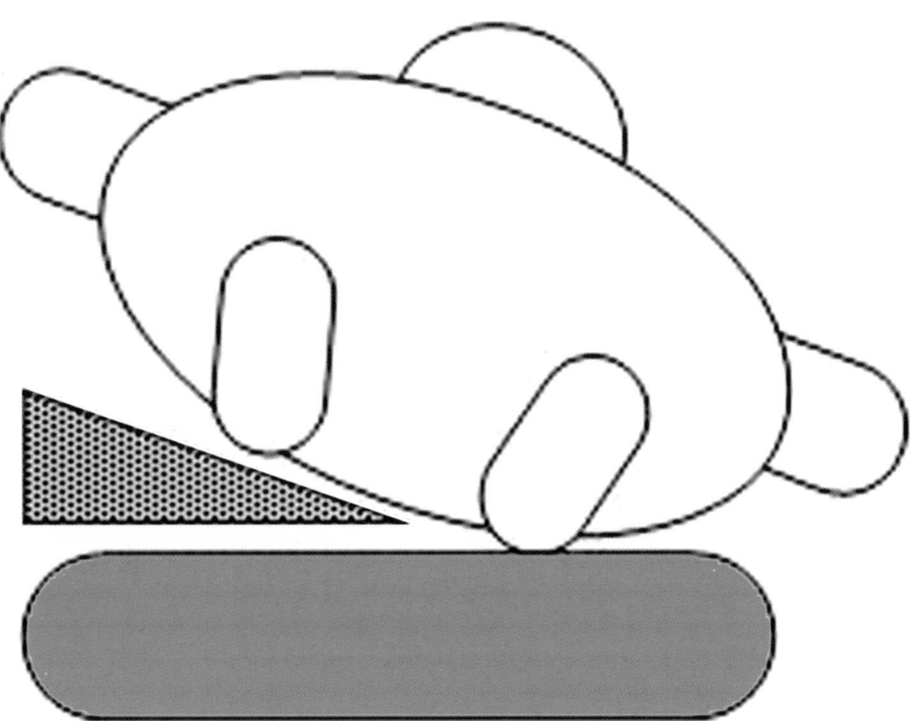

Figure 18.2 Cardiff wedge

Spinal assessment

A log-roll must be performed and is illustrated in Figure 18.3. This is a coordinated, skilled manoeuvre by trained personnel. At least four persons are required to perform this: one to maintain manual inline mobilisation of the patient's head and neck, one for the torso, with two for the hips and legs, with the leader at the head directing the procedure; in order to turn the patient from the supine to the lateral position without causing damage to the spinal cord.

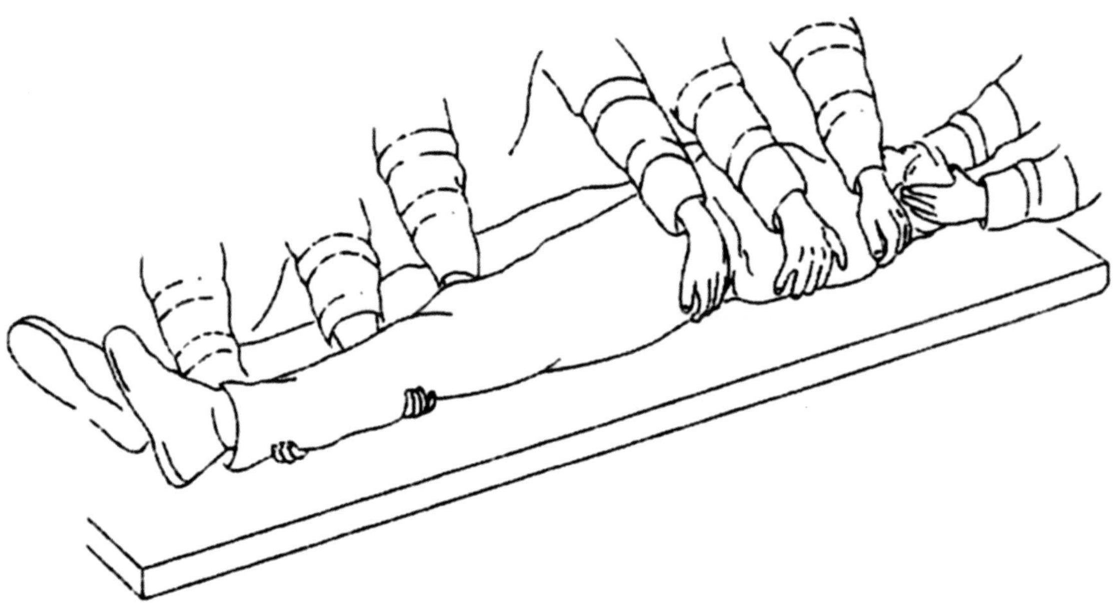

Figure 18.3 Four-person log-roll

Look for bruising, deformity and localised swelling of the vertebral column. Palpate for localised tenderness or gaps between spinous processes. At this point it may be appropriate to carry out a per rectum examination if clinically indicated.

Neurological assessment

Of the many tracts in the spinal cord, the three that can be assessed clinically are:

- corticospinal tract: controls muscle power on the same side of the body and is tested by voluntary movement and involuntary response to painful stimuli
- spinothalamic tract: transmits pain and temperature sensation from the opposite side of the body and is tested generally by pinprick
- posterior columns: carry position sense from the same side.

Each can be injured on one or both sides.

If there is no demonstrable sensory or motor function below a certain level bilaterally, this is referred to as a complete spinal injury. If there is remaining motor or sensory function with some loss this is an incomplete injury (better prognosis). Sparing of sensation in the perianal region may be the only sign of residual function. Sacral sparing is demonstrated by the presence of sensation perianally and/or voluntary contraction of the anal sphincter.

An injury does not qualify as incomplete on the basis of preserved sacral reflexes, e.g. bulbocavernous or anal wink.

The neurological level is the most caudal segment with normal sensory and motor function on both sides. For completeness, the main dermatomes are given in Figure 18.4.

Each nerve root innervates more than one muscle and most muscles have innervation from more than one nerve root. Certain movements, however, are identified as representing a single nerve root.

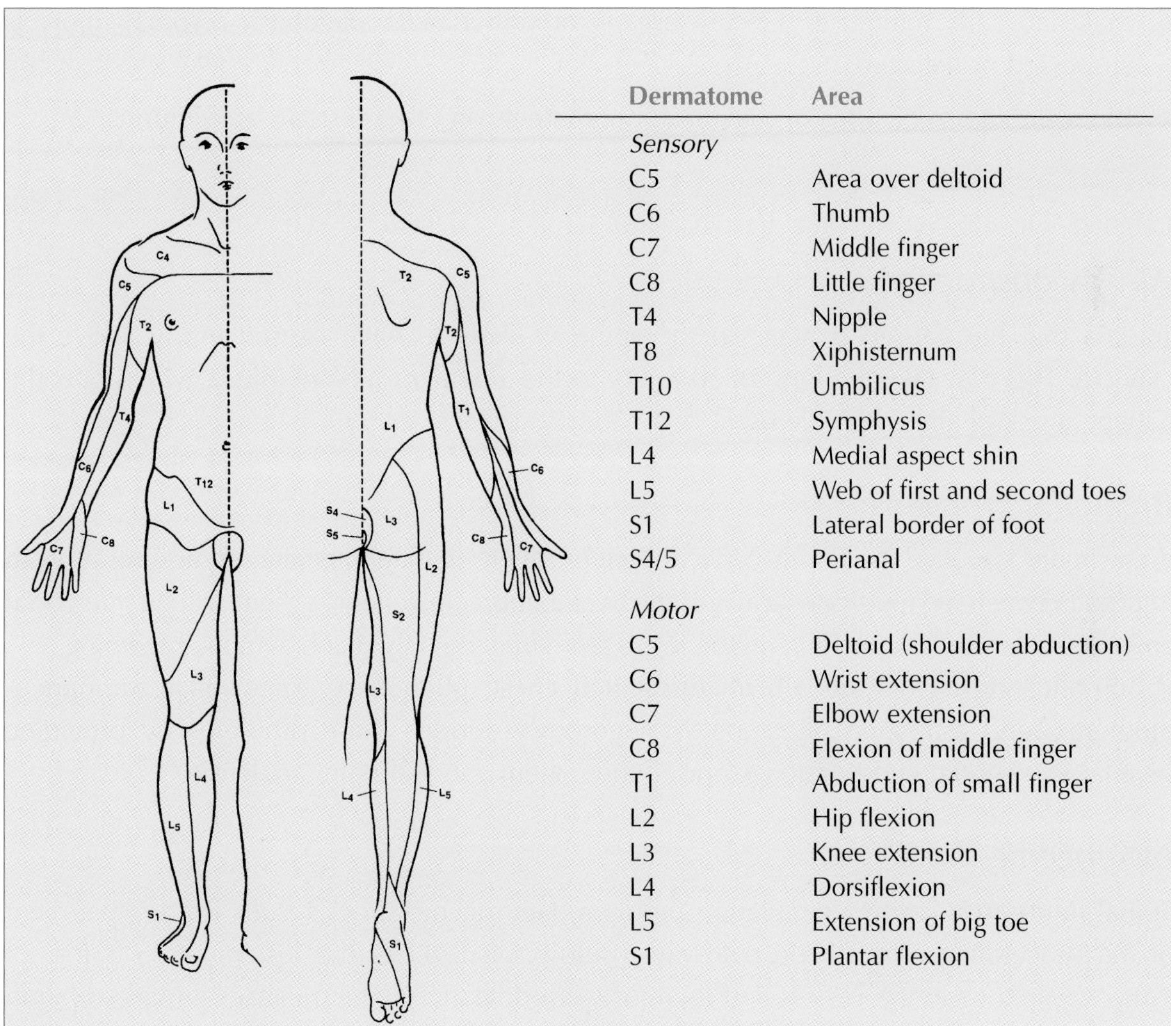

Dermatome	Area
Sensory	
C5	Area over deltoid
C6	Thumb
C7	Middle finger
C8	Little finger
T4	Nipple
T8	Xiphisternum
T10	Umbilicus
T12	Symphysis
L4	Medial aspect shin
L5	Web of first and second toes
S1	Lateral border of foot
S4/5	Perianal
Motor	
C5	Deltoid (shoulder abduction)
C6	Wrist extension
C7	Elbow extension
C8	Flexion of middle finger
T1	Abduction of small finger
L2	Hip flexion
L3	Knee extension
L4	Dorsiflexion
L5	Extension of big toe
S1	Plantar flexion

Figure 18.4 Dermatomes used for sensory and motor testing

A broad distinction can be made between lesions above and lesions below T1 (as determined by sensory and motor testing). Lesions above T1 result in quadriplegia and lesions below T1 result in paraplegia. There is a discrepancy between neurological injury level and level of bony injury because spinal nerves travel up or down the canal from the point of entry through bone to join the spinal cord. The level quoted is the neurological level.

Principles of treatment

The principles of treatment are primary survey and resuscitation, assessment of fetal well-being and viability, then secondary survey and protection from further injury.

A spinal injury may present in either the primary survey or the secondary survey:

- deal with life-threatening conditions according to the A B C but avoid any movement of the spinal column
- establish adequate immobilisation and maintain it until you are certain there is no spinal injury
- make an early referral to a neurosurgeon or orthopaedic surgeon if a spinal injury is suspected or detected
- be aware of associations of spinal injury or effects on other systems and injuries.

Effects or associations identified in the primary survey

Airway obstruction

Trauma that has caused damage to the spine is likely to have caused injury above the clavicle. This may take the form of an injury to the airway or a head injury, which puts the patient at risk of airway problems.

Breathing problems

If the injury is above the fourth cervical vertebra there is diaphragmatic compromise. With injuries between the fourth cervical and the twelfth thoracic vertebrae there will be intercostal embarrassment and, depending on the level, there may be only diaphragmatic breathing.

Complicating factors are: rib fractures; flail chest; pulmonary contusion; haemopneumothorax; and aspiration pneumonitis. Vigorously address these problems by providing ventilatory support, chest drainage and, if the patient can feel pain, analgesia.

Neurogenic shock

Spinal injury may cause a circulation problem. Neurogenic shock results from impairment of the descending sympathetic pathways. Below the level of the lesion, there is loss of sympathetic tone to the vessels and therefore vasodilatation, which causes a marked fall in blood pressure. In this situation, blood pressure is not restored by fluid alone but by the judicious use of vasopressors. Central venous pressure monitoring may be indicated, particularly in the heavily pregnant woman.

Injury above the T4 level causes loss of sympathetic innervation to the heart and therefore bradycardia. With an injury above the T4 level, the combination of vasodilatation below the level of the lesion and the bradycardia caused by impaired sympathetic outflow to the cardiac accelerators can cause profound hypotension.

Atropine may be needed to counteract bradycardia. It may be ineffective and an isoprenaline infusion may be required. Advice from intensivists should be taken.

Abdominal injuries

Abdominal injuries may only present as a C problem. Inability to feel pain due to spinal injury may mask serious intra-abdominal injury that will present as shock. The only symptom pointing to an intra-abdominal problem may be referred shoulder-tip pain. Ileus is usual in a paralysed patient, so a nasogastric tube should be passed.

Locomotor

Musculoskeletal injuries may present with life-threatening hypovolaemia but can be less readily localised in a patient with spinal cord injury, because of the inability to feel pain.

Skin

In a high cord lesion, temperature control function is lost and the patient may become hypothermic or hyperthermic. Spinally injured patients are at severe risk of ischaemic skin loss if not nursed to avoid pressure sores.

Secondary survey

Any injury may be masked by the absence of pain. A vigilant approach to detection is needed. Correct management of upper limb injuries may have a profound effect on the eventual mobility of a quadriplegic.

Bladder

Patients with spinal cord injury and urinary retention need continuous catheter drainage. Urinary output is a good monitor of response to resuscitation.

Recovery and rehabilitation

In a pregnant woman who has sustained severe spinal trauma, the pregnancy may still remain unaffected as long as the vital parameters have been stable. Initial care of the woman with suspected spinal injury determines the outcome of the pregnancy.

Summary

- Appropriate immobilisation of the injured patient during primary resuscitation is a vital part of care until further investigation can be carried out.
- Spinal injuries may be a cause of ABC problems, which should be treated first.
- Hypotension due to spinal shock may require vasopressors rather than excess fluids.

APPENDIX 18A

Practical procedures

Reproduced with permission from the Advanced Life Support Group.

Procedures:

- cervical spine immobilisation
- application of a cervical collar
- application of head blocks and straps
- log-rolling.

Cervical spine immobilisation

All patients with serious trauma (e.g. fall, road traffic accident, assault) must be treated as though they have a cervical spine injury. It is only when adequate investigations have been performed and a neurosurgical or orthopaedic consultation obtained, if necessary, that the decision to remove cervical spine protection should be taken. Manual inline cervical stabilisation should be continued until a hard collar has been applied, and sandbags and tape or head blocks and straps are in position, as described in Figure 18A.1.

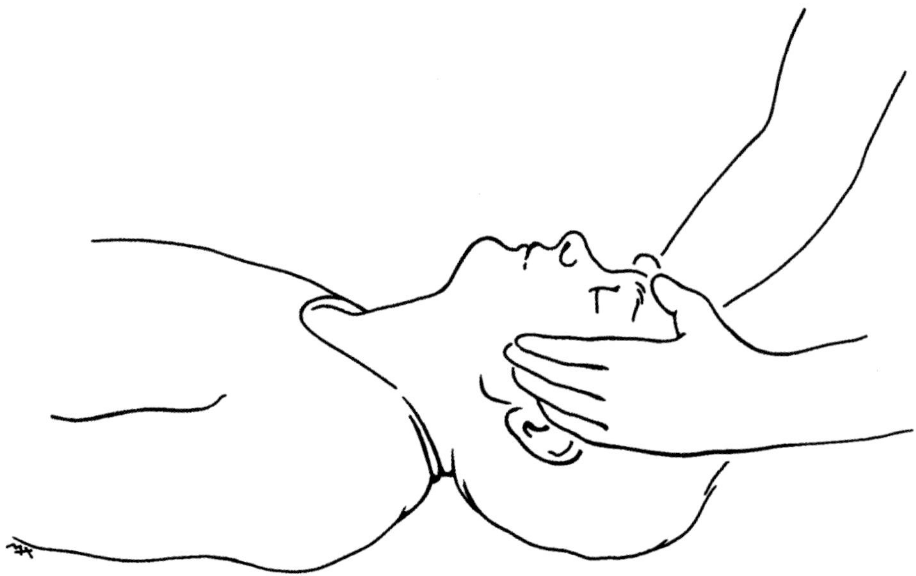

Figure 18A.1 Manual inline cervical spine stabilisation

Once the collar is in place, the neck is largely obscured. Before placing the collar, look for the following signs quickly and without moving the neck:

- distended veins
- tracheal deviation
- wounds
- laryngeal crepitus
- subcutaneous emphysema
- earrings or necklaces (if these are left on they may obscure c-spine radiographs).

Application of a cervical collar

The key to successful, effective, collar application lies in selecting the correct size.

Minimum equipment:

- measuring device
- range of hard collars or a multisized collar.

Method

1 Assess peripheral sensation.
2 Ensure that manual inline cervical stabilisation is maintained throughout by a second person.
3 Using the manufacturer's method, select a correctly sized collar.
4 Assemble the collar as necessary.
5 Taking care not to cause movement, pass the flat part of the collar behind the neck.
6 Fold the shaped part of the collar round and place it under the chin.
7 Fold the flat part of the collar with its integral joining device (usually Velcro® tape) around until it meets the shaped part.
8 Reassess the correct fit of the collar.
9 If the fit is wrong, slip the flat part of the collar out from behind the neck, taking care not to cause movement. Select the correct size and recommence the procedure.
10 If the fit is correct secure the joining device.
11 Ensure that manual inline cervical stabilisation is maintained until head blocks and straps, or sandbags and tape, are in position.

Application of head blocks and straps

Equipment:

- two head blocks
- attachment system.

Method

1. Ensure that manual inline cervical stabilisation is maintained by a second person throughout.
2. Place a head block either side of the head (Figure 18.1).
3. Apply the forehead strap and attach it securely.
4. Apply lower strap across the chin piece of the hard collar and attach it securely.
5. Apply tape across the chin piece of the hard collar and securely attach it to the long spinal board.
6. Attach body straps to the board.
7. Reassess peripheral sensations.

Exception

A patient who is fitting or combative should not be restrained. In such cases, a hard collar should be applied and no attempt made to immobilise the head with head blocks or sandbags and tape.

Log-rolling

In order to minimise the chances of exacerbating unrecognised spinal-cord injury, nonessential movements of the spine must be avoided until adequate examination and investigations have excluded it. If manoeuvres that might cause spinal movement are essential (for example, during examination of the back in the course of the secondary survey), then log-rolling should be performed (Figure 18.3). The aim of log-rolling is to maintain the alignment of the spine during turning of the patient. The basic requirements are an adequate number of carers and good team command.

Method

1. Gather together enough staff to roll the patient. Four people will be required.
2. Place the staff as shown in Table 18A.1.
3. Ensure each member of staff knows what they are going to do as shown in Table 18A.2.
4. Carry out essential manoeuvres as safely as possible.

Table 18A.1 Position of staff in log-rolling an adult

Staff member number	Position
1	Head
2	Chest and flank
3	Pelvis and thigh
4	Lower legs

Table 18A.2 Tasks for individual members of staff

Staff member position and number		Task
1	Head	Hold either side of the head (as for manual inline cervical stabilisation) and maintain the orientation of the head with the body in all planes during turning. Communicate with the patient and explain the procedure to the patient. Control the log-roll by telling other staff when to roll and when to lay the patient back onto the trolley.
2	Chest	Reach over the patient and carefully place one hand over the shoulder and one hand over the flank. When told to roll the patient, support the weight of the chest and torso and maintain stability. Watch the movement of the head at all times and roll the chest and torso at the same rate.
3	Pelvis	Place one hand over the pelvis on the iliac crest and the other under the thigh of the far leg. When told to roll the patient, watch the movement of the head and chest at all times and roll the pelvis at the same rate without adducting the legs.
4	Legs	Support the weight of the far leg by placing both hands under the far leg. When told to roll the patient, watch the movement of the chest and pelvis and roll the leg at the same rate without adducting the legs.

It is vital that staff members 2, 3 and 4 follow the instructions of staff member 1, rolling the patient over or back only on the instruction of staff member 1 who is controlling the head. In addition, they must not remove their hands from the patient until told to do so.

ALGORITHM 19.1 Musculoskeletal trauma

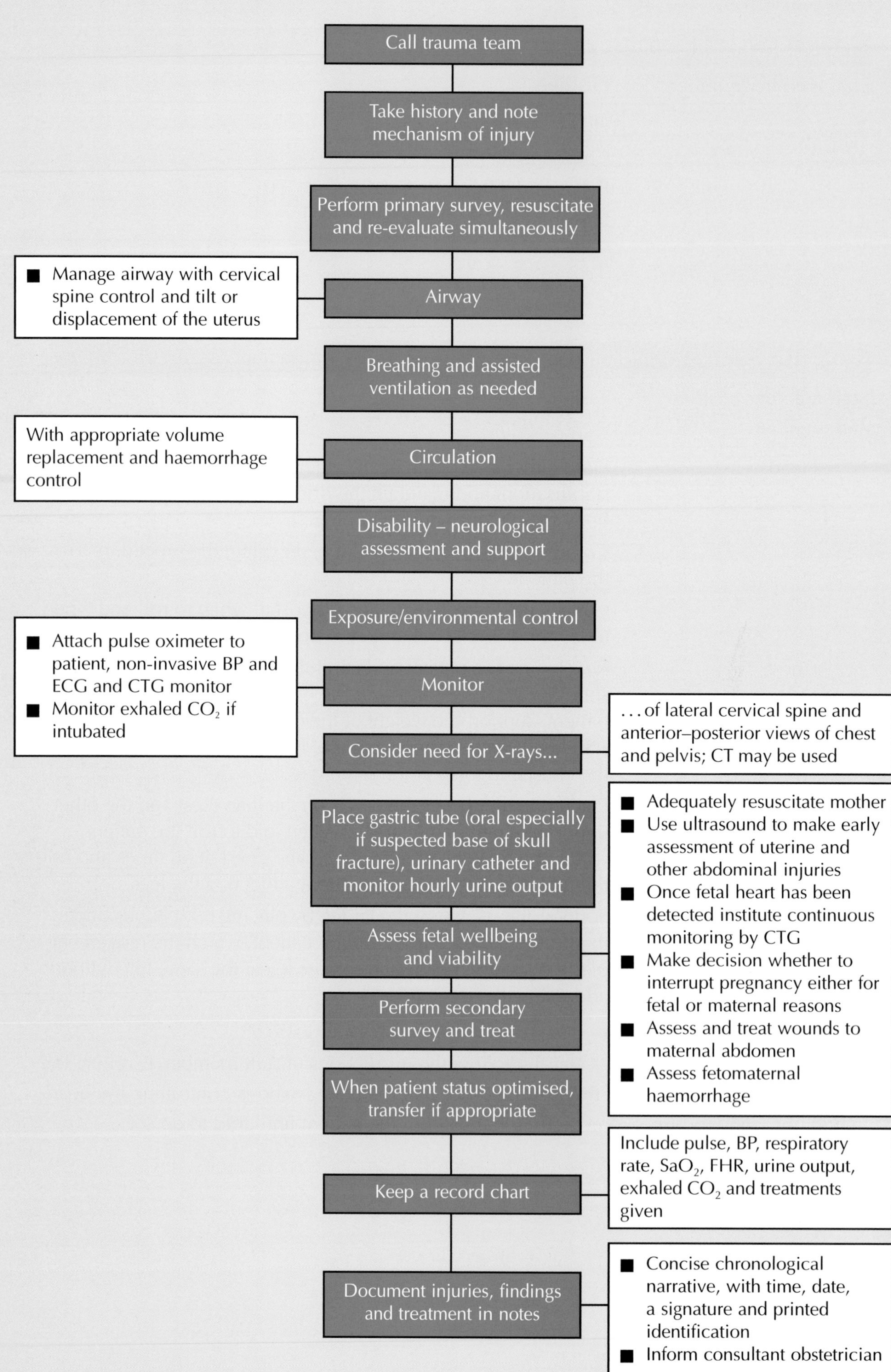

CHAPTER 19

Musculoskeletal trauma

Objectives

On successfully completing this topic, you will be able to:

- understand the principles of management of a patient with musculoskeletal trauma
- be aware of how to identify and treat life-threatening injuries
- be aware of how to identify and treat limb-threatening injuries.

Introduction

Primary survey and resuscitation, secondary survey and definitive care

Within the primary survey, life-threatening injuries are identified and treated. Where musculoskeletal injuries threaten life, it is usually as a circulation problem. There is a need to recognise hypovolaemia, a rapid inspection to identify sites of major bleeding and then measures to stop the bleeding. Beyond the initial resuscitation phase, renal failure can result from traumatic rhabdomyolysis caused by crush injuries; fat embolism is an uncommon, but lethal, complication of long-bone fractures.

It is important to realise that the patient may have multiple injuries. Knowledge of the mechanism of the injury is important in this: a fall from a height can result in cervical spine and other vertebral fractures and/or fractures of the long bones. Some fractures are not easy to detect and are found only after repeated examination. Assistance from an orthopaedic/emergency physician should be summoned immediately.

Life-threatening injuries: primary survey

Life-threatening injuries include:

- major pelvic disruption with haemorrhage
- major arterial haemorrhage

- long-bone fractures
- crush injuries with hyperkalaemic cardiac arrest and later traumatic rhabdomyolysis.

Major pelvic disruption with haemorrhage

There is limited literature concerning serious pelvic injuries in the later stages of pregnancy. However, uncontrolled haemorrhage from pelvic fractures continues to be a cause of potentially avoidable death after major trauma in the nonpregnant population, and the management principles are common to both groups.

Pelvic fractures in pregnant women may cause fracture to the fetal head, especially if the head is engaged. The precise mechanism of injury provides considerable information as to the type of pelvic injury sustained. An anteroposterior radiograph of the pelvis is an important investigation in any major trauma. Serious pelvic injuries are usually obvious, although the pelvis may only be confirmed as the source of bleeding once abdominal, thoracic and external sources have been excluded. Where a pelvic injury is suspected, the patient should be resuscitated and the pelvis immobilised.

Only a very gentle examination of the pelvis should be attempted if a fracture is suspected. This should be by a single experienced person gently pressing inwards on the pelvic bones. Under no circumstances should there be an attempt to demonstrate the 'open book fracture'. Massive retroperitoneal bleeding from pelvic fracture is more likely in pregnancy because of engorgement of the pelvic vessels. Major pelvic disruption tears the pelvic venous plexus.

The input of an orthopaedic surgeon is required urgently as stabilisation of the pelvis by external fixation may be part of resuscitation, in order to 'turn off the tap'.

Venous and arterial haemorrhage should be treated initially with manual attempts to return the pelvis to its anatomical position. The pelvis should be immobilised, preferably with a pelvic binder, but a sheet can be wrapped around the pelvis as a sling. These manoeuvres and the application of an external fixator (required to maintain anatomical reduction) may be difficult in the later stages of pregnancy. Often, delivery by CS will be required to salvage the baby, and to achieve control of pelvic haemorrhage. It may be necessary to empty the uterus by CS, even if the baby is dead, in order to gain access and to control haemorrhage. A high index of suspicion of the pelvis as a potential source of life-threatening bleeding should be maintained until control by other means has been established.

Long-bone fractures

Assess for bleeding and suspect arterial damage if there are changes in colour, temperature or pulse volume in the extremity concerned. Treatment of visible external bleeding comprises compression, resuscitation and immediate orthopaedic input. Haemorrhage from limb injuries is often compressible. Compression is carried out by:

- pressing on an obvious source of bleeding
- immobilising to reduce bleeding, e.g. splinting or definitive surgery/external fixator.

With open limb wounds, the loss may be evident. Loss may be suspected when a limb is swollen and deformed. Equally, loss may only be detected by recognising the signs of hypovolaemia; a closed fracture of the femoral shaft may easily result in the loss of 2litres into the surrounding tissues. Loss into long bones is one of the areas for major occult blood loss (chest, abdomen, pelvis and retroperitoneum and long-bone fractures). This requires resuscitation, immobilisation and immediate orthopaedic input.

Crush injuries with hyperkalaemic cardiac arrest and later traumatic rhabdomyolysis

Crush injuries cause damage to muscle cells, releasing potassium and myoglobin into the circulation. High levels of potassium in the blood can cause cardiac arrest. Myoglobin blocks renal tubules, leading to renal failure. To avoid renal failure, intravenous fluids should be given in sufficient volume to produce a minimum urine of 100 ml/hour. An ECG monitor may give warning of hyperkalaemia (broad, bizarre complexes; tented T-waves). Crush injuries may result in later amputation because of cell damage.

Adjunct to the primary survey is fracture immobilisation, which has the following effects:

- prevents further blood loss
- protects circulation
- prevents further soft tissue damage
- helps to control pain
- reduces the risk of fat embolism.

Radiographs of skeletal injuries: in the main, these are taken as part of the secondary survey. However, an anteroposterior view of the pelvis is taken during the primary survey in all multiply injured patients and other radiographs may be taken during the primary survey depending on initial clinical findings.

Limb-threatening injuries: secondary survey

Limb-threatening injuries are identified in the secondary survey and must be treated promptly. The system of examination of the limbs is look, feel, circulatory assessment, radiographs. Establish the Mechanism of injury, Injuries found, Symptoms and signs and Treatment. The mnemonic is MIST.

Examination

There should be a rapid inspection to identify musculoskeletal injuries.

- *Look* Examine the limbs for obvious wounds, deformity and the presence of any swelling. Note the colour and compare it with the contralateral limb. Note the perfusion of the limb and describe it in the notes; record capillary return time. Describe the wounds (with a sketch if appropriate) and their relationship to any fracture. This will avoid the need for repeated disturbance of the dressings. Note and record any skin loss, especially over fractures.

- *Feel* Palpate for tenderness or crepitus, which will reveal the presence of a fracture. Is there loss of sensation to touch? If so, record the position of sensation loss by drawing a picture.
- *Move* Check all the limbs for active movements where possible. The ability to move all major joints suggests that the joint and nerve muscle unit is intact.
- *Circulatory assessment* Assess, in each limb, the temperature, the capillary refill time, sensation and the peripheral pulses. Alteration in temperature, pulse volume discrepancy, pallor and motor dysfunction may suggest an arterial injury.
- *Fracture assessment* Is the fracture open or closed? Any fracture with a wound adjacent to it must be assumed to be an open fracture. Note any bone protrusion. Splinting may reduce the risk of a closed fracture becoming an open fracture. Surgical toilet of the bone may be required later.
- *Radiographs* Radiographs of the pelvis and other life-threatening injuries are taken during the primary survey; others are taken during the secondary survey.

Types of limb-threatening injuries

These include:

- open fractures and joint injuries
- vascular injuries and traumatic amputations
- compartment syndrome
- nerve injuries secondary to fracture dislocation.

Open fractures and joint injuries

With an open fracture, control haemorrhage by direct pressure, firm compression, bandaging and elevation of the limb. Gross contamination, such as earth and bits of clothing, should be removed and the wound copiously irrigated before applying a dry, sterile compression dressing. Severe soft tissue wounds are immobilised to relieve pain and control haemorrhage. Wounds should be described in the notes to avoid repeated disturbance of the dressing before definitive treatment. A photograph or a drawing is helpful. Repeated wound inspection increases the risk of infection. The fracture is then treated as appropriate.

Dislocations and fracture-dislocations are identified by radiograph. Dislocations are extremely painful when attempts are made to move the joint and this helps early recognition. Such early recognition can allow prompt reduction, especially if there is altered blood supply to the limb, for example, in posterior dislocation of the knee occluding the popliteal artery.

All dislocations are reduced at the earliest opportunity. They are often relatively easy to reduce soon after injury. Distal circulation is checked and the joint immobilised after reduction.

Vascular injuries and traumatic amputations

A major vascular injury may be suspected by:

- obvious arterial or venous haemorrhage from the wound
- an expanding haematoma
- absent distal pulses
- delayed capillary refill
- differing skin colour and temperature compared with the contralateral limb
- increasing pain at the site of the injury
- decreasing sensation.

Repeated assessment of the circulation is necessary.

Vascular injury is more likely if the injury is proximal to the knee or elbow. Fractures or fracture-dislocations around the knee or elbow are commonly associated with injury to the femoral and brachial artery, respectively.

Compartment syndrome

Compartment syndrome occurs when the interstitial pressure in a fascial compartment exceeds the capillary pressure as a result of haemorrhage or oedema within the involved compartment. Initially, venous flow stops and, as the pressure increases, the arterial supply also stops.

The presence of a distal pulse does not exclude a compartment syndrome.

Ischaemia of nerves and muscles occurs with rapid and irreversible damage. The distal pulses may be present throughout. The compartments most commonly affected are the anterior tibial compartment and the flexor compartment of the forearm.

Causes include crush injuries, prolonged limb compression, open or closed fractures, ischaemia of the limb and tight plasters or dressings.

In an obstetric rather than trauma context, *there are reports of compartment syndrome associated with the Lloyd Davies position and the lithotomy position.* This is possibly caused by arterial hypo-perfusion due to the leg being above the level of the heart. Other factors might include venous obstruction from kinking of the veins at the groin, or external pressure from stirrups or compression cuffs. There could also be an increase in compartment pressure due to weight of limb in stirrups or passive plantar flexion of foot.

The main presenting symptom is severe pain in an injured limb that is adequately immobilised. The pain is aggravated by passive stretching of the muscles in the involved compartment. Active movements are absent. The compartments may be swollen and tense with reduced distal sensation (although this is not always obvious clinically), but they are tender and the pain is out of proportion to the clinical findings.

Untreated, this will lead to rapid loss of the limb and permanent disability. Prompt recognition and emergency surgery are needed. If the limb is in plaster, or has circumferential dressings, split them completely down to the skin and open them widely. If symptoms do not improve within 15 minutes, any dressings overlying open wounds should be removed and the underlying muscle examined (see also Chapter 20 on burns and escharotomy). Its colour should look like raw, red meat; if it does not, suspect compartment syndrome. Such a limb requires urgent fasciotomy.

Nerve injuries secondary to fracture dislocation

Some injuries are often associated with neurological damage; for example, a dislocated hip and sciatic nerve injury or a dislocated elbow and median nerve injury. Altered sensation or motor power, or both, suggests nerve involvement. Orthopaedic surgeons must be involved immediately.

Definitive care

Definitive care continues in the hands of the orthopaedic surgeons.

Summary

- Manage life-threatening injuries first; they usually present as a circulation problem.
- Call orthopaedic surgeons.
- Suspect, detect and treat limb-threatening injuries.

Further reading

1 Browner BD, Jupiter JB, Levine AM, Trafton PG (editors). *Skeletal Trauma*. Philadelphia, PA: WB Saunders 1991.

2 Hansen ST, Swiotkowski MF. *Orthopaedic Trauma Protocols*. New York: Raven Press 1993.

ALGORITHM 20.1 Burns

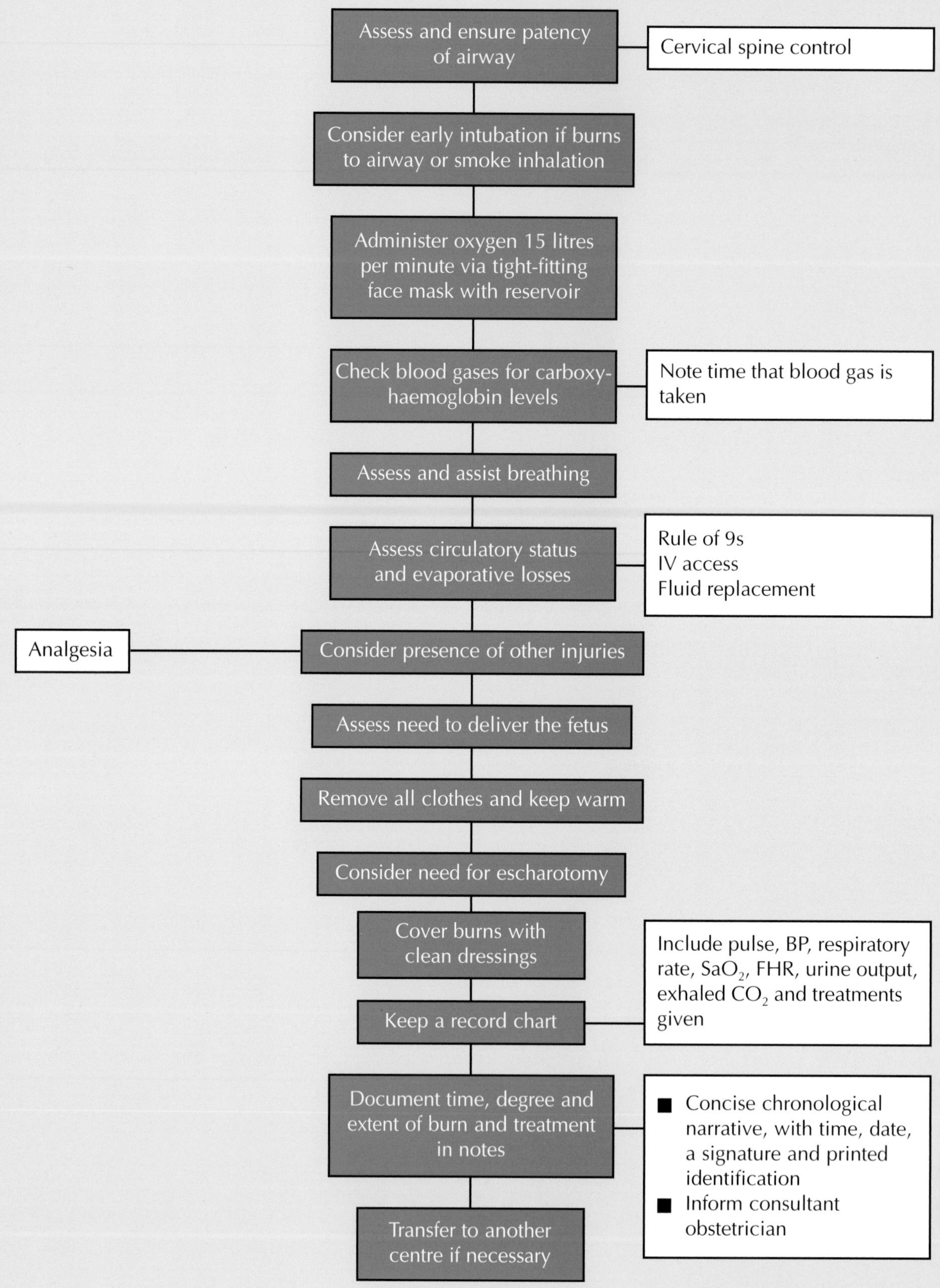

CHAPTER 20

Burns

Objectives

On successfully completing this topic, you will be able to:

- understand the impact of a thermal injury on the airway, breathing and circulation
- describe the immediate management of airway breathing and circulation in a patient with burns
- assess the severity of burns
- discuss the management of the fetus in the pregnant patient with burns.

Introduction

The incidence of pregnancy in women admitted to hospital with burn injuries has been found to be 6.8–7.8%. The burned pregnant woman should be managed jointly by the burns team and obstetricians. This may necessitate transfer to a burns centre with appropriate transfer of care to a local obstetrician. Most burns are caused by thermal injury but chemical, electrical and radiation burns also occur.

The severity of the injury is chacterised by the area and depth of the burn and the effect on the vital functions (the 'ABCs'). Burns may cause immediately life-threatening problems that need to be identified and simultaneously treated in the primary survey. A surface area burn of 25–50% has a mortality rate of 63% for both mother and fetus.

Pathophysiology of burns

Airway obstruction

Airway burns may result in airway obstruction due to oedema as a direct response to thermal injury (heat). Obstruction of the lower airways may be caused by deposition of soot particles. Airway injury from burns can be immediate or delayed, so the airway must be continually observed and early intubation should be considered, particularly if the patient is to be transferred. The maximum oedema is likely to occur at 24 hours after injury, but changes in airway patency can be rapid and disastrous. Clinical changes of impending airway obstruction will be seen, i.e. stridor, increased work of breathing with falling SaO_2 and decreasing conscious level. Stridor is therefore a 'red flag' symptom in the context of burn injury.

Impaired gas exchange

Respiratory injury to the lung parenchyma may be caused directly by hot gas or steam and may result in critically impaired gas exchange. However, impairment of respiratory function can occur in the burns patient in the absence of obvious respiratory injury. The mechanism for this may be unclear, but can involve ventilation/perfusion mismatch, secondary infection or adult respiratory distress syndrome (ARDS) and may occur up to 2 weeks after the initial injury.

Inhalation of carbon monoxide

Inhalation of carbon monoxide is common if the burn has been sustained in an enclosed area. It can occur without any burn injury due to inhalation from, for example, exhaust fumes or faulty household heaters. Oxygen delivery relies on haemoglobin binding to oxygen. Carbon monoxide has a greater affinity for haemoglobin than oxygen so displaces oxygen from the binding sites on the haemoglobin molecule, resulting in reduced oxygen delivery to the tissues.

A carboxyhaemoglobin level of greater than 10% indicates significant inhalation of carbon monoxide. There are, however, usually no physical symptoms at less than 20% hence the danger in this condition, and the risk of failing to make a diagnosis. Carboxyhaemoglobin levels should be measured routinely in patients exposed to burning materials in an enclosed space. In addition, a reversible period of relative hypoxia for the mother may have consequences for the fetus, depending on the period of time and the gestation, as for any other cause of inadequate fetal oxygen delivery. Carbon monoxide levels of 60% are likely to result in death.

Circulatory effects

Localised tissue damage causes oedema and fluid leak into the tissues. In addition, circulating inflammatory mediators cause an increase in systemic capillary permeability. This leads to a generalised extravasation of fluid from the intravascular compartment into the tissues, producing massive peripheral and pulmonary oedema. These inflammatory mediators can have a direct effect on cardiac function, which, when combined with relative hypovolaemia, vasodilatation, vascular stasis and tissue oedema, produces a marked reduction in tissue perfusion. A summary of these effects can also be simply defined as 'shock', which in the case of a severe burn may be classified as hypovolaemic, cardiogenic and distributive shock.

Immediate first aid

The burning process must be stopped: extinguish the flames by laying the affected patient on the ground and wrapping them in a blanket or equivalent. Gently remove burned clothing and any jewellery, unless stuck to the burnt skin. Small burns can be cooled with clean, cold water. Burns should be covered to avoid hypothermia. Nonsterile, domestic cling film is useful as a first aid dressing: it allows visualisation of the wound, but protects it from contamination and fluid loss while reducing pain.

Primary survey and resuscitation

Airway and breathing

Airway and breathing injuries should be suspected particularly if:

- the burn was sustained in an enclosed space
- there is hoarseness, loss of voice, stridor or wheeze
- there is evidence of burns around the lips, mouth and nose
- there is singeing to the nasal hair or eyebrows
- there is soot around the mouth or nose, or the patient is coughing up carbonaceous sputum
- there is respiratory distress and alteration in level of consciousness
- in the presence of carbon monoxide poisoning.

If there is a suspicion of an airway and breathing problem, or in the presence of carbon monoxide poisoning, advice from an anaesthetist is required as early intubation and ventilation may be indicated.

Management of suspected carbon monoxide inhalation

High-flow oxygen should be administered until adequate monitoring is established, including arterial blood gases and carboxyhaemoglobin levels are known.

In the presence of significant carboxyhaemoglobin, oxygen saturation monitoring may be an inaccurate and a falsely reassuring measure of maternal oxygenation. The woman may look pink or even 'cherry red'. Diagnosis is made by laboratory measurements of carboxyhaemoglobin. Note the time of the burn and the time that the arterial sample for carboxyhaemoglobin level is taken.

Oxygen will compete with carbon monoxide at the binding sites within the haemoglobin molecule, so in severe cases hyperbaric oxygen therapy may be required to increase the oxygen carriage in the blood.

Carbon monoxide poisoning in the mother results in relatively more serious effects for the fetus. It crosses the placental barrier and binds with even higher affinity to fetal haemoglobin leading to fetal tissue hypoxia. This may result in fetal death, injury, miscarriage or preterm labour even if the mother's injury appears mild.

Cyanide may also be absorbed by inhalation as a product of combustion of certain materials, and impairs respiration at the cellular level with equivalent reduction in cellular oxygenation.

Circulation

Circulatory losses should be suspected and fluid requirements calculated based on the time elapsed since the burn, the weight of the patient and the severity of burns using the 'rule of nines' (see Table 20.1), taking account of the increased abdominal girth of pregnancy (the area of the patient's palm represents about 1% of the body surface area) and any other injuries.

Table 20.1 The 'rule of nines'

Body surface area	Area burned (%)
Head and neck	9
Each upper limb	9
Front of trunk*	18
Back of trunk	18
Each lower limb	18
Perineum	1

*The gravid abdomen would represent a larger proportion of the total body surface area. The area of the patient's palm represents about 1% of the body surface area.

Monitor circulatory status and evaporative losses by heart rate, urine output, blood pressure and haematocrit. Fluid replacement should result in a urine output of at least 50 ml/hour.

Secure intravenous access, through nonburned skin, where possible. It is difficult to secure intravenous lines in burned areas and may increase the risk of infection, but on occasions may be the only option. In extreme difficulty with intravenous access, central venous lines or intraosseous cannulae may be required.

Replace fluids with warmed crystalloid solution. The patient requires 2–4ml/kg/percentage of body surface area burned in the first 24 hours from the time of the burn. Half of this volume is given in the first 8 hours following the burn and half in the next 16 hours. Further fluid replacement may be needed in the presence of myoglobinuria (secondary to rhabdomyolysis), under guidance from the intensive care teams.

Pain relief

As soon as resuscitation treatment allows, offer pain relief. Covering of the burn wounds, where practicable, with a transparent film will help to relieve pain while maintaining wound visibility. Opiates will be necessary for most cases, usually fentanyl or morphine intravenously, titrated to achieve satisfactory pain relief.

Severity of the burn

Severity of the burn depends on the:

- body surface area burned
- depth of the burn.

Depth of the burn

First degree burns are characterised by erythema and pain without blisters.

Second degree (partial thickness) burns are red, mottled, blistered, swollen, may look wet and are very painful.

Third degree (full-thickness) burns are dark and leathery, mottled or translucent. They are painless, usually dry and are hard to the touch.

Secondary survey and definitive care

It is important to recognise that a burned patient may have any other injury and that these may be masked by the pain of the burn. Especially for patients rescued from house fires, there may be major internal or musculoskeletal injuries caused by attempts to escape the building.

A full top-to-toe secondary survey is necessary to identify injuries that have not been apparent in the primary survey.

Escharotomy – Burned tissue may constrict the blood supply to the limbs. Check peripheral circulation by capillary refill and estimating perfusion. Call for general/plastic surgical assistance for assessment and treatment. The procedure of cutting through burned tissue to restore blood supply (and prevent rhabdomyolysis) is called escharotomy.

Sepsis – prevention of sepsis by appropriate dressings, early excision and grafting is important. Sepsis is the major cause of death due to burns in pregnancy. Prophylactic systemic antibiotics are not usually recommended.

Thrombosis – There should be a high index of suspicion for venous thrombosis.

Coagulation – There may be disturbance of coagulation either by dilutional effects where there is large fluid loss or by development of DIC. Manage in conjunction with haematological advice.

Assess need to deliver the fetus

Obstetric management has to be individualised. Within hours, the mother becomes hypermetabolic causing hyperthermia, has an increased oxygen consumption, develops tachypnoea, tachycardia and an increase in serum catecholamine levels. Maternal acidosis is a predictive factor with regard to progression of metabolic insult. In burns of 50% or greater, urgent delivery should be carried out if second- or third-trimester pregnancy, as fetal survival is not improved by waiting, and the additional metabolic requirements may compromise the mother.

Earlier in pregnancy there appears no evidence that pregnancy affects the maternal survival after a burn injury. However, with increasing burn injury there will be an increased risk of miscarriage, preterm labour or fetal death.

If the burn is less than 30% body surface area, the prognosis is good for both mother and fetus (dependent upon gestational age) and depends on the prevention of complications such as hypoxia, hypovolaemia and sepsis.

There are limited data on the management of electrical burns in pregnancy. The amniotic fluid and uterus are good conductors of electricity. There are reports of long-term oligohydramnios and intrauterine growth restriction. However, it is generally felt that there is an 'all or nothing' effect on the fetus: either death results, or the prognosis is comparatively good.

Summary

- Management of the burned pregnant woman involves the joint working of burns surgeons and obstetricians.
- Assess the actual or potential effect of the burn on the ABCs and treat.
- Assess the severity and depth of surface burns and treat.
- Arrange the timely delivery of the fetus when appropriate.
- Conduct secondary survey and definitive care.

Further reading

1 Chama CM, Na'Aya HU. Severe burn injury in pregnancy. *J Obstet Gynaecol* 2002;22:20–2.
2 Deitch EA, Rightmire DA, Clothier J, Blass N. Management of burns in pregnant women. *Surg Gynecol Obstet* 1985;161:1–4.
3 Matthews RN. Obstetric implications of burns in pregnancy. *Br J Obstet Gynaecol* 1982;89:603–9.
4 Polko LE, McMahon MJ. Burns in pregnancy. *Obstet Gynecol Surv* 1998;53:50–6.
5 Schmitz JT. Pregnant patients with burns. *Am J Obstet Gynecol* 1971;110:57.

SECTION 5

Other medical and surgical emergencies

ALGORITHM 21.1 Abdominal emergencies in pregnancy

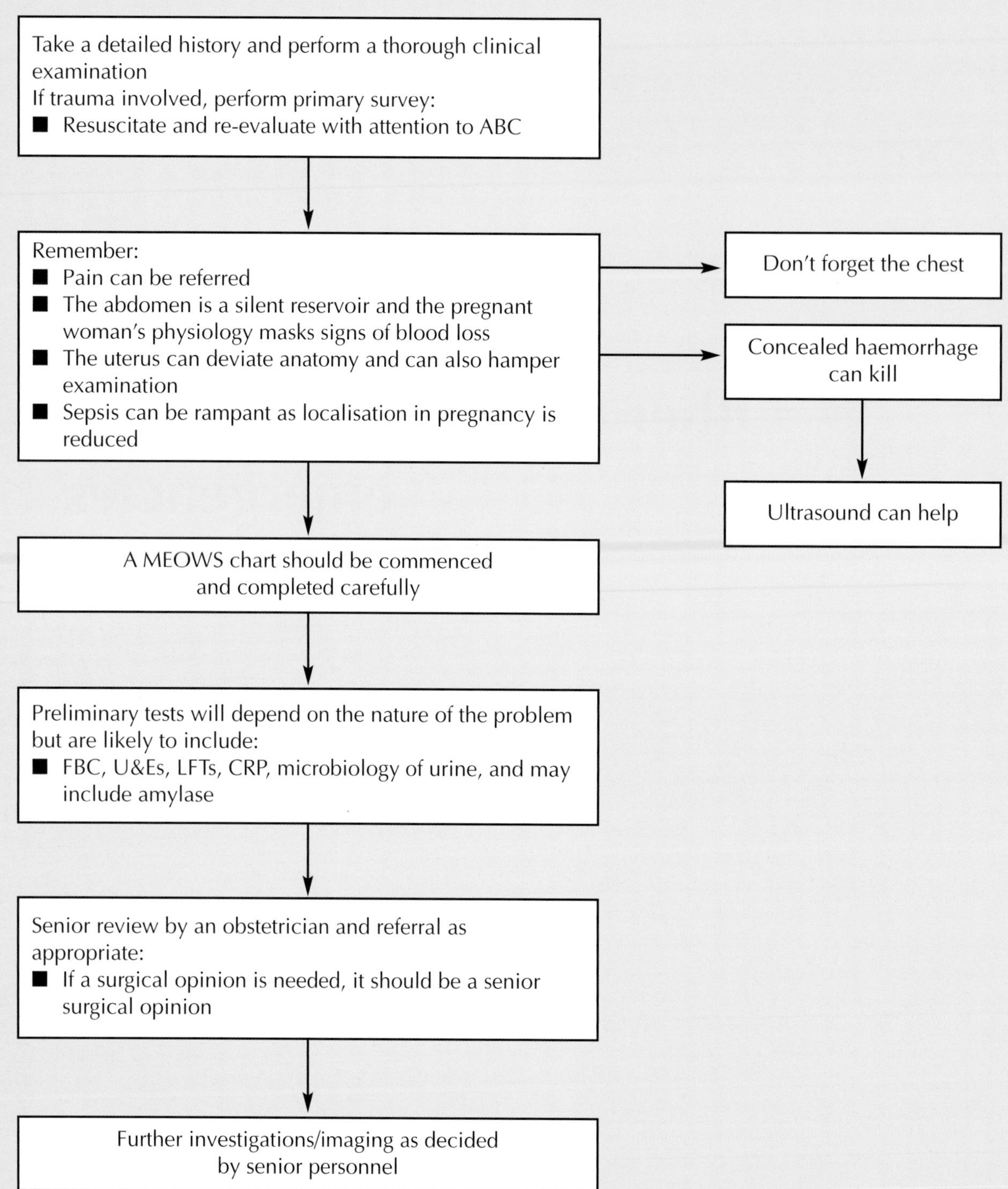

CHAPTER 21

Abdominal emergencies in pregnancy

Objectives

On successfully completing this topic, you will be able to:

- understand how to assess the pregnant woman with abdominal pain
- appreciate how to suspect and promptly diagnose potentially life-threatening conditions
- appreciate the changes in anatomy and physiology that occur in pregnancy and understand how these may affect the response to, and presentation of, acute abdominal conditions
- understand the investigation and treatment of abdominal pain in pregnancy.

Background and incidence

Abdominal discomfort in pregnancy is common, but any abdominal pain should be taken seriously. Frequently, minor ailments such as urinary tract infections are found to be the cause, but significant serious pathology does occur and can present in subtle ways. This can result in serious diagnoses being missed or delayed which can, in turn, result in death of the mother and/or fetus. In the UK all maternal deaths in pregnancy are reported and there are approximately three deaths each year due to intra-abdominal pathology (Table 21.1).

Information for intra-uterine deaths from maternal disease/peritonitis is not systematically collected, so this aspect of mortality is unmeasured. Many of the women who died received substandard care which often included a delay in diagnosis. Recurrent problems highlighted throughout the confidential reports include:

- failure to entertain the possibility of a nonobstetric diagnosis
- readmission or multiple admissions with no consultant input
- repeated doses of pethidine given for analgesia without consultant review or an adequate cause for pain being established

- high-risk women being looked after in a disjointed way by junior clinicians with lack of communication between services
- anxiety and confusion too readily being attributed to a psychiatric cause rather than the underlying (undiagnosed) organic disease.

Table 21.1 UK deaths due to nonobstetric abdominal pathology (1997–08)

Cause of death	1997–99	2000–02	2003–05	2006–08	Total
Intestinal obstruction	3 (small bowel)	3 (+1 late death)	0	0	7
Pancreatitis	2	1+1 pancreatic cyst	2 (+2 late deaths)	0	8
Splenic artery aneurysm	1	0	0	0	1
Intra-abdominal bleeding	1	0	0	0	1
Liver failure	1	0	3	4	8
Liver rupture	1	0	1	0	2
Peritonitis	0	1	1 appendicitis 1 faecal peritonitis	0	3
Duodenal ulceration	0	0	0	2 (1 bled; 1 perforated)	2
Ruptured oesophagus	0	1	0	0	1
Pseudo-membranous colitis	0	0	0	1	1
Crohn's disease	0	0	0	2	2
Total	9	7 (+1 late death)	8 (+2 late deaths)	9	36

Pathophysiology of abdominal pain in pregnancy

Abdominal pain, especially of acute onset, in the pregnant woman is a medical emergency that requires urgent assessment. As pregnancy advances, the assessment of the abdomen becomes more challenging:

- areas of maximum pain or tenderness may shift due to organ displacement
- the uterus inhibits abdominal palpation
- the peritoneum is less sensitive.

The other problem produced by the gravid uterus is that of hampering the omentum from its role as 'policeman' of the intra-abdominal contents, with the consequence of an inability to contain local inflammation; in turn, this results in more rampant progression of conditions such as appendicitis or perforation.

Intra-abdominal bleeding can also confuse the clinician as the mother, especially in later pregnancy, tolerates blood loss well. The reader is referred to Chapter 5 (Shock) and Chapter 25 (obstetric haemorrhage), and reminded that the signs of bleeding, including tachycardia, narrowing of the pulse pressure, oliguria and confusion, all occur after significantly more blood is lost in the pregnant than the nonpregnant woman, and that hypotension is an *extremely* late sign. What does help with assessment in pregnancy is that the fetus tolerates maternal blood loss very badly and is a good 'monitor' of maternal hypovolaemia, demonstrating heart rate abnormalities on monitoring. Early fetal heart rate monitoring is therefore extremely useful in women presenting with abdominal pain from the late second trimester onwards.

Clinical approach to diagnosis: history, examination, investigation

History

A detailed history around the *nature of the pain* is a vital step in beginning the diagnostic process, and is especially important in pregnancy where abdominal examination can be so inhibited by the gravid uterus. The following should be found from general and then direct enquiry.

Pain onset: acute versus gradual

- ***Acute*** onset with *persistent severe pain* suggests rupturing or tearing including ruptured ectopic, ruptured uterus, ruptured aneurysm (splenic, renal, epigastric or aortic), rupture of an abscess or perforation of an ulcer. Acute abruption also presents with severe acute abdominal pain and should be the presumptive diagnosis until ruled out. Acute onset with *colicky pain* suggests either intestinal or ureteric obstruction. Hernial orifices should be checked (sometimes difficult in a heavily pregnant and/or obese woman). If colicky pain becomes constant then the possibility of underlying ischaemia must be considered (e.g. bowel or ovary).
- ***Gradual*** onset increasing over a comparatively short time is more characteristic of 'inflammation' such as might occur with acute appendicitis, acute degeneration of a fibroid, acute cholecystitis, acute pancreatitis and acute diverticulitis.

Other important characteristics

- ***Quality*** and severity (colicky pain suggests an obstruction or something twisting, while continuous pain is more likely to suggest inflammation/infection).
- ***Location*** (think uterine, intraperitoneal, retroperitoneal and referred).
- ***Radiation*** (remembering diaphragm to shoulder, renal to groin and ovary down inner thigh).
- ***Exacerbating or relieving factors*** (movement, coughing, voiding, position).
- ***Associated symptoms*** (anorexia, nausea, vomiting, constipation, dysuria, haematuria, frequency).

Location of the pain and its likely cause

Uterine pain: abruption, degeneration of fibroids, chorioamnionitis or uterine contractions

The location of this is usually straightforward and confirmed by tenderness on palpation of the uterus but fibroids can lie posteriorly and be inaccessible to palpation, and a posteriorly located placenta can abrupt without producing local tenderness. Remember to check:

- the placental location relative to any uterine pain or tenderness
- the fetal heart rate pattern.

Intraperitoneal (abdominal) pain

Visceral peritoneal, compared with parietal peritoneal, irritation stimulates the afferent nerve fibres running within the sympathetic part of the autonomic system back to the sympathetic chain and spinal cord. This, therefore, produces a vague 'referred pain', usually in the central region, corresponding to the cutaneous nerves that arise from the corresponding level of the spinal cord. For example, in appendicitis this produces pain in the region of T10, which is around the umbilicus.

Once the parietal peritoneum becomes involved, segmental somatic innervation comes into play and produces sensation in the location of the problem, hence vague pains 'move' to localise as the disease process progresses. Inflammation and infection tend to produce constant pain that evolves as described above, but is also usually associated with constitutional upsets of nausea, anorexia, vomiting and fever. In many conditions, initial inflammation leads to subsequent infection, such as in appendicitis and cholecystitis.

Obstruction produces colicky pain that can be severe, and can also be associated with nausea and vomiting if the obstruction is in the small intestine. There may be a change in bowel habit depending if the distal small bowel or colon is involved. Perforation of a viscus usually follows deterioration of the above conditions or more directly from a peptic ulcer, or sigmoid diverticulum. This leads to the severe constant pain of generalised peritonitis, worsened by movement of any sort.

- Examples of inflammation without infection include oesophagitis (heartburn) and (simple) peptic ulceration. These lead to epigastric pain, whereas a flare up of either Crohn's disease or ulcerative colitis leads to more central abdominal pain, which may be colicky and usually associated with diarrhoea. It is worth noting that the administration of steroids, either to promote fetal lung maturation, or as treatment for inflammatory bowel disease, can not only exacerbate peptic ulceration, but also, importantly and dangerously, mask intra-abdominal signs and add to confusion in the diagnostic process.
- Examples of inflammation, which lead to infection, include cholecystitis and appendicitis. Both these conditions present with increasing pain that settles into a specific location. The appendix migrates superiorly with advancing gestation, progressing from the right iliac fossa upwards to the right paraumbilical region and can even reach the right hypochondrium.

- Examples of obstruction include sigmoid volvulus and pseudo-obstruction, the latter often occurs post-CS. While a sigmoid volvulus is usually associated with absolute constipation, pseudo-obstruction may not be so, and small amounts of liquid stool are not uncommon. Colonic neoplasms, although rare, can also occur.
- Perforations from peptic ulceration arise de novo and are rarely associated with any prodromal symptoms of an underlying ulcer. Perforations from appendicitis, sigmoid volvulus or pseudo-obstruction occur due to delay in both diagnosis and management.
- Rupture or torsion of an ovarian cyst can also produce a colicky pain, which can progress to a constant pain with constitutional upset once ischaemia develops. While this pain is located in an iliac fossa early in early pregnancy, as with appendicitis, it can occur relatively higher in later pregnancy.

Inflammation and swelling of an organ (liver)

- Hepatic pain from inflammation or infection can be severe and even result in spontaneous rupture secondary to gross swelling: the pain is often epigastric rather than right subcostal and this, together with local tenderness in the pre-eclamptic patient should alert to the possibility of HELLP syndrome.

Vascular accident

- Spontaneous rupture of an artery can occur. Most commonly this is a splenic artery aneurysm that produces sudden onset of severe pain rapidly progressing to collapse. This is usually mistaken for an acute abruption and the diagnosis only realised after blood is discovered free in the abdominal cavity at CS. In its less dramatic form it can present with left upper-quadrant pain; this is a very unusual location for pain in pregnancy and should always be taken seriously.
- Deep vein thrombosis of the pelvic vessels can produce a vague, generalised abdominal pain.
- A bleeding peptic ulcer is not associated with abdominal pain unless there is a concomitant anterior perforation. It usually presents with haematemesis and/or melaena along with hypovolaemia. A history of indigestion may give a clue as to the cause. If the bleed is catastrophic, collapse and death may occur before melaena is ever passed.

Retroperitoneal

- Loin pain is usually due to pyelonephritis and, because of the dextro-rotation of the uterus, this is invariably on the right side (serious consideration should be given to the accuracy of this 'diagnosis' if pain is left-sided). The pain tends to be constant and is usually associated with a fever although the urine may be clear. Loin tenderness can also occur with cholecystitis, but anterior tenderness in this condition helps to distinguish it from renal pain.
- Colicky pain commencing in the loin, but migrating towards the groin may be produced by renal/ureteric colic and the passage of a stone. Haematuria may be present.

- Pancreatitis causes constant, severe, epigastric pain that radiates through to the back. It is sometimes relieved by leaning forward.

Referred and neurological pain

- Pathology in the chest can present with abdominal discomfort. Examples include: myocardial ischaemia, pneumonia, pulmonary embolus and aortic dissection.
- Cholecystitis is commonly referred to the area of the lower ribs posteriorly or between the shoulder blades; hyperaesthesia may be present over the lower ribs to the right (Boas's sign).
- Irritation under the diaphragm (usually from sepsis or blood) will produce pain in the shoulder region. This is more common on the left than the right, due to the presence of the liver on the right-hand side.
- Herpes zoster can produce abdominal pain before the vesicular eruption occurs.

Examination

Obstetricians tend to forget to perform a general examination and instead go straight to the abdomen. This must be avoided and a systematic, thorough general examination is needed, including assessment of:

- pulse rate, pulse character and vascular perfusion
- colour, temperature, hydration and fetor oris
- lymphadenopathy and jugular venous pressure
- chest, including respiratory rate
- legs.

Abdominal examination will then include:

- looking – do they move or lie still? shallow breathing?
- palpation for tenderness with guarding or rebound
- auscultation for the presence and character of the bowel sounds.

Abdominal examination is further confounded by obesity, which is an ever-increasing problem in the pregnant population.

Investigations

Cardiotocography

Cardiotocography should be performed early to assess uterine activity and fetal condition.

Blood tests

Blood tests can help make a diagnosis in patients with abdominal pathology, for example, a grossly elevated amylase in acute pancreatitis or deranged liver function tests in HELLP. More commonly, however, they can be less useful and even on occasions misleading. An elevated white cell count can be a normal finding in pregnancy due to a neutrophilia (typically white cells rise from about 7 x 10^9 to 15 x 10^9/litre). Therefore the danger here is for obstetricians to assume an elevated count is normal, while surgeons might read too much into it. Inflammatory and infective conditions can occur with remarkably normal white cells. Elevated C-reactive protein levels are a good indication of an underlying inflammatory condition and these levels do not change in normal pregnancy. D-dimers are unhelpful in diagnosing thrombosis in pregnancy.

Ultrasound

This is useful to check on the viability of the pregnancy, the location of the placenta and any fibroids, and can also be useful to check for intra-abdominal bleeding. It may, however, fail to identify small amounts of intraperitoneal fluid, or other pathology and a negative exam - ination should be viewed with caution. It is not good at diagnosing an early, or evolving, abruption.

Radiographs

Chest radiographs can be helpful for cardiac and chest pathology and for excluding air under the diaphragm from a visceral perforation (the latter is unhelpful in women who have had a recent CS).

Abdominal plain radiographs are rarely used during pregnancy, but can be very useful post-delivery in assessing colonic dilatation in pseudo-obstruction.

CT and MRI

CT provides a highly sensitive and specific examination for abdominal pain; however, in pregnancy the radiation involved to both mother and fetus must be taken into account. For this reason MRI is often preferred and, although it is not as sensitive as CT in the assessment of intra-abdominal pathology, in cases of diagnostic uncertainty MRI may still be useful and reveal the cause. In such circumstances, it is best to discuss imaging with the radiologist. One problem with these advanced imaging modalities is that the pregnant woman may not fit into the scanner. Care should be taken during these tests that the woman be placed tilted in the left lateral position, to avoid caval compression during the scan.

Clinical management

Having taken a history and performed a thorough examination, if the diagnosis is not obviously obstetric related, the consultant obstetrician should be called for an opinion. This focuses attention on the problem, helps to identify who is the best specialist to involve, and adds weight to the referral – which in most circumstances should be on a consultant to consultant basis. These are high-risk women and making a diagnosis can not only be extremely difficult, but the cost of failure is high for both mother and baby, not to mention the hospital. Assessment and referral between junior doctors is fraught with potential errors and should cease. In cases where the diagnosis is not clear, but surgical intervention is required, a midline incision is advisable.

Acute appendicitis

Acute appendicitis is more common in the first two trimesters, but perforation is more common in the third, probably due to the difficulties in establishing an early diagnosis. It has long been recognised that there is a higher morbidity for mother and baby in pregnancy and therefore a relatively high negative operation rate is acceptable. Laparoscopy may be helpful in early pregnancy and laparoscopic appendectomy is usually possible. Later in pregnancy, the position of the appendix shifts upwards and laterally and because of access difficulties due to the enlarged uterus, a muscle-splitting incision should be made over the site of maximum tenderness. This is often in the right upper quadrant.

Acute cholecystitis

In the general population, acute cholecystitis is best managed by early laparoscopic cholecystectomy in patients fit for surgery. In pregnant patients, the severity of symptoms needs to be weighed up against the risk of losing the pregnancy from either surgery or sepsis. Patients who have simple biliary colic without obvious signs of acute inflammation (ultrasonographic features of a thickened gall bladder wall, localised tenderness and free fluid) are better treated nonoperatively as the symptoms are usually short lived and the gall bladder can be removed at some stage after the pregnancy has been completed. Patients who develop significant and recurrent biliary colic during pregnancy should be considered for laparoscopic cholecystectomy, preferably in the second trimester, as this is associated with less risk to the fetus than in the first or third trimesters. In patients with obvious acute cholecystitis, the decision is more difficult and other factors will need to be taken into account such as the state of the patient and the stage of the pregnancy.

In general, because of the risk of fetal loss during surgery, nonoperative management should be attempted in the first instance. However, persistence of symptoms and/or progression of disease should lead to laparoscopic cholecystectomy. In the advanced stages of pregnancy laparoscopic access may again be difficult and open surgery may be required.

Acute pancreatitis

Acute pancreatitis is not rare in pregnancy, occurring in approximately 3 in 10 000 pregnancies. It is most commonly due to cholelithiasis, but the oestrogenic effects of hyperlipidaemia can also be responsible. If severe, it is associated with a maternal and perinatal mortality rate of almost 40%. While symptoms are usually gastrointestinal with pain, nausea and vomiting, 10% of cases are associated with respiratory effects, which can progress to ARDS.

Acute pancreatitis should be considered in any women with unexplained abdominal pain and early clinical suspicion should lead to laboratory assessments. Oxygen saturations should also be measured. Once a diagnosis is made, prompt multidisciplinary care should follow. When caused by gall stones, early laparoscopic cholecystectomy is recommended, again, taking into account the various factors discussed above. Otherwise, management is essentially nonoperative and supportive in the initial period, and in the severe form this may require critical care support. In such circumstances early delivery will be required.

Colonic pseudo-obstruction

This was first described secondary to retro-peritoneal malignancy by Ogilvie and is sometimes referred to as Ogilvie's syndrome (incorrectly, unless malignancy is the cause).

This functional (i.e. nonmechanical) colonic obstruction can be a complication of pregnancy and delivery, most commonly caesarean section, but many (especially junior) surgeons will not be familiar with it in young women. The main features are:

- increasing abdominal distension, which may be dramatic
- bowel sounds may sound obstructive
- constipation is rarely absolute.

Investigation and treatment includes the following:

- Abdominal radiographs will show generalised, and often relatively nonspecific, distension of the colon. There is often, but not invariably, a cut-off seen in the region of the splenic flexure (where the parasympathetic fibres of the vagus nerve distribution and those ascending from the pelvic nerves meet). Distension of the small bowel may also be present. As the condition progresses, the caecum will enlarge to a greater extent than the rest of the colon and if greater than 9 cm the risk of perforation is high. Patients may or may not complain of right iliac fossa pain. Tenderness, almost always present in the normal population, may be masked by the enlarged uterus. This is an absolute surgical emergency and immediate colonoscopic decompression is indicated.
- Water-soluble contrast enema can aid diagnosis and colonoscopy may be used to decompress the bowel if simple measures to manage the ileus are not successful.
- Opiate analgesia is often used to keep these patients comfortable and this can compound the problem. Avoiding opiates and administering metochlopramide can help. While neostigmine can be useful in the nonpregnant or postpartum woman, it is contraindicated in pregnancy, as its stimulant effect on the myometrium can precipitate preterm labour.
- A defunctioning colostomy is never required. If the caecum cannot be adequately decompressed by an experienced colonoscopist, surgical decompression through a right-sided abdominal incision should be performed. In such cases, a tube caecostomy should be inserted.

- If diagnosis has been delayed and perforation has occurred with faecal peritonitis, a right hemicolectomy will be required with or without primary anastomosis (an end ileostomy with a mucous fistula or with closure of the distal colon may be needed in advanced cases when the baby is likely to need to be delivered at the same time).

Sigmoid volvulus

The incidence of volvulus is increased in pregnancy. Pain is left-sided and colicky in nature, examination confirms an obstructive picture. A plain abdominal radiograph is usually diagnostic and a flexible sigmoidoscopy is therapeutic.

Intestinal obstruction

Intestinal obstruction can be due to small or large bowel pathology. Small bowel obstruction is primarily related to adhesions, which can either be congenital or follow previous abdominal surgery. External hernias should always be searched for and, if present, surgery will be required. Always check the femoral canal. Causes of large bowel obstruction are more likely to require intervention. Volvulus and pseudo-obstruction have already been discussed. Neoplasms and diverticular strictures can still occur in the more elderly pregnant patients and adequate investigation of suspected 'pseudo-obstruction' is essential to avoid missing an underlying mechanical cause, which will require either colonoscopic stenting or surgical resection. The management of small bowel obstruction due to suspected adhesions is non-operative, with a high chance of success. The patient is made "nil by mouth', nasogastric aspiration is commenced and intravenous fluids administered. Failure to settle within 24–48 hours may indicate that a laparotomy will be required and, depending on the gestation and fetal assessment, the baby may need to be delivered at the time of laparotomy. Administration of water-soluble oral contrast material with plain abdominal radiographs after 90 minutes and 4 hours are useful in assessing whether the obstruction is likely to settle without surgery, and can indeed be therapeutic in precipitating bowel activity. Obviously if there are any signs of possible underlying bowel ischaemia, urgent laparotomy should be undertaken.

Summary

- Acute abdominal problems in pregnancy are difficult to diagnose and can be associated with a high morbidity and mortality to mother and baby. Prompt diagnosis and treatment is therefore essential.
- A high index of suspicion is required in all patients together with early obstetric and general surgical consultant input.
- When nonobstetric conditions are suspected, obstetricians should call on other specialists for advice, while remembering that few specialists have experience of dealing with pregnancy. The obstetrician must therefore ensure that a specialist of appropriate seniority is involved and the consultant obstetrician must coordinate any multidisciplinary input.

- It must always be remembered how well young, fit, pregnant women compensate for blood loss.
- Be aware that obesity adds greatly to the diagnostic challenge.

Further reading

1 Eddy JJ, Gideonsen MD, Song JY, *et al.* Pancreatitis in pregnancy. *Obstet Gynecol* 2008;112(5):1075–81.

2 Kakarla A, Posnett H, Jain A, Ash A. Acute colonic pseudo-obstruction after CS. *The Obstetrician & Gynaecologist* 2006;8(4):207–13.

3 Taylor D. Acute abdomen in pregnancy, updated 2009 (http://emedicine.medscape.com/article/195976-overview).

ALGORITHM 22.1 Management of diabetic ketoacidosis

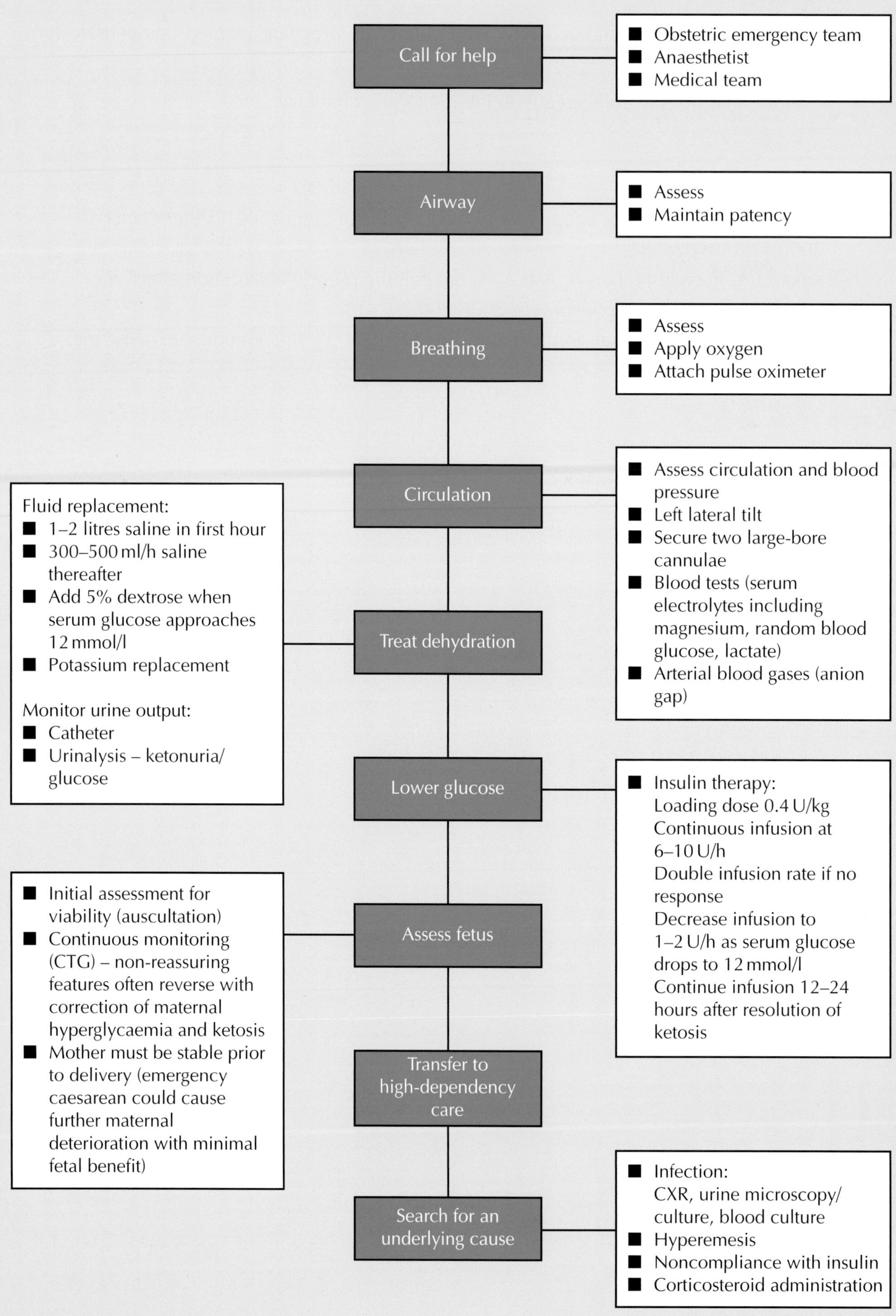

CHAPTER 22

Cardiac, diabetic and neurological emergencies in pregnancy

Objectives

On successfully completing this topic, you will be able to:

- understand the serious cardiac, diabetic and neurological problems that can affect pregnant women
- anticipate the health problems of women with pre-existing disease
- appreciate the critical diagnostic features heralding emergencies in pre-existing and new conditions
- take part in the urgent multidisciplinary care of pregnant and puerperal women with complex disorders
- understand important aspects of service provision for such women with complex disorders.

Introduction and incidence

The 2006–08 Triennial Confidential Enquiry into maternal deaths (*Saving Mothers' Lives*) reported a total of 53 deaths from heart disease related to pregnancy.[1] This was an increase from the previous triennium when 48 deaths were reported. Cardiac disease remains the commonest cause of indirect maternal death and also the commonest cause of maternal death overall. Some degree of substandard care was present in 51% of cases.

The same enquiry reported three deaths of women with diabetes mellitus, 0.13 per 100 000 maternities, all probably due to hypoglycaemia. The mortality from diabetes is stable with one death reported in the previous triennium and three in the triennium prior to that. Diabetes is an uncommon cause of indirect maternal death, but the burden of disease is high and growing and emergency complications must be recognised and appropriately managed.

Neurological disease in pregnancy and the puerperium is not singled out in the report as a separate entity. However, the overall recommendations of *Saving Mothers' Lives* are pertinent.

Especially so are the recommendations to take due note of pre-existing disease and to work within a multidisciplinary, specialist team, both to avoid and to treat emergencies in complex cases.

Cardiac disease

Cardiac disease can be divided into congenital heart disease and acquired heart disease, with maternal deaths from acquired heart disease greatly exceeding those from congenital heart disease. However, since more women with congenital heart disease are now surviving into their childbearing years, the number of women with congenital heart disease seen in antenatal clinics is increasing with a prevalence estimated to be around 0.8% in the antenatal population.

The main cardiac causes of maternal death are sudden adult death syndrome (SADS), peripartum cardiomyopathy, aortic dissection, myocardial infarction and myocardial ischaemia.

Acquired heart disease

SADS

The case definition for SADS is a sudden unexpected cardiac death (i.e. presumed fatal arrhythmia) where all other causes of sudden collapse are excluded, including a drug screen for stimulant drugs such as cocaine. Ten women died of SADS in the 2006–08 triennium, more than in any previous triennium. Six of the women were obese. Obesity appears to be associated with cardiac hypertrophy, and both obesity and cardiac hypertrophy are risk factors for arrhythmia.

Cardiomyopathy

There are different types of cardiomyopathy – peripartum, dilated and hypertrophic.

Peripartum cardiomyopathy typically presents either as a woman approaches term or in the first few weeks after delivery, although it can occur up to five months postpartum. While it is commoner in older, obese, black or hypertensive women, it can present in women with no risk factors who have previously been well. Unexplained breathlessness, tachycardia, gross oedema or supraventricular tachycardia should prompt a chest radiograph, ECG and echocardiography. Prior to delivery, peripartum cardiomyopathy can be treated with diuretics and beta-blockers, with angiotensin-converting enzyme (ACE) inhibitors being added after delivery or in very severe cases. There is a high recurrence risk in future pregnancies and women with cardiomyopathy should receive preconceptual counselling prior to embarking on further pregnancies.

If dilated cardiomyopathy is considered, anticoagulation should be instigated to prevent intracardiac thrombus formation.

Hypertrophic obstructive cardiomyopathy (HOCM) is an autosomal dominant condition which shows anticipation (gets worse in each subsequent generation). Usually pregnancy outcome is good unless there is severe diastolic dysfunction. Output may be compromised by:

- bleeding – prevent/treat blood loss aggressively
- tachycardia – consider beta-blockers to prolong diastole and allow adequate ventricular filling
- vasodilatation – avoid nifedipine as a tocolytic
- arrhythmias – treat arrhythmia and consider anticoagulation.

Acute myocardial infarction (MI) and ischaemic heart disease

Mortality from acute coronary syndromes has been estimated at 11% and is highest in peripartum women. The majority of women who die from acute MI or ischaemic heart disease have identifiable risk factors relating to lifestyle, such as increased maternal age (odds ratio (OR) = 6.7 for age >30 years), diabetes, obesity or smoking. Other risk factors include hypertensive disorders and existing thrombophilias. Infection in the third trimester and postpartum seems to heighten the risks further.

Pathophysiology

The predominant mechanism for MI in the nonpregnant population is rupture of an atheromatous plaque causing coronary occlusion. In pregnancy, 50% of MIs are thought to be caused by coronary artery dissection resulting in coronary artery occlusion. This is rare in the nonpregnant population. Coronary thrombosis may occur without underlying atherosclerosis, due to the hypercoagulable state that naturally exists in pregnancy.

The demands on the cardiovascular system increase with the rising oxygen demands of the developing fetus and uterus. Labour adds a further cardiovascular challenge, with increasing catecholamine stimulus due to pain. The highest incidence of coronary dissection occurs immediately after delivery.

Presentation

Chest pain should always be taken extremely seriously in pregnancy, as should other symptoms of cardiac disease, such as fatigue, dyspnoea, palpitations and syncope.

Diagnosis

Failure to consider the diagnosis of ischaemic heart disease in women presenting with chest pain during pregnancy is a common failing. There should be a high index of suspicion, particularly if the woman requires opiate analgesia for the chest pain, and there should be a low threshold for further investigation.

ECG

The diagnostic ECG criteria are the same as in the nonpregnant state with elevated ST segments and Q waves. Cardiac enzymes will also be raised. However some difficulties may be encountered in the interpretation of ECG results. ST elevation may be a normal finding in the third trimester, along with left axis deviation. Q waves may be seen along with mildly inverted T waves in lead III in normal pregnancy (ST segment depression is also commonly seen in women undergoing anaesthesia for CS).

Blood tests

In general, troponin is the preferred biochemical diagnostic marker for cardiac disease in pregnancy, although it can be elevated in pre-eclampsia or gestational hypertension; it is not affected by labour or surgery. Additionally, serum creatine kinase-MB may be raised in association with uterine contractions.

Imaging

A coronary angiogram can be performed with effective abdominal shielding to reduce fetal irradiation (see Chapter 4: Appendix 'Radiology in the pregnant woman'). Echocardiography is usually not used as a definitive test, but may be used in pregnancy due to its noninvasive nature, at least to look at ventricular function and wall motion abnormalities. It is also useful in excluding valvular problems or aortic dissection.

Treatment

Modern treatment of acute MI requires prompt diagnosis, oxygen via facemask if SaO_2 readings are below 95%, pain relief e.g. intravenous diamorphine, and urgent referral to a cardiac team with the intention of achieving rapid reperfusion. This may be achieved either by the provision of thrombolytic drugs, or by primary percutaneous coronary intervention (PCI), often with the provision of a coronary stent. The current thinking is to prefer PCI.

Difficulties in planning treatment in pregnancy include the hazards of the fetus requiring urgent delivery and also the risks of haemorrhage in the peripartum period.

PCI may have some radiation risk to the fetus but also requires prolonged antiplatelet therapy. Drug requirements are relatively much greater when drug-eluting stents are used as opposed to bare metal stents. Consideration of whether to stop these drugs or not has to be addressed in the context of CS and regional anaesthesia. Bare metal stents would be the treatment of choice in pregnancy.

Thrombolytic therapy has been traditionally thought of as contraindicated in pregnant women although, of course, they were naturally excluded from all clinical trials. There has been some clinical experience suggesting that haemorrhage remains a real threat, particularly in the peripartum and postpartum period. However, during pregnancy it is thought that there is little transplacental passage of streptokinase and other similar agents, so these may not pose a risk to the fetus. In association with a coronary dissection, the use of thrombolytic therapy could worsen the bleeding. As this is a common cause of acute MI in pregnancy, it is likely that PCI, where available, will be preferred over thrombolytic therapy.

Coronary artery or other cardiac surgery is only performed when there are complications such as coronary dissections or catastrophic valvular dysfunction. If still pregnant, it is recommended that fetal heart monitoring should be conducted to ensure adequate bypass pump flow. Depending on the stage of pregnancy, a choice may be made to deliver the fetus at the time of coronary surgery.

Drug therapy after MI

In the nonpregnant population, follow-up therapy would include a wide variety of drugs, many of which are aimed at vasodilatation or suppression of platelet activity (see Table 22.1). Planning therapy in a pregnant woman has to take account of the varied side effects on the fetus and passage into breast milk for the lactating mother.

Table 22.1 Cardiac drugs and their adverse effects in pregnancy, labour and lactation

Drugs used post-MI	Potential problems in pregnancy and postpartum
Beta-blockers	Bradycardia, hypoglycaemia, hyperbilirubinaemia, apnoea in neonate Accumulate in breast milk Labetalol well used in pregnancy
Organic nitrates	Used in pregnancy for hypertension and preterm labour Also used to relax uterus for breech version or placental retention Avoid hypotension if fetus undelivered
Calcium channel blockers	Nifedipine well known in pregnancy Diltiazem possibly teratogenic Excreted in breast milk, so not advised
ACE inhibitors (also angiotensin-receptor antagonists)	Used to decrease afterload to heart Teratogenic so not advised if pregnant May affect uterine blood flow Disrupts development of fetal kidneys
Statins	Used to reduce low-density lipoprotein (LDL) levels; unclear if they contribute to fetal abnormalities, as same patients likely to be obese or diabetic, so have added risk factors for fetal abnormalities
LMWH	Molecule too large to cross placenta Well known in pregnancy Reduced risk of bleeding compared with unfractionated heparin Need to be discontinued 24 hours before labour/surgery
Antiplatelet therapy	Aspirin in first trimester may be associated with birth defects Low-dose aspirin in second and third trimester appears safe for fetus and mother; high dose may result in fetal haemorrhage, intrauterine growth restriction and premature closure of ductus arteriosus Clopidogrel and glycoprotein IIb/IIIa inhibitors are frequently used in association with PCI in non-pregnant women; little known on use in pregnancy or breastfeeding

Choice of delivery

Where possible, the delivery should be delayed to allow time for healing of the myocardium. This will not always be possible. There appears to be no evidence that either method of delivery is better than the other and each has its risks. Care to reduce cardiac work, in the form of adequate pain relief and minimal pushing, will be needed as for other women with cardiac disorders. Great care should be taken with syntocinon due to the vasodilatation, and ergometrine is contraindicated due to the possible spike in blood pressure it might provoke.

Aortic dissection

Of the disorders affecting the aorta during pregnancy, Marfan's syndrome and Ehlers–Danlos Type IV are the most important. Women with bicuspid aortic valves are also at increased risk of aortic dissection. Approximately 80% of women with Marfan's have some cardiac involvement, the majority having mitral valve prolapse. Patients with Marfan's should have regular echocardiograms during pregnancy to look for an increase in the aortic root diameter.

Risk of aortic dissection:

- aortic root diameter less than 4cm 1%
- aortic root diameter more than 4cm 10%.

The time of greatest risk is in labour and immediately postpartum when cardiac output is increased. Hypertension increases the risk of dissection and the systolic blood pressure should be carefully monitored and controlled. Women with Ehlers–Danlos Type IV are known to be at risk of aortic dissection even if the aortic root is of normal size.

Consider the diagnosis in women with:

- central chest, jaw or interscapular pain – i.e. remember not all chest pain is due to pulmonary embolism
- family history (Marfan's and Ehlers–Danlos IV are usually autosomal dominant)
- women with a known bicuspid aortic valve.

Valve disease

Regurgitant valve disease

Although cardiac output increases in pregnancy, the reduction in systemic vascular resistance compensates in part for this, and pregnancy is generally well tolerated.

Stenotic valve disease

Increased cardiac output across the stenosed valve will increase the transvalvular gradient and pregnancy may be poorly tolerated. The onset of functional deterioration occurs most frequently during the second trimester.

Prosthetic valves

Women with mechanical prostheses require anticoagulation throughout pregnancy. There is debate as to which anticoagulant regimen to use. LMWH does not cross the placenta and is therefore safer for the fetus, but may be associated with a higher risk of valve thrombosis, particularly if patient noncompliance is a concern. Whatever the anticoagulation regime, pregnancy in a patient with a mechanical prosthesis is associated with a maternal mortality between 1 and 4%, mainly due to valve thrombosis.

Congenital heart disease

Congenital heart disease accounts for <10% of all maternal deaths due to cardiac causes. However, more women with congenital heart disease are now surviving until their child-bearing years and are the group of women most commonly seen antenatally in a joint obstetric cardiac clinic. Since this group of women are known to the healthcare services prior to pregnancy, there is an opportunity to offer preconceptual counselling. Pre-pregnancy counselling should include a frank discussion of the risks to enable a woman to make an informed choice about whether to embark on pregnancy or not.

At the time of booking for antenatal care, it is important to define the lesion and determine what surgery has been done previously. Women with surgically corrected congenital heart disease are still at risk, as there may be a residual defect. A specific recommendation from the most recent maternal mortality report is that, *'Women with a known history of cardiac disease must be referred for consultant-led obstetric care in a maternity unit where there is a joint obstetric/cardiology clinic or a cardiologist with expertise in the care of women with heart disease in pregnancy.'*

Service provision for women with heart disease

Preconceptual care

If women are known to have heart disease prior to pregnancy, pre-pregnancy counselling should be offered and is ideally performed jointly by an obstetrician and a cardiologist including:

- a frank discussion of the risks involved to enable the woman to make an informed choice as to whether to embark on pregnancy or not
- optimising cardiac function (medically, e.g. control arrhythmias, or surgically, e.g. valvotomy)
- review and adjust medication, avoiding teratogens
- contraception advice if the woman decides against embarking on pregnancy
- contact numbers to facilitate early referral once pregnant.

Women undergoing assisted conception often have additional risk factors such as increased age, the risk of ovarian hyperstimulation and multiple pregnancy.

Early pregnancy

Ideally, women with heart disease should be referred to a joint obstetric cardiac clinic. There should be:

- easy access to facilitate prompt referral
- accurate information gathered about the type and severity of the cardiac disease, previous and current treatments
- a frank discussion of the risks involved to enable the woman to make an informed choice whether to continue with the pregnancy or not
- professional interpreter (if needed) to ensure that relevant history is disclosed. Interpreters from within the family should not be used as, in the family's desire to help the woman have a successful pregnancy, risks may not be accurately relayed to the patient
- for women who choose not to continue the pregnancy, there should be easy access to termination of pregnancy in a hospital that can care for a woman with heart disease. Infection, bleeding and the need for an anaesthetic are recognised complications of termination and will pose a more significant risk to a woman with cardiac disease.

Awareness of cardiac disease in the antenatal population

Recognition of relevant history, important signs and symptoms which may prompt referral to a cardiologist:

- unexplained breathlessness
- isolated systolic hypertension
- interscapular pain
- severe chest pain not due to thromboembolism
- polycythaemia
- tachycardia.

Guidelines are needed locally to enable:

- recognition of risk factors at the time of the initial antenatal visit and facilitate appropriate referral
- the appropriate pattern of care to be initiated that would ideally be hospital-based care with a joint cardiac obstetric clinic for high-risk women
- follow up of women with heart disease who do not attend for care
- multidisciplinary management of women with heart disease to plan delivery or to facilitate prompt attention if their condition deteriorates.

Appropriate response to cardiac arrest is needed:

- knowing how to call the arrest team for an obstetric patient
- efficient bleep system to ensure that the appropriate people, including an obstetrician and a paediatrician, are called
- resuscitation training and drills specifically directed at cardiac arrest in a pregnant woman, for example, Advanced Life Support in Obstetrics (ALSO) and MOET courses
- well-maintained equipment with which staff are familiar.

Inherited cardiac disease:

- family members may also be at risk of cardiac disease and may need to be screened, for example, for Marfan's disease, HOCM and possibly SADS
- fetal echocardiography may be indicated if either parent had congenital heart disease
- The 22q11 deletion in either parent would increase the risk of congenital heart disease in the fetus.

Multidisciplinary care plan

This should include a plan for management during pregnancy, intrapartum and postpartum. It should include contingency planning for such conditions as preterm labour and postpartum haemorrhage; and contact numbers for members of the multidisciplinary team.

Delivery

Generally aim for a vaginal delivery, unless a woman cannot raise her cardiac output sufficiently for labour safely. Women where CS for cardiac indications may be appropriate include those with severely stenotic valves, poor ventricular function, ischaemia, cyanosis, some women with pulmonary hypertension and women with a dilated aortic root. During labour avoid hypotension, provide good analgesia and ensure careful fluid balance. Syntocinon given by an infusion over 10–20 minutes may be preferable to a bolus of syntocinon for management of third stage, and this should be specified in the individualised care plan. Ergometrine should also be used with great care and may be contraindicated in some obstetric conditions.

Postpartum

The majority of maternal deaths from cardiac causes occur postpartum. This is a time when increased vigilance is required, but when complacency often occurs. Maternal observations must be monitored regularly, by strict attention to and recording of fluid balance, with an appropriate response if abnormal.

Contraception

Appropriate contraceptive advice *must* be provided after any pregnancy. This allows time for reassessment of cardiac function and treatment to improve function, for example valvotomy. One successful pregnancy must not engender complacency. Some conditions, such as peripartum cardiomyopathy, have a high recurrence risk and assessment and discussion should occur prior to embarking on a further pregnancy. Other conditions worsen with age and in each subsequent pregnancy the risks would be higher.

Diabetes in pregnancy

Diabetes complicates 2–5% of pregnancies. It has been predicted that there will be a 35% increase in 30 years. Diabetes may affect women prior to pregnancy, or develop during pregnancy.

Aspects of diabetes that are affected by pregnancy include:

- diabetic ketoacidosis (see Algorithm 22.1)
- retinopathy – 50% risk of progression in pregnancy
- nephropathy – 6% of women with pre-existing diabetes have nephropathy prior to conception. If moderate/severe renal impairment is present in early pregnancy, there is significant risk of deterioration.
- hypertension – pre-existing hypertension is common; 12–40% develop pre-eclampsia
- infection – more common in women with diabetes; in patients with type 1 diabetes who are pregnant, 80% will experience at least one infection, plus there is associated increased risk of preterm labour and ketoacidoisis
- other associated endocrine problems, e.g. thyroid dysfunction.

Recent classification of diabetes in pregnancy is into five types:

- type I diabetes mellitus (0.2–0.5% of pregnancies) inadequate insulin production
- type II diabetes mellitus (0.2–2% of pregnancies) insulin resistance
- impaired glucose homeostasis
- gestational diabetes (1–6% of pregnancies, with 20–50% subsequently developing type II diabetes)
- diabetes due to specific aetiologies, including genetic, endocrine (Cushing's), drug and infection induced.

Pregnancy is a state of physiological insulin resistance and glucose handling is significantly altered, especially in late pregnancy. Insulin requirement is likely to increase by 50% or more. Many complications are associated with maternal diabetes. Most of these are caused directly by persistent maternal hyperglycaemia. These complications include:

Maternal:

- hypoglycaemia
- caesarean rates range from 25 to 80% in women with diabetes

Fetal:

- congenital abnormalities, affecting 3–8% of infants of women with pre-existing diabetes; risk is directly related to glycaemic control around conception and is correlated with glycated haemoglobin (HbA_1C):
  - less than 8% has risk of 5%; >10% has risk up to 25%; abnormalities include neural tube defects and cardiac malformations
- early pregnancy loss, directly related to glucose control
- spontaneous preterm labour, up to 20%
- macrosomia, 20–40% have birthweight over 90th centile (>4.5 kg), with more adipose tissue and larger shoulders; macrosomia is associated with shoulder dystocia and birth trauma
- perinatal mortality, up to tenfold increase; rates have fallen with improved diabetic management
- polyhydramnios, with risk of cord prolapse and premature rupture of membranes
- neonatal complications of an infant of a diabetic mother include fetal hyperinsulinaemia, which results in risk of neonatal hypoglycaemia and respiratory distress syndrome.

Diabetic emergencies in pregnancy

- Hypoglycaemia
- Diabetic ketoacidosis (Algorithm 22.1).

Hypoglycaemia

Tight glucose control results in a 33% increase in hypoglycaemic attacks for every 1% decrease in HbA_1C. Mild hypoglycaemic episodes (home blood glucose <4.0 mmol/litre) become more frequent in pregnancy and this, combined with a loss of warning symptoms, result in an increased risk of severe hypoglycaemic episodes requiring someone else to manage the symptoms. Signs and symptoms of hypoglycaemia have rapid onset with sudden loss of consciousness, particularly if the mother has taken insulin, but then not eaten.

Women experiencing hypoglycaemic episodes must discuss this with the team.

Family members should be educated to use glucagon injections and Glucogel (formerly Hypostop) for emergency treatment of hypoglycaemia. Intramuscular or subcutaneous injection of 1 mg glucagon in a readymade 'rescue kit', followed by a sugary snack or drink should be given in the event of hypoglycaemia.

Medical management of hypoglycaemia

Making a diagnosis:

- suspect in any patient with diabetes who is behaving oddly, is confused or lethargic and check their blood glucose
- suspect in any patient who is unconscious or fitting and do a blood glucose.

Treatment:

- the patient needs glucose urgently
- if conscious and can tolerate it, give her something sugary orally (food or oral glucose gel) and review
- if too drowsy for the above, or unconscious, then administer 25–50 ml intravenous glucose 50% via a large vein or intramuscular or subcutaneous glucagon 1 mg.

Discontinue any insulin-containing solution if they have been on a sliding scale and then reassess further requirements for insulin and dextrose.

Diabetic ketoacidosis

In established diabetes, ketoacidosis is rare, particularly with the tighter glucose control. Thirty percent of ketoacidosis cases in pregnancy are probably due to unrecognised new onset type I diabetes. Precipitating factors, such as hyperemesis, infection, tocolytic therapy and corticosteroid administration, as well as noncompliance with insulin can predispose to ketoacidosis, which has been recognised in patients with type II diabetes and gestational diabetes, as well as type I diabetes. Symptoms and signs of ketoacidosis include: gradual onset of drowsiness and polyuria; polydipsia; dehydration; nausea; vomiting; abdominal pain; hyperventilation; tachycardia; hypotension; ketotic breath; disorientation and coma.

Ketoacidosis in pregnancy tends to occur with lower glucose levels than usually expected, including rarely with normoglycaemia. Management of these women should be multiprofessional, including obstetricians, anaesthetists, midwives, neonatologists (if delivery anticipated), diabetologists and diabetic nurses. Algorithm 22.1 gives the management of diabetic ketoacidosis.

Service provision for women with diabetes

The St Vincent Declaration, ratified by the World Health Organization Regional Committee for Europe in 1991,[11] set a 5-year target to: 'Achieve pregnancy outcome in the diabetic that approximates to that of the non-diabetic woman.' The findings of a CEMACH report (2007) showed that women with diabetes do not appear to be receiving enough support.[12] Preconception care was often poor and uncoordinated. There was evidence that the care provided to women with type II diabetes was of a lower standard than that provided to women with type I diabetes. Pregnancies in women with pre-existing diabetes continue to have perinatal mortality rates that are five times higher than the general population.

The Department of Health published a National Framework for Diabetes[13] with a standard: 'To achieve a good outcome and experience of pregnancy and childbirth for women with pre-existing diabetes and for those who develop diabetes in pregnancy.' NICE published the guideline *Diabetes in Pregnancy*.[14]

Pre-existing diabetes

Preconceptual care

If women have diabetes prior to pregnancy, pre-pregnancy counselling should be offered. The importance of avoiding unplanned pregnancy should be an essential component of diabetes education from adolescence for women with diabetes.

Pre-pregnancy information should include:

- information that establishing good glycaemic control before conception and continuation through pregnancy will reduce the risk of miscarriage, congenital malformation, stillbirth and neonatal death
- the role of diet, bodyweight and exercise
- risks of hypoglycaemia and hypoglycaemia awareness
- how nausea and vomiting can affect glycaemic control
- the increased risk of having a baby who is large for gestational age
- the possibility of transient neonatal morbidity
- risk of the baby developing obesity and/or diabetes in later life.

There should be a review of medications (women with type II diabetes are increasingly being managed with oral hypoglycaemic agents) and a medical review, with a view to commencing folic acid 5 mg daily at least one cycle before attempted conception and establishing good glycaemic control. A relative should receive education to be able to manage hypoglycaemic episodes.

Antenatal care

Women should be managed by a multidisciplinary team, ideally in a joint clinic. Individual targets for glucose control should be established (Table 22.2). A specific antenatal care plan should be established within each unit and should include:

Glycaemic control during labour and birth. In an otherwise uncomplicated pregnancy, vaginal birth between 38–40 weeks should be advocated. The unit should have care pathways for management of women with diabetes during labour and birth. Capillary blood glucose should be monitored on an hourly basis and maintained between 4 and 7 mmol/l, and the urine should be checked for ketones. In women with type I diabetes there should be an intravenous dextrose and insulin infusion (sliding scale) from the onset of established labour/peridelivery if CS is planned. Women with other types of diabetes will vary in their needs for a sliding scale approach depending on their insulin requirements in the antenatal

Table 22.2 Plan for antenatal assessment and advice for diabetic mothers

Appointment	Care for women with diabetes
First appointment (joint diabetes and antenatal clinic)	Offer information, advice and support in relation to optimising glycaemic control Take a clinical history to establish the extent of diabetes-related complications Review medications for diabetes and its complications Offer retinal and/or renal assessment if these have not been undertaken in the previous 12 months
7–9 weeks	Confirm viability of pregnancy and gestational age
Booking appointment (ideally by 10 weeks)	Discuss information, education and advice about how diabetes will affect the pregnancy, birth and early parenting (such as breastfeeding and initial care of the baby)
16 weeks	Offer retinal assessment at 16–20 weeks to women with pre-existing diabetes who showed signs of diabetic retinopathy at the first antenatal appointment
20 weeks	Offer four-chamber view of the fetal heart and outflow tracts plus scans that would be offered at 18–20 weeks as part of routine antenatal care
28 weeks	Offer ultrasound monitoring of fetal growth and amniotic fluid volume Offer retinal assessment to women with pre-existing diabetes who showed no diabetic retinopathy at their first antenatal clinic visit
32 weeks	Offer ultrasound monitoring of fetal growth and amniotic fluid volume Offer nulliparous women all investigations that would be offered at 32 weeks as part of routine antenatal care
36 weeks	Offer ultrasound monitoring of fetal growth and amniotic fluid volume Offer information and advice about: ● timing, mode and management of birth ● analgesia and anaesthesia ● changes to hypoglycaemic therapy during and after birth ● management of the baby after birth ● initiation of breastfeeding and the effect of breastfeeding on glycaemic control ● contraception and follow-up
38 weeks	Offer induction of labour, or CS if indicated, and start regular tests of fetal wellbeing for women with diabetes who are awaiting spontaneous labour
From 39 weeks	Offer tests of fetal wellbeing if induction of labour is declined

period, and this should be clearly documented in their individual care plan. Those who are not on a sliding scale but who develop a raised glucose stick recording will need to be converted to a sliding scale.

Neonatal care. Babies of women with diabetes should be kept with their mothers unless there is a clinical complication or there are abnormal clinical signs that warrant admission for intensive or special care. Maternity units should have a written policy for the prevention, detection and management of hypoglycaemia in babies of women with diabetes.

Postpartum care. Women with insulin-treated diabetes pre-pregnancy should reduce their insulin immediately after birth back to pre-pregnancy requirements and monitor glucose levels to check or establish the appropriate dose. Women should be informed that they are at increased risk of hypoglycaemia, especially during breastfeeding. Insulin requirement drops rapidly after birth.

Contraception should be discussed.

Gestational diabetes

There are independent risk factors for developing gestational diabetes. NICE recommend testing for diabetes with a glucose tolerance test (GTT) in the following:

- body mass index above 30kg/m^2
- previous macrosomic baby weighing 4.5kg or above
- previous gestational diabetes
- family history of diabetes (first-degree relative with diabetes)
- family origin with a high prevalence of diabetes:
  - South Asian (specifically women whose country of family origin is India, Pakistan or Bangladesh)
  - Black Caribbean
  - Middle Eastern (specifically women whose country of family origin is Saudi Arabia, United Arab Emirates, Iraq, Jordan, Syria, Oman, Qatar, Kuwait, Lebanon or Egypt).

There is no clear consensus in the UK regarding testing for and diagnosing gestational diabetes. NICE recommend the WHO criteria: following a 75 g oral GTT, gestational diabetes exists if fasting glucose >7.0 mmol/l or 2-hour glucose level >7.8 mmol/l. Individual units should establish written policies for testing.

Close collaboration between the obstetric and diabetic teams is required. In most women, gestational diabetes will respond to changes in diet and exercise; 10–20% of women will need oral hypoglycaemic agents or insulin.

Women who were diagnosed with gestational diabetes should be offered lifestyle advice (including weight control, diet and exercise) and offered a fasting plasma glucose measurement (but not an oral glucose tolerance test) at the 6-week postnatal check and annually thereafter.

Neurological emergencies in pregnancy

Some catastrophic neurological emergencies do arise during pregnancy, many of which may be related to previous underlying disease, while some are related to the physiological changes of pregnancy.

The majority of neurological emergencies will present with headaches or seizures, with varying levels of alteration in consciousness from mild confusion to coma. Occasionally, acute problems in the spinal cord or peripheral nerves will give rise to serious concerns.

Problems in diagnosis and management may occur if multidisciplinary team management is not used for these patients. Neurologists and neurosurgeons may not be aware of all the changes occurring in pregnancy that affect the mother, and obstetricians may not appreciate all the complex factors surrounding the neurological conditions. Obstetric physicians (when available) and obstetric anaesthetists may help to bridge this gap.

Headache

Headache has been mentioned in Chapter 4 with major features representing red flag symptoms; these include:

- sudden onset
- associated neck stiffness
- described as 'the worst headache ever'
- any neurological sign on examination.

Headache requiring opiates should always be considered potentially serious. It is unlikely to be a postdural puncture headache (see Table 22.3), and urgent imaging to make a diagnosis should be thought necessary in most circumstances. Multidisciplinary discussion will help decide what imaging is most appropriate for the symptoms involved and the diagnoses suspected.

Table 22.3 Types of headache and confusion in pregnancy with features, investigations and immediate treatment

	Features	Investigation and immediate treatment
Vascular		
Migraine	Usually a preceding history. Can have alarming features suggestive of CVA	• diagnosis of exclusion • involve neurologist if in doubt • consider a low threshold for imaging • pain relief
Subarachnoid haemorrhage	Sudden onset of severe headache; may be hypertensive in response to this event. May have altered conscious level, confusion or coma	• ABC • CT scan • lumbar puncture when appropriate • involve neurologist/ neurosurgeon • interventional radiology for intravascular coiling or surgery
Cerebral thrombosis (arterial thrombosis or haemorrhage)	Headache, fitting or neurological deficit suggestive of CVA. Altered conscious level	• ABC • CT/MRI scan • involve neurologist
Cerebral venous sinus thrombosis	Significant/severe headache Confusion, altered conscious level, coma. Signs of focal neurological dysfunction, e.g. hemiparesis	• CT venogram • MR angiography • involve neurologist • anticoagulation after cerebral haemorrhage excluded
Pre-eclampsia and eclampsia	Pregnancy-related hypertension and proteinuria Features may include: headache, flashing lights, epigastric pain, nausea. Vascular spasm responsible initially although can lead on to cerebral oedema if left untreated	• circumstantial history • ABC • uric acid, renal function, liver function • magnesium sulphate and blood pressure control • (management discussed elsewhere)
Infection		
Meningitis	Headache, neck stiffness, vomiting, photophobia, confusion, altered conscious level, fitting, pyrexia	• blood cultures, FBC, PCR for meningococcal/pneumococcal antigen (remember TB) • lumbar puncture depending on absence of signs of raised intracranial pressure or major clotting problems • antibiotics

Table 22.3 Continued

	Features	Investigation and immediate treatment
Infection (continued)		
Overwhelming sepsis	Confusion due to hypotension or tissue hypoxia. May have fever and other signs of CVS compromise	• ABC • FBC, blood gases to detect metabolic acidosis, blood cultures, U&E, LFT, clotting • involve senior anaesthetic/ICU support • fluids, inotropes, antibiotics
Altered intracranial pressure		
Dural puncture headache (or spontaneous CSF leak)	Follows an epidural or spinal anaesthetic. Occipital/ frontal headache ± neck stiffness; postural headache; can be severe	• diagnosis from history and exclusion of other causes • relieved largely by lying down, so does not require opiate analgesia • inform anaesthetist • blood patch may be offered
Raised intracranial pressure due to tumour, blocked shunt, benign intracranial hypertension	Headache; may be associated with early morning headache and vomiting if cerebral oedema. Altered conscious level if severe. May present with new-onset epilepsy.	• examination of fundi • involve neurologist • CT scan • mannitol in acute emergency • dexamethasone • possible surgery
Epilepsy	Usually known history that can be confusing if other organic cause is also present Careful note from patient or family of unusual features, escalation of fits or other clinical signs	• diagnosis from history • involve neurologist • CT/MRI scan if doubts. • danger from aspiration during fits • ABC • involve anaesthetist for airway management • drug protocol for controlling convulsions if prolonged

Table 22.3 Continued

	Features	Investigation and immediate treatment
Other causes of confusion or altered mental state		
Encephalopathy	Altered mental state for usually metabolic reasons, e.g. liver failure, hyponatraemia Viral hepatitis leading to liver failure Rare causes of congenital metabolic disorders usually associated with hypoglycaemia and metabolic acidosis Rare infections such as viral encephalitis, cerebral malaria.	• check renal and hepatic function, glucose, blood gases and clotting, plasma sodium • blood film • treat as appropriate • involve medical teams • maintain blood glucose • antiviral agents • malarial treatment
Hypoxia	Any respiratory or circulatory disturbance leading to brain hypoxia	• SaO_2 • blood gases • vital signs • CXR • ABC • O_2
Diabetic hypoglycaemia	Confusion, eventually leading to coma if not treated	• blood glucose • give food, dextrose or glucagon as emergency if IV access not available
Diabetic hyperglycaemia/ ketoacidosis	Thirst, dehydration, rapid breathing, abdominal pain, confusion leading to coma if not treated	• blood glucose, arterial blood gas, infection screen • fluids/insulin/glucose (see Chapter 22)
Acute intermittent porphyria (inherited enzyme disorder)	Seizures, confusion, quadriparesis (peripheral motor neuropathy) abdominal pain, hypertension (autonomic involvement)	• urine testing for porphobilinogen • sodium levels as hyponatraemia may occur • can be provoked by drugs used for seizures so resistant status epilepticus may occur • high glucose load required • haematin (derived from red blood cells) corrects metabolic fault
Psychiatric causes		
Puerperal psychosis or pre-pregnancy known morbidity Drugs or alcohol	Altered and often paranoid behaviour	• exclude organic causes • involve psychiatric team • awareness of suicide risk • high-level supervision of mother and baby

Diagnosis

In many of the above conditions, an urgent brain scan may be required. MRI has added much useful information to the diagnosis of acute brain conditions and avoids the need for imaging with radiation. However, it should be remembered that for antenatal women in the third trimester in particular, some attempt should be made to tilt the pelvis to avoid aorto-caval compression. Many pregnant women near term find supine lying extremely unpleasant and may find the position required to achieve a scan very difficult if this effort is not made.

CT scan can be achieved with reduced dose to the baby by effective abdominal shielding (see Chapter 4, Appendix: Radiology in the pregnant woman).

Iodinated radiological contrast media and gadolinium contrast media both cross the placenta and the effects on the fetus are not clear. It is therefore recommended that these modalities are avoided unless the risks to the mother are greater, and informed consent is obtained where possible.

Seizures

Many of the illnesses in Table 22.3 could have a seizure as part of their presentation. The majority of women who fit during pregnancy will be known to have epilepsy. New-onset epilepsy during pregnancy is likely to require further investigation.

The common differential diagnosis is eclampsia with all its other associated features. In the absence of these features, the possibilities include metabolic disturbances such as hypoglycaemia, intoxicating drugs, space-occupying lesions, infective illnesses such as meningitis or cerebral malaria or an underlying vascular accident such as venous sinus thrombosis. Even a faint or vasovagal event can be associated with a brief convulsive episode.

Management of status epilepticus

Up to 30% of women with known epilepsy may experience an increase in fits during pregnancy, possibly due to altered pharmacokinetics of the anticonvulsant medication in pregnancy, or due to poor compliance with treatment.

Status epilepticus is fairly rare during pregnancy as most convulsions are self-limiting. Standard treatment should be used, with the added urgency of establishing a left lateral position to reduce both the risk of acid aspiration and aortocaval compression. A prolonged seizure may lead to hypoxia and acidosis, both of which will be a risk for both mother and baby. Maintaining an airway, avoiding further physical harm, giving oxygen and the use of intravenous anticonvulsants may all be needed. Any seizure longer than 5–10 minutes should be terminated as quickly as possible, as outcome is related to the length of seizure.

Fetal monitoring should be started when feasible, as both fetal distress related to acidosis or even placental abruption may occur due to any trauma sustained.

If the diagnosis is not clear, then consideration needs to be made as to choice of the first-line drug, magnesium sulphate in eclampsia and lorazepam in known epilepsy. It will be important to check for metabolic causes, in particular blood glucose and sodium levels, followed by neuroimaging when the mother is stable, to help with diagnosis.

In the event of the clinician being unable to access a vein for giving intravenous anticonvulsants for a prolonged seizure, the buccal (or nasal if there is much salivation) or rectal routes can be considered. A preparation of midazolam for buccal or nasal use is available, but not licensed. The intravenous preparation of midazolam can also be used, but is similarly not licensed. The dose is 10 mg and the onset of action is within minutes. Rectal diazepam is a licensed preparation and available in 2.5 ml tubes of rectal solution containing the dose of 10 mg. Its onset of action is similar to midazolam. When treating any patient with benzodizepines for seizures, monitor respiration and intervene with bag/mask support in the event of apnoea or hypoventilation. These respiratory events are usually short lived, but anaesthetic help should be gained.

If the fit is prolonged, or treatment with benzodiazepines affects the respiratory efforts or mental state of the mother, then early help should be sought from the anaesthetic team. They may need to induce anaesthesia to both control the convulsion and protect the airway by the use of rapid sequence induction using thiopental.

Other causes of headache

Postdural puncture headache

If a woman has received an epidural or spinal anaesthetic during labour or delivery, a postpartum headache is commonly attributed to these. However, care must be taken not to miss other organic causes of headache, with particular reference to the red flag symptoms, which will not be present in a postdural puncture headache. As mentioned earlier, a need for opiates for a postdural puncture headache should signal concern.

The postdural puncture headache characteristically comes on in the first 24–72 hours following the procedure (see also Chapter 38). It can be almost immediate, or delayed for up to a week. It is usually a frontal or occipital headache. It may be described as a very sudden onset headache leading to confusion with a subarachnoid haemorrhage, but should be relieved by lying down. It may be described as neck pain rather than a headache.

Other symptoms can include double vision and difficulty hearing, described as 'hearing as though underwater'. Nausea or vomiting may occur and it is worth trying anti-emetics, as well as ensuring an adequate fluid intake, as the headache will be worsened by dehydration. There is no benefit in trying to overcome the headache by being upright.

Further management should be guided by the senior obstetric anaesthetist, who may choose to obtain a neurological opinion. Various treatments aimed at relieving postdural puncture headache have been tried, such as caffeine, and antimigraine analgesia such as sumatriptan, which is safe in breastfeeding mothers.

The headache is caused by CSF leakage through the hole in the dura into the epidural space, resulting in a lower pressure inside the CSF, so-called 'low-pressure headache' syndrome. In the acute stage, there are no diagnostic features seen on MRI scan and the diagnosis is usually made clinically. It is mostly a self-limiting headache, settling within 10 days to 2 weeks, but may involve spending a large amount of time lying down, which has obvious disadvantages for both looking after a new baby, and also the requirement for thromboprophylaxis in a nonmobile mother.

Rare complications can include subdural haematoma, thought to be caused by the stretching of the bridging veins as the brain sags when upright. It is important for follow up to occur until the headache is resolved, and the mother to be encouraged to report any change in characteristics of the headache or any newly occurring neurological signs. Such changes might be an indication for investigation by neuroimaging.

An epidural blood patch may be used to treat the headache, as advised by the anaesthetist. Obstetric and anaesthetic staff will need to coordinate over timing of thromboprophylaxis to allow this procedure to occur.

Cerebral venous sinus thrombosis

This may present with an insidious headache, seizure, altered level of consciousness, neurological symptoms and signs, or as an acute cerebrovascular accident or 'stroke'. A high index of suspicion is needed, as symptoms may be vague.

Diagnosis has increased in recent years, probably due to improvements in imaging. Most cerebral venous sinus thrombosis occurs postpartum, although any thrombosis may be a feature at any stage of pregnancy. Risk factors include any factors leading to dehydration, plus specific thrombophilias.

Diagnosis is best with MRI including MRV and MRA (venography and angiography). Treatment will usually involve anticoagulation and supportive therapy, although more recent advances in interventional radiology have used localised thrombolysis via a catheter in the superior sagittal sinus.

Meningitis

Diagnosis will be similar to the nonpregnant woman with regard to presentation of fever, headache, possible seizure or confusion leading to deteriorating levels of consciousness.

A rare iatrogenic risk in pregnancy relates to the breach of the dura with the use of spinal anaesthesia or accidental dural tap during epidural placement. Any breach of the dura has the potential for introducing infection into the CSF, leading to meningitis. From the case reports, onset may be very rapid, but recovery does also appear rapid if effective antibiotics are given. Serious morbidity and death have also been reported. It is important to realise that the anaesthetic procedure may be the source of the organism, as this may aid the neurologist/ microbiologist in choosing the correct tests to identify an organism, and guide the choice of antibiotic therapy. In particular, *S. salivarius* has been found responsible in these circumstances, and may require an unusual choice of antibiotics taking into account the current spectrum of antibiotic resistance to this organism, as well as the usual more commonly recognised pathogens.

Intracranial neoplasms

Although there is no specific link between pregnancy and brain tumours, most brain tumours will expand during pregnancy, either because of the overall increase in extracellular fluid which worsens oedema around the lesion, or because some tumours have hormonal receptors. In particular, meningiomas and acoustic neuromas, which are characteristically slow growing, may have oestrogen or progesterone receptors, or both, which will encourage a more rapid expansion in the hormone rich environment of pregnancy. The classic presenting features of headache, nausea and vomiting may be ascribed to 'early morning sickness', 'hyperemesis' or, later in pregnancy, confused with pre-eclampsia. Features such as a new-onset seizure without other features suggestive of pre-eclampsia, or focal neurological deficit should prompt urgent neuroimaging.

Steroids can be used urgently to reduce tumour oedema. Anticonvulsants may be required. Further management may be conservative or operative, includes consideration of best timing for delivery and will depend on a balance of risks to both the mother and fetus. In particular:

- diagnostic difficulties concerning ionising radiation, and the relative contraindications to the use of contrast media for accurate imaging in both CT scans and MRI imaging during pregnancy (see Chapter 4 Appendix – Radiology in the pregnant woman)
- surgical success may be better after embolisation of the tumour, again requiring interventional radiography
- aggressive tumours will need to be treated sooner
- many less-aggressive tumours would regress in the puerperium as the hormonal levels drop, allowing easier surgical treatment
- delivery may need to take into account the need to avoid raising the intracranial pressure further due to pain or pushing at delivery
- anaesthesia has risks due to inability to perform regional anaesthesia in the face of raised intracranial pressure, but the known rise in intracranial pressure associated with intubation requires careful management when combined with the requirement for rapid sequence induction.

Cerebral malaria

Plasmodium falciparum, the causative protozoan, is mainly seen in the tropics, but travellers from nonimmune areas are vulnerable, and may present on return to their own country. Women may present with high fever, rigors and headache leading on to drowsiness, seizures and coma. Investigations will show the parasite in the blood film with severe anaemia due to haemolysis and thrombocytopenia. Further progression may lead to liver and renal impairment and ARDS. Supportive intensive care may be needed together with intravenous quinine. Mortality from this severe infection is high.

Summary

- Women with pre-existing disease of any sort should have pre-pregnancy counselling about the risks of pregnancy to themselves and their infants.
- Women with pre-existing disease and those in whom disease develops during pregnancy should have easy and timely access to multidisciplinary clinics for the management and planning of their pregnancy and labour to achieve the best outcome both for themselves and for their infants.
- Clinical staff caring for pregnant and labouring women should be aware of 'red flag signs', make and record appropriate observations and consult early with seniors and specialists when problems arise.
- Pregnancy and labour are a time of risk for women with pre-existing disease and for those who develop new illnesses in the vulnerability of pregnancy. The prevention of unnecessary morbidity and mortality is best achieved by careful observation and communication between the woman and her clinicians and then prompt, close multidisciplinary partnership working by relevant clinical teams in the event of emergencies.

References and further reading

General

1 *Saving Mothers' Lives*: Reviewing maternal deaths to make motherhood safer: 2006–2008. *BJOG*: 2011; 118:1–203.

2 Lewis, G (ed.) The Confidential Enquiry into Maternal and Child Health (CEMACH). *Saving Mothers' Lives: reviewing maternal deaths to make motherhood safer – 2003–2005. The Seventh Report on Confidential Enquiries into Maternal Deaths in the United Kingdom.* London: CEMACH 2007.

Cardiac

3 Pearson GD, Veille JC, Rahimtoola S, *et al.* Peripartum Cardiomyopathy National Heart, Lung, and Blood Institute and Office of Rare Diseases (National Institutes of Health) Workshop Recommendations and Review. *JAMA* 2000;283:1183–8.

4 The Task Force on the Management of Cardiovascular Diseases during Pregnancy of the European Society of Cardiology. Expert consensus document on management of cardiovascular diseases during pregnancy. *Eur Heart J* 2003;24:761–81.

5 Rossiter JP, Repke JT, Morales AJ, *et al.* A prospective longitudinal evaluation of pregnancy in the Marfan syndrome. *Am J Obstet Gynecol* 1995;173:1599–1606.

6 Lipscomb KJ, Smith JC, Clarke B, *et al.* Outcome of pregnancy in women with Marfan syndrome. *BJOG* 1997;104:201–6.

7 Hameed A, Karaalp IS, Tummala PP, *et al.* The effect of valvular heart disease on maternal and fetal outcome of pregnancy. *J Am Coll Cardiol* 2001;37:893–9.

8 Hanania G. Management of anticoagulants during pregnancy. *Heart* 2001;86:125–6.

9 McLintock C, McCowan L, North R. Maternal complications and pregnancy outcome in women with mechanical prosthetic heart valves treated with enoxaparin. *BJOG* 2009;116:1585–92.

10 RCOG. *Cardiac Disease in Pregnancy. Good practice No 13.* London: RCOG 2011.

Diabetic

11 Workshop report. Diabetes Care and Research in Europe: The Saint Vincent Declaration. *Diabetic Med* 1990:7;360.

12 *Confidential Enquiry into Maternal and Child Health. Diabetes in Pregnancy: Are we providing the best care? Findings of a national enquiry. England, Wales and Northern Ireland.* London: CEMACH 2007.

13 Department of Health. *National Service Framework for Diabetes Standards.* London: COI 2001.

14 National Institute for Health and Clinical Excellence. *Diabetes in Pregnancy: Management of diabetes and its complications from pre-conception to the postnatal period.* London: NICE 2008.

15 Black RS, Gillmer MDG. Diabetes in pregnancy. *The Obstetrician & Gynaecologist* 2003;5:143–8.

16 Fraser R. Achieving euglycaemia in pregnancy: evidence based management. *The Obstetrician & Gynaecologist* 2011;13:149–53.

17 Kamalakannan D, Baskar V, Barton DM, Abdu TAM. Diabetic ketoacidoisis in pregnancy. *Postgrad Med J* 2003;79:454–7.

Neurological

18 Karnad DR, Guntupalli KK. Neurologic disorders in pregnancy. *Crit Care Med* 2005:10;S362–71.

19 Lowe SA, Sen RC. Neurological disease in pregnancy. *Obstetrics, Gynaecology and Reproductive Medicine* 18:7; 187–92.

20 Alvis SA, Hicks RJ. Pregnancy-induced acute neurological emergencies and neurologic conditions encountered in pregnancy. *Semin Ultrasound CT MR.* 2012;33(1):46–54.

21 Basurto Ona X, Martínez García L, Solà I, Bonfill Cosp X. Drug therapy for treating post-dural puncture headache. *Cochrane Database Syst Rev* 2011;(8):CD007887.

CHAPTER 23

Perinatal psychiatric illness

Objectives

On successfully completing this topic, you will be able to:

- acknowledge the prevalence of mental health problems in the pregnant population
- recognise the importance of identifying the at-risk woman
- be aware of the need for team working with mental health teams
- be prepared for the onset of acute mental health problems after delivery
- understand the effects on the infant of maternal mental health medications and the need to collaborate with other specialties, both in pregnancy and after birth.

Introduction

Mental health problems are common in the community at large, with an incidence of at least 20%. The most common mental health problems are mixed anxiety and depression. Women are at least twice as likely to suffer from these conditions as men and they are most prevalent among younger women with children under the age of 5 years. Serious mental illnesses, such as schizophrenia and bipolar disorder (manic depressive illness), are less common, with a prevalence of approximately 1% for each condition and are no more common in women than in men.

Mental health problems in pregnancy

Conception rates in women with mental disorder (with the exception of severe learning disability and anorexia nervosa) are the same as the general population. Antenatal depression and anxiety are therefore common and as common as after delivery, affecting 10–20% of all women. In addition, women with personality disorders, panic disorder, obsessive compulsive disorder, psychoses, substance misuse and eating disorders will become pregnant.

The incidence (new onset) of serious mental illness (schizophrenia, psychoses and bipolar disorder) during pregnancy is markedly reduced compared with other times. However, serious mental illness does sometimes occur for the first time during pregnancy and poses particular management problems. A more frequent situation is that of a woman who already has a chronic serious mental illness and becomes pregnant. Approximately two per 1000 births are to women with chronic serious mental illness. Pregnancy is not protective against a relapse of these conditions, particularly if patients stop taking their medication. However, continuing medication may pose problems for management during labour and for the care of the newborn, and a careful risk–benefit analysis must be undertaken before any decision is made whether to continue or not.

Mental health problems after delivery

By contrast, there is a dramatic increase in the incidence of serious affective illness following delivery. Women face a relative risk of 32 of developing a psychotic illness in the first 3 months following delivery. These illnesses are thought to belong to the bipolar group of illnesses. There is also an increased risk (relative risk 10) of developing a severe unipolar depressive illness. There is no increase in risk of developing schizophrenia. Women who have a previous history of bipolar illness, schizoaffective disorder, puerperal psychosis or severe postnatal depression (PND) have at least a 50% risk of recurrence of this condition following delivery, even if they have been well for many years and are in comfortable social circumstances. Fifty percent of puerperal psychoses will have presented by day 7, 75% by day 14 and all by 42 days. Women without a personal history but with a family history of bipolar illness, particularly if it is of postpartum onset or who have a first-degree relative who has had a puerperal psychosis, also face an elevated risk of developing a serious mental illness following delivery.

These serious postpartum mental illnesses, which become manifest in the early days following delivery, are life threatening. Although the early symptoms can be nonspecific (e.g. insomnia, irritability and/or agitation), women can very quickly become acutely disturbed, very frightened and bewildered, and the illness poses a risk both to their physical health and safety. They require urgent psychiatric assessment and treatment and should be admitted to a mother and baby unit rather than to a general psychiatry ward.

Severe, but nonpsychotic, depressive illness tends to develop more gradually and present later in the first 12 weeks following delivery. While it benefits from specialist psychiatric care, it can frequently be managed at home with the usual treatments for severe depressive illness, modified by whether or not the woman is breastfeeding.

The more common mild to moderate depressive illness, often associated with marked features of anxiety (PND), is in fact no more common following childbirth than in women who have not given birth. These conditions usually present later in the postpartum year, after 3months, and are best managed in primary care involving the local Improving Access to Psychological Treatment Service (or equivalent) where appropriate. For these conditions, psychosocial treatments are often as effective as antidepressants.

Confidential Enquiries into Maternal Deaths

The triennial reports of the CEMD over the period from 1997 to 2005 revealed that if late deaths are included, then up to 25% of maternal deaths were caused by psychiatric disorder and 15% by suicide, with suicide identified as the leading cause of maternal death in the UK. The 2006–08 report only includes late deaths up to 6 months, so direct comparisons cannot be made with previous figures. This most recent report also highlighted the fact that many of the psychiatric deaths that occurred took place shortly after a child protection case conference, or a child being removed into care, and a third of the women who committed suicide, and half of the women who were substance misusers, appeared to be avoiding maternity care. Furthermore, substandard care associated with psychiatric deaths is present in approximately 50% of patients.

The most important findings from these enquiries for obstetricians and midwives are:

1 Women who died from suicide were in the main older, more socially advantaged and better educated than in other causes of maternal death. Suicide is not associated with the same socio-economic factors as other causes of maternal death.

2 The majority were seriously mentally ill before they died. They had been well during pregnancy and developed either a puerperal psychosis, or very severe depressive illness. Over 50% of these women had had a previous episode requiring inpatient psychiatric treatment, even though they had been well for some time before giving birth. This identifiable risk factor had, in the majority of cases, neither been identified at booking, nor had the management of this risk been planned during pregnancy. Both psychiatric and maternity services had failed to take the opportunity to anticipate the risk following delivery. The rapid deterioration of a sudden onset illness appears to have taken all by surprise.

3 There was little evidence of communication taking place between psychiatric and maternity teams and the lack of planning was reflected in the lack of information that was passed between involved professionals.

4 The remainder of the psychiatric deaths, those not due to suicide, were due to women dying from physical illness that could either be directly attributable to their psychiatric disorder (in half the cases, the consequences of alcohol or drug misuse) or because their life-threatening illness was missed or misattributed to psychiatric disorder. Obstetricians and midwives are reminded that serious physical illness can present as, complicate, or coexist with, psychiatric disorder.

5 Women who are substance misusers should have integrated specialist care. They should not be managed solely by their GP or midwife. Integrated care should include addiction professionals, child safeguarding and specialist midwifery and obstetric care. Care of the mother should continue once a child has been removed.

Implications for obstetric practice

The long-standing knowledge of the epidemiology and distinctive clinical features of perinatal psychiatric disorder, together with the findings of the CMACE, provide the evidence base for obstetric and midwifery practice and for the psychiatric care of pregnant and post-partum women.

1. All women with serious mental illness, and those taking psychotropic medication, should discuss with their general practitioner, psychiatrist or obstetrician their plans for becoming pregnant, with regard to the risks to their mental health and the risks to the developing fetus of their medication. Specialist perinatal mental health services offer pre-conceptual counselling and advice.
2. All women should be asked in a systematic and sensitive way about their previous, as well as current, psychiatric history at booking in early pregnancy. These questions should be structured so that those with a previous or current history of serious mental illness, previous psychiatric care and/or admission can be identified. Those responsible for booking should receive training to enable them to distinguish between serious psychiatric disorders and common mental health problems.
3. Women with serious mental health problems currently, or those with a past history of a serious psychiatric disorder, should have a written management plan shared between the woman, the general practitioner, obstetrician and psychiatrist, with regard to her peripartum management and the management of her risk in the early weeks following delivery.
4. Women with serious mental health problems complicating pregnancy and the early postpartum period should have access to a specialist psychiatrist in perinatal mental health, supported by a specialist multidisciplinary team and if this is not available, to general psychiatric services.
5. In child protection cases, while the needs of the child must remain paramount, extra support and vigilance is needed for the mother and communication between all agencies involved in her care is essential. Further efforts are required to retain women who are substance misusers in treatment programmes after their child has been removed. Social workers should liaise with, and refer pregnant women in their care to, the local maternity services if necessary.

Despite many national recommendations, specialist perinatal mental health teams have yet to be developed in the majority of maternity localities and there are insufficient mother and baby units in the UK to ensure equity of access for all. In addition, both the psychiatric and maternity professions have yet to fully acknowledge and implement the need for screening and proactive management of this high-risk group of women. Therefore, sadly, midwives and obstetricians will still be presented with women in late pregnancy and shortly after delivery, with serious psychiatric disorders who have not been previously identified, as well as those who develop illnesses at this time that could not have been anticipated.

Management of well 'at-risk' women

The well 'at-risk' woman will have been well often for many years, but will have a previous history of either puerperal psychosis or severe PND or a previous episode of bipolar illness. She may not have been in contact with psychiatric services for some time, will not be taking any medication and may be in very comfortable social circumstances and well educated. Ideally, she should have been detected at the booking clinic and should have been seen by a specialist psychiatrist during pregnancy. The risk of a recurrence of the condition and a management plan should have been drawn up during pregnancy. However, often this has not happened and the risk may be identified only in late pregnancy or on admission to the labour suite.

There are no particular management concerns during labour. If no management plan is in place then the risk of recurrence of the puerperal psychosis or bipolar illness should be explained to the woman and her family. She should be seen by the psychiatrist serving the maternity hospital as soon as possible following delivery, preferably before she is discharged. The maximum risk of a recurrence of the condition is in the first 2 weeks following delivery, so early contact is essential. The minimum requirement will be that the community midwife and GP are alerted and that, together with the psychiatric team, the woman's mental health should be closely monitored over the first 6 weeks following delivery. Ideally, there should be a specialist perinatal mental health team involved, but these are not available to all maternity services. The psychiatrist may consider using prophylactic medication, such as lithium carbonate or an antipsychotic (small dose of typical or atypical antipsychotic), if this is acceptable to the woman. In these circumstances she should not breastfeed. The evidence for the prophylactic effect of antidepressants is less strong, but many women may wish to consider it.

Management of women with chronic severe mental illness

Women with chronic severe mental illness are usually still under the care of psychiatric services. They may be suffering from either chronic schizophrenia and receiving antipsychotic medication, or from recurrent bipolar illness and receiving mood stabilisers, antidepressants or antipsychotic medication. Ideally, these women should not present unannounced. There should have been frequent communication and joint management during the pregnancy, consideration given to the choice of medication and its management during pregnancy. There should also be clear, written management plans for both the peripartum period and for her care following delivery.

Women with bipolar illness may be taking lithium carbonate or other mood stabilisers. The haemodynamics of later pregnancy and increased clearance of lithium may well have resulted in increasing oral doses of lithium in order to maintain a therapeutic lithium level (0.6–0.9 mmol/l) during pregnancy. During labour, this situation will alter and the woman will need a reduction of her dose of lithium and frequent monitoring of her serum lithium levels, at least twice in 24 hours during labour and daily for the first 3–4 days following delivery, to guard against increasing levels and the possibility of lithium toxicity (levels higher than 1.5 mmol/l). Following delivery, the dosage of lithium carbonate will need to be reinstated at her usual prepregnancy dose. The neonatal paediatricians will need to be alerted.

Many women with bipolar disorder will be taking an anticonvulsant mood stabiliser as an alternative to lithium. The most common preparation in use for the management of bipolar illness is divalproex semisodium. Despite clear guidance, from the National Institute for Health and Clinical Excellence, on the management of both epilepsy and bipolar disorder – that sodium valproate should not be used in pregnancy and in women of reproductive age, unless there is no reasonable alternative – this situation still arises. The neonatal paediatrician should be alerted. Following delivery, the dose of sodium valproate should be adjusted back to the prepregnancy dose and continued, because of the high risk of a relapse of the bipolar disorder following delivery. If the woman wishes to breastfeed, then sodium valproate, or other antiepileptic mood stabiliser, should be given in divided dosage and the infant monitored for drowsiness and rashes.

A variety of antipsychotic medications may be taken by women with chronic serious mental illness. Some will still be taking the older antipsychotics (such as trifluoperazine and haloperidol). These preparations do not appear to be associated either with an increased risk of major congenital abnormalities or any particular problems during pregnancy. Most women will be taking atypical antipsychotics (including olanzapine, quetiapine, risperidone and aripiprazole). There are fewer data available on these newer drugs. There is a potential concern that olanzapine may be associated with an increased risk of gestational diabetes. In an ideal world, these concerns will have been discussed by the psychiatrist and obstetricians prior to delivery and consideration given to switching medication and the possibility of tapering before delivery. If this has not happened, the neonatal paediatricians will need to be alerted because of the possibility of withdrawal effects in the infant. Following delivery, the prepregnancy dose will need to be reinstated because of the risk of relapse postpartum.

Many women, both those suffering from serious mental illness and milder mental illness, are taking antidepressants during pregnancy. These may be the older tricyclic antidepressants (e.g. imipramine or amitriptyline), but most will be taking selective serotonin re-uptake inhibitors (SSRIs) such as paroxetine, citalopram and fluoxetine or some newer drugs such as venlafaxine, reboxetine, duloxetine and mirtazepine. There has been some concern that antidepressants may be associated with an increased risk of ventricular septal defect and pulmonary hyperplasia with first-trimester exposure. There is more robust evidence that their use at term is associated with the neonatal adaptation syndrome. Previously, if time allowed and the woman's mental health was stable, tapering the dose of antidepressants prior to delivery was considered. However, recent data have shown that this does not reduce the incidence of neonatal adaptation syndrome. In either case, the neonate should be observed for withdrawal symptoms. Following delivery, the maternal medication should be continued.

Labour ward crises

True psychiatric emergencies occurring in the labour ward are extremely uncommon. Women with chronic serious mental illness who are under the care of psychiatric teams should probably be accompanied during labour by a familiar mental healthcare professional if they are frightened, unable to fully comprehend what is happening to them or if they are symptomatic. Women who are well, but at risk because of a previous history, should be managed as other women are, but attention paid following delivery to their need for close surveillance in the early postpartum period. If a woman's mental health is predicted to be likely to be unstable around delivery, consider discussing advance directives during pregnancy when her mental state is stable.

Occasionally, acute episodes of distress may occur in women either in early labour or in the minutes and hours following delivery. These acute episodes of distress will usually be understandable (if not proportional) to the contextual meaning of events or procedures in the light of previous experience. Examples would be: previous sexual abuse, previous experience of a traumatic delivery or loss of a baby, misattribution of sensations or procedures, to name but a few. Women will be more vulnerable to the possibility of this occurring if they have previous experience of panic attacks, if they cannot speak English or if they are frightened for a wide variety of reasons.

The overwhelming majority of these situations will respond to calm kindness and reassurance. However, some women will be suffering from panic attacks. These will usually be evident because of hyperventilation and are associated with feelings of imminent disaster, a fear of dying or suffocation, losing control or even imminent insanity. Panic attacks are the great imitators. The CMACE describes individual cases where women with cardiac and respiratory disease were mistaken for panic attacks, but, conversely, panic attacks can be mistaken for pulmonary embolus and other physical emergencies. Swift differential diagnosis is therefore necessary. In many cases, encouragement to control hyperventilation would be sufficient, together with an explanation to the woman of what is happening to her. However, on other occasions, *after excluding physical disease*, it may be necessary to use a short-acting benzodiazepine tranquilliser. Lorazepam 0.5–1.0 mg is best suited to use in labour because of its swift action and short duration.

Neonatal paediatrician

The neonatal paediatrician needs to be alerted in the following circumstances:

1 Lithium – Infants born to mothers taking lithium during pregnancy are at increased risk of suffering from cardiac abnormalities. Ebstein's anomaly is rare (approximately 2 per 1000 exposed pregnancies), but other cardiac abnormalities are more common (up to 10% of all exposed pregnancies). Continuing use throughout pregnancy is associated with an increased risk of: hypothyroidism; large-weight infants; nephrogenic diabetes insipidus; and the floppy baby syndrome following delivery.

2 Sodium valproate – Infants born to mothers taking sodium valproate are at increased risk of: neural tube defects; fetal valproate syndrome; and cardiac abnormalities following first trimester exposure. Continuing use throughout pregnancy is associated with an increased risk of neurodevelopmental and cognitive problems in later childhood.

3 Antipsychotic medication – Infants born to mothers receiving antipsychotic medication may experience withdrawal symptoms, jitteriness and convulsions, as well as short-term and reversible extrapyramidal symptoms if taking atypical antipsychotics.

4 Antidepressants – Infants born to mothers receiving tricyclic antidepressants at full therapeutic dosage may be at risk of withdrawal symptoms, neonatal jitteriness and convulsions, as well as anticholinergic adverse effects.

5 Infants born to mothers receiving SSRI medication may experience: withdrawal effects; jitteriness; irritability; feeding difficulties and problems maintaining blood sugar and temperature.

Summary

- Most perinatal psychiatric crises can be predicted and avoided by identification of potential psychiatric problems in early pregnancy, proactive management and collaborative perinatal management plans between psychiatry and obstetrics.
- Occasionally crises and emergencies do arise during labour and more frequently in the early days following delivery. The effective management of these requires the rapid response of a specialist perinatal mental health team.
- The possibility of neonatal consequences of maternal psychiatric medication needs to be borne in mind following delivery.

Further reading

1 Henshaw C, Cox J, Barton, J. *Modern Management of Perinatal Psychiatric Disorders.* London: RCPsych Publications 2009.

2 Lewis G (editor). *The Confidential Enquiry into Maternal and Child Health (CEMACH). Saving Mothers' Lives: Reviewing Maternal Deaths to make Motherhood Safer — 2003–2005. The Seventh Report on Confidential Enquiries into Maternal Deaths in the United Kingdom.* London: CEMACH 2007.

3 Centre for Maternal and Child Enquiries (CMACE). Saving Mothers' Lives: reviewing maternal deaths to make motherhood safer: 2006–08. The Eighth Report on Confidential Enquiries into Maternal Deaths in the United Kingdom. *BJOG* 2011;118(Suppl. 1):1–203.

4 National Institute for Health and Clinical Excellence. *Antenatal and Postnatal Mental Health.* London: NICE 2007.

5 Royal College of Obstetricians and Gynaecologists. *Management of Women with Mental Health Issues during Pregnancy and the Postnatal Period. Good Practice No.14.* London: RCOG 2011.

6 Scottish Inter-Collegiate Guidelines Network. *Guideline 127: Management of Perinatal Mood Disorders.* Glasgow: Scottish Inter-Collegiate Network, 2012.

SECTION 6

Obstetric emergencies

ALGORITHM 24.1 Pre-eclampsia/eclampsia

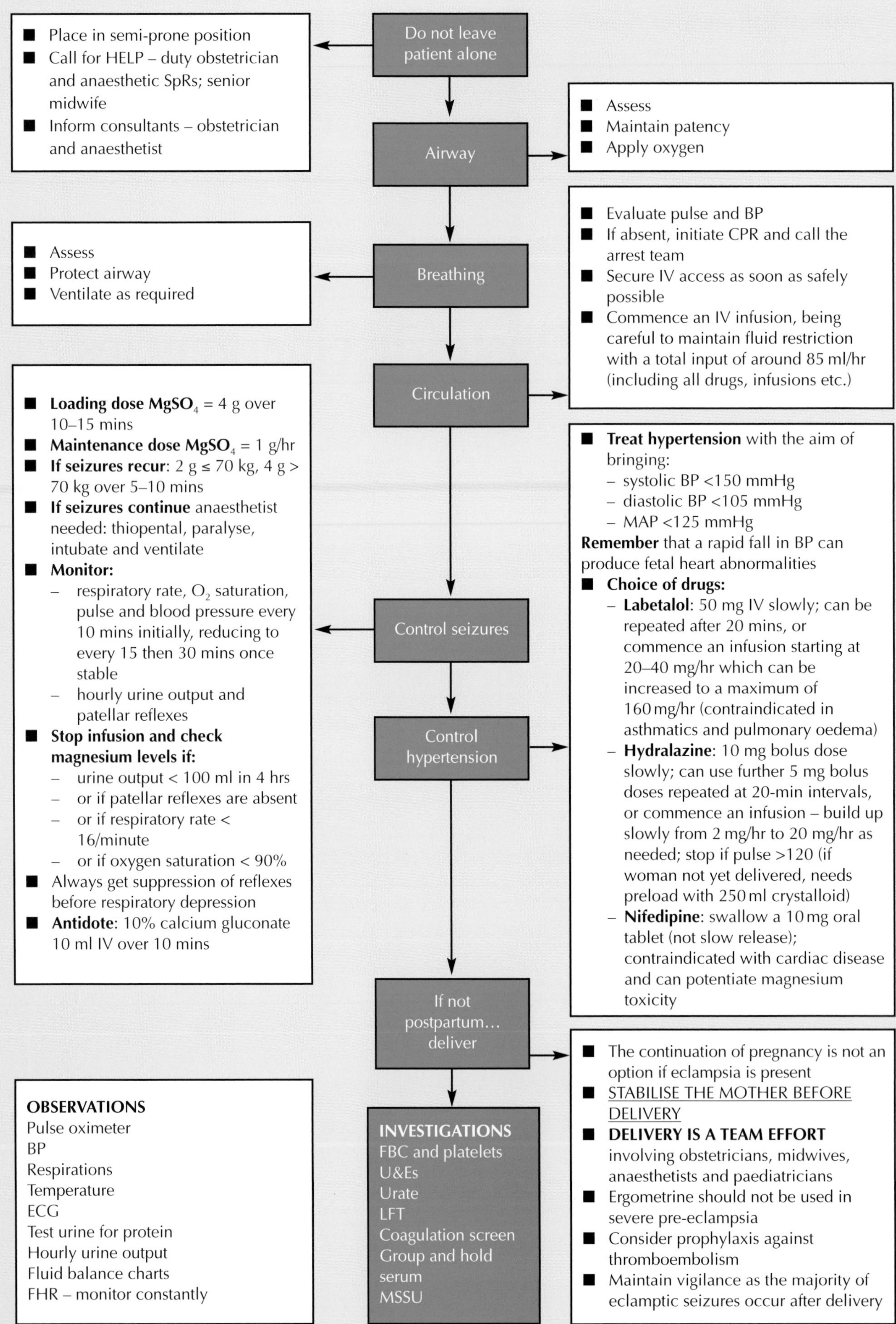

CHAPTER 24

Pre-eclampsia and eclampsia

Objectives

On successfully completing this topic, you will be able to:

- understand the management of severe hypertension in pregnancy
- prevent and treat eclamptic fits
- manage fluid balance in pre-eclampsia/eclampsia
- investigate, recognise and treat the complications of the condition.

Introduction

Definitions: pre-eclampsia and eclampsia

Pre-eclampsia is pregnancy-induced hypertension in association with proteinuria or oedema or both. Virtually any organ system may be effected.

The Magpie trial defined severe pre-eclampsia as:

- diastolic blood pressure greater than 110 mmHg on two occasions or systolic blood pressure greater than 170 mmHg on two occasions and proteinuria greater than 3+ or
- diastolic blood pressure greater than 100 mmHg on two occasions and proteinuria greater than 2+ and at least two signs or symptoms of imminent eclampsia.

Eclampsia is defined as the occurrence of one or more convulsions during pregnancy or the first 10 days postpartum, together with at least two of the following features within 24 hours of the convulsions:

- hypertension
- proteinuria
- thrombocytopenia
- elevated liver enzymes.

HELLP (haemolysis, elevated liver enzymes and low platelets) syndrome is an important variant of pre-eclampsia. Strictly, a diagnosis of HELLP syndrome needs confirmation of haemolysis, either by measuring lactate dehydrogenase (LDH) levels, as commonly carried out in the US, or by blood film to look for fragmented red cells. Alanine aminotransferase (ALT) levels above 75IU/l are seen as significant and levels above 150 IU/l are associated with increased morbidity to the mother. The platelet count should be below 100 x 10^9/litre to support the diagnosis.

Epidemiology

Eclampsia rates have fallen since the introduction of magnesium sulphate. The UK Obstetric Surveillance study in 2005 reported a rate of 2.7 cases per 10 000 births, compared with 4.9 cases per 10,000 births in the 1992 survey. There were no deaths in the 2005 study. Sixty-three percent of the women did not have established pre-eclampsia, and over 20% had their first fits at home.

However, the latest CMACE report identified 19 deaths from pre-eclampsia and eclampsia. Fourteen died from cerebral causes, five of these were directly associated with eclamptic seizures. Particular areas of care highlighted for improvement were:

- control of systolic hypertension (aim for <150 mmHg)
- management of the third stage as three women developed hypertension after administration of syntometrine.

Management of severe pre-eclampsia and eclampsia

The general principles are outlined below.

Senior and multidisciplinary involvement including:

- obstetrician
- midwife
- anaesthetist
- haematologist
- intensivist
- paediatrician.

All must be working to a standardised pattern of management (guidelines) that should only be deviated from rarely and then only by senior staff (consultants) and should undertake:

- regular review of all parameters with an awareness of complications
- prompt control of hypertension (especially systolic)
- meticulous fluid balance to avoid iatrogenic fluid overload
- seizure prophylaxis.

Note: Automated blood pressure recording systems can systematically underestimate blood pressure in pre-eclampsia, to a serious degree. Blood pressure values should be compared at the beginning of treatment, with those obtained by conventional sphygmomanometers and, if different, manual recording should be made subsequently.

Symptoms and signs

Pre-eclampsia is a multisystem disorder and its clinical presentation reflects this. Awareness of the complications (see Table 24.1) that can occur allows anticipation and prompt management.

The following should raise concern:

- headache, visual disturbances
- vomiting, epigastric pain
- nondependent (especially facial) or pulmonary oedema
- right upper-quadrant or epigastric abdominal tenderness
- recently developed hypertension greater than 160/110 mmHg with proteinuria greater than 1g in 24 hours
- hyper-reflexia with clonus
- rapidly changing biochemical/haematological picture.

Initial assessment of the woman

Antenatal history

A major aim of antenatal care is to detect women at risk of or with early signs of pre-eclampsia and increase the level of care. The Pre-eclampsia Community Guideline (PRECOG) emphasises the importance of investigating women with either new hypertension or new proteinuria.[1]

Table 24.1 Complications of pre-eclampsia/eclampsia

Maternal	Fetal
Severe hypertension	Prematurity
Risk of cerebrovascular accident	Intrauterine growth restriction
Oliguria, renal failure	Respiratory distress syndrome
Liver failure or rupture	Acute fetal distress (particularly with lowering of blood pressure)
DIC	
HELLP syndrome	Intrauterine death
Placental abruption	
Pulmonary oedema, ARDS	
Pulmonary oedema/haemorrhage	
Aspiration pneumonia	
Retinal detachment	

Acute management

The maternal and fetal condition should be assessed. As these are potentially sick women, it is appropriate that senior obstetric and anaesthetic staff should be involved in their assessment and management early.

The classification of severity is primarily based on the level of blood pressure and the presence of proteinuria. However, after making an initial diagnosis, other organ involvement becomes important in assessing maternal risk and this includes fetal assessment.

Atypical presentations of pre-eclampsia include women presenting initially with convulsions, abdominal pain or general malaise. In these cases, pre-eclampsia should always be considered and the blood pressure should be measured, the urine analysed and blood sent for analysis. A deterioration in clinical condition, particularly headache and abdominal pain, indicates worsening disease. Increasing oedema is not in itself a sign that should determine management. Maternal tendon reflexes are difficult to perform in a reproducible way, so are not of value to assess the risk of convulsion, although the presence of exaggerated clonus may be helpful.

NB: Tendon reflexes are of help when assessing magnesium toxicity: in this case they are reduced or absent.

Taking the blood pressure

Automated methods can systematically underestimate blood pressure, particularly the systolic blood pressure. It has been suggested that mercury sphygmomanometers should be used to establish baseline values. However these are no longer available in many units and a baseline check with another device, validated for use in pregnancy, is recommended, although such devices are limited.

While taking the blood pressure, the woman should be in a comfortable position, if possible, sitting at a 45° angle. The blood pressure cuff must be of the appropriate size. Too small a cuff over reads and too large will under read. Table 24.2 gives the correct-sized cuff to use, based on the circumference of the middle of the upper arm.

Table 24.2 Appropriate cuff sizes

Upper arm circumference	Sphygmomanometer cuff size
18–23 cm	Small adult cuff
23–33 cm	Standard adult cuff
33–42 cm	Large adult cuff

The cuff should be at the level of the heart. There are fluctuations in blood pressure in normal circumstances so multiple readings are needed to confirm the diagnosis. There is now a consensus that Korotkoff phase 5 is the preferable measurement of diastolic blood pressure.

As part of the initial assessment, blood pressure should be checked every 15 minutes until the woman is stabilised and then repeated half hourly. If intravenous antihypertensive drugs are administered, the blood pressure may need to be measured every 5 minutes in order to titrate treatment against the response.

Measuring proteinuria

Proteinuria is classically associated with the pathological lesion, glomeruloendotheliosis. Proteinuria per se is not a sign of renal damage and will usually recover after delivery. The widely used visual dipstick assessment as a screening test produces significant rates of false negative as well as false positive results. 2+ protein on dipstick testing is evidence of proteinuria but a more accurate test, such as 24-hour urine, should be undertaken to confirm this. In circumstances where immediate delivery is required, newer techniques such as protein/creatinine ratios can be performed quickly but have not yet been fully evaluated. A level of 30 mg/mmol urinary protein/creatinine appears to be equivalent to 0.3 g protein/24 hours.

Basic investigations

Blood should be sent for:

Serum electrolytes:	Na, K, urea, creatinine, urate
Liver function tests:	albumin, ALT, aspartate aminotransferase (AST), bilirubin
Full blood count:	haemoglobin, white cell count, platelets
Clotting factors:	prothrombin time (PT), APTT + fibrinogen, fibrin/fibrinogen degradation products (FDPs)

Group-and-save serum

Urine should be tested for protein and sent for culture.

All tests should be checked daily or more frequently if abnormal.

Coagulation

If the platelet count is above 100 x 10^9/litre and liver function tests are normal, the likelihood that the clotting results will be abnormal is very low and some units choose not to perform clotting tests without an abnormal platelet count. If the woman is clinically unwell, a coagulation screen should be sent to establish baseline values. There is no direct correlation between platelet count and liver damage and assessment of liver enzyme levels (usually by AST and ALT) is required. An AST level of above 75 IU/litre is seen as significant and a level above 150 IU/ litre is associated with increased maternal morbidity.

A diagnosis of HELLP syndrome must not be made on liver function tests alone – there needs to be confirmation of haemolysis, either increased LDH levels (commonly measured in the USA) or by visual examination of the blood film to look for fragmented red cells.

Renal function

Although, in pre-eclampsia, a rise in urate correlates with a poorer outcome for both mother and baby, the levels, in themselves, are not useful for clinical decision-making.

Renal function is generally maintained in pre-eclampsia until the late stage. Elevated creatinine at presentation should lead to suspicion of an underlying renal problem. In severe disease, rising serum creatinine is associated with a worsening outcome. Renal failure requiring support is now uncommon in pre-eclampsia in the developed, but and when it occurs it is usually associated with haemorrhage or sepsis.

Monitoring of clinical signs

The following should be monitored:

- blood pressure (see above for details) and pulse rate
- respiratory rate should be measured hourly particularly in women on magnesium
- oxygen saturation should be measured continuously and charted hourly; if oxygen saturation falls, then medical review is essential to consider the possible differential diagnosis, with a high index of suspicion of early pulmonary oedema
- fluid balance should be monitored very carefully and detailed input and output recordings should be charted
- urine output should be measured carefully and hourly rates calculated; in more severe disease, and when delivery is planned or intravenous fluids are being given, this should be via an indwelling catheter
- urine should be tested for proteinuria 4-hourly, if conservative management is planned, then a 24-hour assessment of urinary protein is helpful in assessing the disease
- temperature should be measured 4-hourly, especially in those women with pre-eclampsia who are in labour, postpartum or immediately postoperative
- optic fundi should be examined to assess for any signs of haemorrhage or papilloedema.

Assessment of the fetus

The fetus is at risk of growth restriction. Ultrasound assessment of fetal growth and liquor volume may be appropriate. Umbilical artery Doppler is a valuable noninvasive test of fetal wellbeing but is gestation dependent and needs careful interpretation in the very preterm pregnancy (below 30 weeks). Doppler of fetal vessels can be used but requires expert assessment and evaluation.

Cardiotocography (CTG) is the most widely used technique for the initial assessment of fetal wellbeing but it has little predictive value. If the woman is in labour, continuous electronic fetal monitoring is required.

Antepartum and intrapartum management

Control of blood pressure

The level of blood pressure that requires treatment is still unclear.

The 2006–08 CMACE report suggests that treatment should be instituted if the systolic blood pressure is over 150 mmHg.[2] The previous confidential maternal mortality report had suggested treating systolic pressures of 160 mmHg. Previously, the Magpie study definition of severe hypertension (systolic over 170 mmHg or diastolic 110 mmHg or mean arterial pressure [MAP] above 125 mmHg) was considered a clear threshold for treatment.[3]

The aim of therapy should be to stabilise the woman's blood pressure. As a guide, this means:

- maintaining systolic blood pressure at less than 150 mmHg
- reducing diastolic blood pressure by 10 mmHg and bringing it below 105 mmHg in the first instance
- maintaining the blood pressure at or below these levels.

Rapid drops in blood pressure should be avoided, particularly when the fetus is undelivered as this can potentially trigger acute fetal compromise.

Drug treatment

Labetalol

Labetalol is a combined alpha and beta blocker and is less likely to decrease uteroplacental blood flow than pure beta-blockers. It may improve cerebral perfusion, thereby reducing the risk of eclampsia.

Oral

If the woman can tolerate oral therapy, an initial 200 mg dose can be given. This can be given immediately, before venous access is established, to achieve as quick a result as an initial intravenous dose. There should be a reduction in blood pressure in about half an hour. A second oral dose can be given, if needed, after 1 hour. Over 50% of women requiring antihypertensive treatment can be controlled with oral therapy.

Intravenous

- If there is no initial response to oral therapy, or if it cannot be tolerated, control should be by repeated bolus of labetalol followed by a labetalol infusion. Over 90% of women can be controlled with labetalol alone.
- Bolus dose is 50 mg (10 ml labetalol 5 mg/ml) given over at least 1minute. This should have an effect by 5 minutes and should be repeated if diastolic blood pressure has not been reduced. This can be repeated to a maximum dose of 200 mg. The pulse rate should remain over 60 beats/minute.
- Following this or as initial treatment in moderate hypertension, a labetalol infusion should be commenced. An infusion of (neat) labetalol 5 mg/ml at a rate of 4 ml/hour via a syringe pump should be started. The infusion rate should be doubled every half-hour to a maximum of 32 ml (160 mg)/hour until the blood pressure has dropped and then stabilised at an acceptable level.

- It should be remembered that women who are on beta-blockers can fail to mount a tachycardia, therefore this should be highlighted to clinicians and on the patient's MEOWS chart, otherwise signs of haemorrhage may be missed by a falsely reassuring 'normal pulse rate'. If unrecognised, the first signs of a significant blood loss may be a complete collapse.

Vasodilators

As hydralazine and nifedipine are vasodilators, expansion of the circulating blood volume prior to treatment is frequently recommended in antenatal patients to reduce the likelihood of a precipitous drop in blood pressure, which may trigger fetal distress. A 250 ml bolus of crystalloid is commonly used prior to the use of these vasodilators to achieve volume expansion.

Nifedipine

If labetalol is contraindicated or fails to control the blood pressure, then nifedipine is an alternative agent. Theoretically the effect of nifedipine might be exacerbated by magnesium sulphate (and vice versa). Clinically, this is rarely a problem. In the Magpie study, large numbers of women were treated with no adverse events reported.

Dose: 10 mg oral tablet swallowed (not sublingual and not a slow-release tablet). If this controls blood pressure it should be repeated 6-hourly initially, although the dose may be changed postnatally to a slow-release preparation which lasts 12 hours. Blood pressure should be measured every 10 minutes during the first half-hour after administration, as often there can be a very marked drop in pressure and the fetal heart rate should be carefully monitored. Oral antihypertensive treatment should be commenced once intravenous treatment has been discontinued.

Hydralazine

Initial dose is 10 mg, as a slow bolus with repeated doses of 5mg at 20-minute intervals (as long as the pulse stays below 120). The effects last up to 6 hours. An infusion of 2 mg/hour can be established for maintenance, increasing by increments of 0.5 mg/hour to a maximum of 20 mg/hour.

Choice of antihypertensive

A systematic review of hydralazine and labetalol revealed that hydralazine was associated with more maternal hypotension (odds ratio [OR] 3.29, 95% confidence interval [CI] 1.50–7.13), more caesarean sections (OR 1.30, 95% CI 1.08–1.59), more placental abruptions (OR 4.17, 95% CI 1.19–14.28), more maternal oliguria (OR 4.0, 95% CI 1.22–12.50) and more adverse effects on fetal heart rate (OR 2.04, 95% CI 1.32–3.16). Compared with labetalol, there were overall more maternal adverse effects (OR 1.5, 95% CI 1.16–1.94) but with less neonatal bradycardia (OR –0.24, 95% CI –0.42 to –0.06). It was suggested that, although the results were not robust, they did not support hydralazine as a first-line treatment. However, there is a wealth of experience in the use of hydralazine and it remains in use in many units. The NICE guidelines on hypertension in pregnancy support the use of all three treatments described above.

Fluid management prior to delivery

Fluid balance should be recorded in all inpatients with pre-eclampsia and once a decision has been made to deliver, modest fluid restriction should occur to avoid fluid overload, particularly when intravenous fluids are being given.

Total intravenous input should be limited to 85ml/hour (approximately 1ml/kg/hour). If Syntocinon is used, a high concentration should be given via a syringe driver (rather than the more commonly dilute solution given by volumetric infusion pump. The hourly input should include all other infusions such as magnesium sulphate and Syntocinon. During labour, oliguria does not require any specific intervention, except to ensure progress to delivery is being achieved and that magnesium levels are not rising towards toxic levels. As women with pre-eclampsia are at high risk of CS, oral intake should be limited appropriately.

Anaesthesia and fluids

Women suffering from moderate or severe pre-eclampsia have a relatively reduced intravascular circulating volume, and it *may* be appropriate to give a cautious fluid load prior to establishing a regional block.

Factors to consider prior to fluid loading include:

- previous fluid balance, in particular whether a recent fluid load has been given (e.g. prior to administering antihypertensive treatment)
- examination to detect signs of fluid overload or cardiac dysfunction (e.g. pulmonary oedema)
- degree of vasodilatation likely to be achieved by the block: a cautious low-dose technique for labour or incremental technique for CS should cause little haemodynamic disturbance and fluid load may be unnecessary and may complicate fluid balance.

Monitoring of fetal heart rate is an indicator of adequate perfusion to the placenta.

Controlled fluid loading can be achieved either by use of a pump to control volume or by the simple precaution of using only small bags of intravenous fluids. In this way, an accidental litre of crystalloid cannot run in during the anaesthetic procedure or at any other time.

Hypotension, if it occurs, can be controlled with very small doses of a vasopressor. Prophylactic vasopressors are not recommended.

For CS, regional anaesthesia is now the preferred choice in pre-eclampsia as it avoids many of the hazards of general anaesthesia in these women. In the past, regional anaesthesia, especially spinal block, was assumed to result in severe hypotension, but in practice this is rarely the case. By contrast, general anaesthesia can be very challenging. The surge in blood pressure in response to intubation is very marked and difficult to control. When general anaesthesia cannot be avoided, then extra care and drugs are required to control this rise in blood pressure.

Seizure prophylaxis

The risk of eclampsia is low, at around 1% even in women with severe pre-eclampsia. The Magpie trial, designed to establish the clinical efficacy of magnesium sulphate in pre-eclampsia, has shown that treatment with magnesium sulphate reduced the risk of seizures by 58%. Overall, 11 per 1000 fewer women had seizures when treated with magnesium sulphate. There was a trend towards a reduction in mortality, with a relative risk of 0.55 (95% CI 0.26–1.14). Overall, the number needed to treat (NNT) to prevent a seizure was 63 (range 38–181) in severe pre-eclampsia and 109 (range 72–225) without. In countries with a low mortality rate, the NNT may be over 300. Adverse effects were more common with magnesium sulphate (25% versus 8%) but were mostly mild; the intravenous route gave fewer problems.

In the UK, the decision to use prophylactic magnesium sulphate should be based on consideration of risk–benefit and cost. As the drug is relatively cheap, the main cost is the closer observation required during the infusion period. For women already being cared for on a high-dependency basis, there is little extra cost to magnesium sulphate. It would seem logical to use it in these circumstances.

Magnesium sulphate protocol

Clinicians need to be aware that there are differing concentrations of magnesium sulphate available and therefore to avoid confusion over dosing, each unit should have access to one stock only and clear guidelines on how to draw it up. The easiest and least confusing preparation to use is ampoules of 1 g in 10 ml (i.e. 10% solution). Magnesium sulphate is given as a loading dose of 4 g, followed by a continuous infusion of 1 g/hour for 24 hours or until 24 hours after delivery, whichever is the later. In cases where it is used for prophylaxis, it may be discontinued before 24 hours if all the other features of pre-eclampsia have settled.

Important observations

When magnesium sulphate is in progress, assessment of the patient needs to occur before each new dose. The following observations should be performed:

- continuous pulse oximetry
- hourly urine output
- hourly respiratory rate
- deep tendon reflexes.

Consider reducing magnesium sulphate infusion (to 0.5 g/hr) and check magnesium levels if:

- urine output is less than 100 ml in 4 hours.

Stop magnesium sulphate infusion and check levels if:

- patellar reflexes are absent (assuming this is not due to a regional block) or if
- respiratory rate is fewer than 16 breaths/minute or if
- oxygen saturation is less than 90% ON AIR.

Ninety-seven percent of magnesium is excreted in the urine and there is a significant risk of toxic levels occurring when oliguria is present. If magnesium is not being excreted, then the levels should not fall and no other anticonvulsant is needed. Magnesium should be re-introduced once urine output improves.

Adverse effects

Muscle weakness, absent tendon reflexes, respiratory depression and cardiac arrhythmias (increased conduction time) may all occur (Table 24.3). The risk can be minimised by the slow administration of magnesium and close monitoring. Overdose of magnesium (whether relative or absolute) should be treated with 10 ml of 10% calcium gluconate, given as a slow intravenous bolus.

There is no need to measure magnesium levels with the following protocol, as long as urine output is maintained.

Dose of magnesium sulphate

If using 10% magnesium:

- loading dose: 4 g (40 ml) over 10–20 minutes (each 10 ml ampoule contains 1 g magnesium sulphate; therefore 4 ampoules needed = 40 ml) administered via syringe pump over 20 minutes (i.e. rate of 120 ml/hour) according to local protocol
- maintenance dose is then 10 ml/hour via syringe pump.

If using 20% magnesium:

- loading dose: 4 g slow infusion over 10–20 minutes (20 ml magnesium sulphate 20%) according to local protocol administered via a syringe pump (over 20 minutes needs an infusion rate of 60 ml/hour)
- maintenance dose: 1g/hour intravenously for 24 hours; magnesium sulphate 20% via a syringe pump at an infusion rate of 5 ml/hour.

If using 50% magnesium:

- loading dose: 4 g slow infusion over 10–20 minutes: 8ml magnesium sulphate 50% added to 12 ml physiological saline (= 20 ml) according to local protocol administered via a syringe pump over 20 minutes (needs infusion rate of 60 ml/hour)
- maintenance dose: 1 g/hour intravenously for 24 hours, add 50 ml magnesium sulphate 50% to 250 ml physiological saline, draw 60 ml out of the bag and administer via a syringe pump at an infusion rate of 12 ml/hour; repeat appropriately.

Table 24.3 Levels of magnesium sulphate at which adverse effects occur

Symptoms	$MgSO_4$ levels (mmol/litre)
Feeling of warmth, flushing, double vision, slurred speech	3.8–5.0
Loss of tendon reflexes	>5.0
Respiratory depression	>6.0
Respiratory arrest	6.3–7.0
Cardiac arrest	>12.0

Antenatal steroids

If the pregnancy is preterm and can be prolonged beyond 24 hours, steroids may help to mature the fetal lungs. The maximum benefit from steroid therapy is probably 48 hours after administration. Since the benefits to the fetus peak between 48 hours and 6 days, delaying delivery beyond 48 hours may not be advantageous to the baby or mother.

Planning delivery

'Planned delivery on the best day in the best way'

The delivery should be well planned, done on the best day, performed in the best place, by the best route and with the best support team. Timing affects the outcome for both mother and baby. If the mother is unstable then delivery increases her risk. Once stabilised with anti-hypertensive drugs and magnesium sulphate as indicated, then a decision should be made in terms of timing and route of delivery. In the absence of convulsions or other major complications, prolonging the pregnancy may be possible to improve the outcome of a premature fetus, but only if the mother remains stable. Continued close monitoring of mother and baby is needed.

Delivery, particularly of premature infants, should be undertaken during normal working hours if at all possible.

Mode of delivery

The mode of delivery should be discussed with the consultant obstetrician. Fetal wellbeing and the likelihood of successful labour are important in determining mode of delivery. If gestation is under 32 weeks, CS is the recommended mode of delivery. After 34 weeks, vaginal delivery should be considered in a cephalic presentation. Vaginal prostaglandins will increase the chance of success.

Antihypertensive treatment should be continued throughout assessment and labour. If vaginal delivery is planned, then the second stage should be kept short with consideration given to operative vaginal delivery if active pushing raises the blood pressure.

The third stage should be managed with 5 units intravenous Syntocinon. Ergometrine or syntometrine are absolutely contraindicated because of the risk of precipitating a rapid rise in blood pressure.

Regional analgesia may be helpful in preventing any further rises in blood pressure caused by labour pains, as long as coagulopathy is not present.

Appropriate thromboprophylaxis should be given to all women who are immobilised.

Organisation and transfer

Even a few hours' warning of imminent delivery may enable the neonatal unit to organise a cot, or to transfer a reasonably stable mother to a place where a cot is available.

If a maternity unit does not have access to a high-dependency unit (HDU)/intensive care unit (ICU), is unable to cope with maternal complications or is unable to cope with preterm babies, it may be appropriate to consider antenatal transfer of the mother.

Maternal safety must not be jeopardised and she must be stabilised prior to transfer. In some cases it is safer to deliver the mother and then transfer the infant and mother too, if she is well enough.

Stabilisation before transfer

The following are necessary prior to transfer:

- blood pressure should be stabilised at an acceptable level
- all basic investigations should have been performed and the results clearly recorded in the accompanying notes or telephoned through as soon as available
- fetal wellbeing has been assessed to be certain that transfer is in the fetal interest before delivery; steroids should be given if the woman is preterm (see above)
- appropriate personnel are available to transfer the woman; this will normally mean at least a senior midwife with medical staff as appropriate
- transfer has been discussed with appropriate consultant medical staff and all the relevant people at the receiving unit: the neonatal unit and neonatal medical staff, the resident obstetrician, the midwife in charge of delivery suite, the anaesthetist covering labour ward and the intensive care team where appropriate (see also Chapter 40 on transfer).

Postpartum fluid management

In the immediate postdelivery phase, women commonly have a degree of oliguria. Women with severe pre-eclampsia should remain fluid restricted until a natural diuresis occurs, 36–48 hours following delivery. Prior to this, there is a risk of iatrogenic fluid overload, so careful fluid balance is needed. The total intravenous fluid that should be given is approximately 85 ml/hour (1 ml/kg/hour): Hartmann's solution or equivalent crystalloid plus other infusions of drugs. Urine output should be recorded hourly. It is not necessary to be aggressive in maintaining urine output.

Responding to significant oliguria over an 8-hour period should follow local guidance which should include the type of approach below:

- assess urine output in 4-hour blocks and record it on the observation chart
- each 4-hour block has a target urine output total in excess of 80–100 ml
- if one 4-hour block fails to achieve this target, review the patient and her fluid input and output to check care has been appropriate and that she is otherwise well.

Only 2% of women will fail to achieve this target in *two* consecutive blocks and the rate of renal compromise in this group is no higher than in the women without oliguria, but in such cases further action is needed based on the clinical findings and the difference between input and output:

- if input is significantly more than output since delivery or in the last 'time period' (this volume and time period should be specified), then 20 mg furosemide is given intravenously
- if the diuretic fails to increase urine output, consultant review should occur with intensivist input/regional support.

If total input is less than this specified excess compared with output in the specified given time period, then an infusion of 250 ml of colloid over 20 minutes is given. If output remains low, furosemide can then be given, but if there is still no response, discussion and review at a senior level is needed as mentioned above.

When there is oliguria requiring a fluid challenge or furosemide, then the electrolytes need to be carefully assessed and should be checked 6-hourly. If there is concern over a rising creatinine and/or potassium, the case should be discussed with a renal physician or regional centre.

If oxygen saturation levels fall, this may indicate pulmonary oedema, which may be caused or exacerbated by fluid overload. Input and output should be assessed, together with clinical assessment of the fluid balance, and supplemented if necessary by invasive (central or cardiac output) monitoring. The chest should be carefully examined and a chest radiograph should be performed. Appropriate treatment may include sitting the patient upright, furosemide and oxygen. If there is no diuresis and the oxygen saturation does not rise then intensive care/renal referral should be considered.

Indications for central venous pressure (CVP) monitoring

CVP monitoring is usually not necessary and may be misleading. This is because pulmonary oedema can occur in the presence of a low CVP because of left ventricular dysfunction and increased pulmonary interstitial fluid.

CVP monitoring may be indicated:

- at CS, particularly if blood loss is excessive
- if blood loss is excessive or if delivery is complicated by other factors such as placental abruption.

Patients requiring large volumes of colloid, such as FFP, blood or platelets, can suffer from fluid overload and are a particular challenge. It is not difficult putting more fluid in, but getting it out can be a real problem. Senior clinicians should be involved early on.

In cases where close fluid balance measurements are likely to be inaccurate, owing to the difficulties of measuring blood loss, early recourse to central monitoring may be appropriate. This should be a multidisciplinary decision as CVP insertion may be difficult or hazardous (e.g. in the presence of coagulopathy, or if lying head down is impossible due to severe pulmonary oedema) and the consultant anaesthetist and obstetrician should be involved.

Management of imminent eclampsia or eclampsia

Immediate resuscitation

Management should follow the basic principles of airway, breathing and circulation.

Do not leave the woman alone, but call for help including appropriate personnel such as the senior midwife, anaesthetist and senior obstetrician.

Aim to prevent maternal injury during the convulsion.

A Place the woman in the left lateral position and assess and, if necessary, maintain the airway.

B Administer high-flow oxygen and assess breathing. Pulse oximetry is helpful once the fit has stopped. Lungs should always be auscultated after the convulsion has ended to detect aspiration or pulmonary oedema.

C Check pulse and blood pressure.

Establish a fluid balance record if this has not already been done, including urinary catheter.

Once the woman is stabilised, plans should be made to deliver the baby, but there is no particular hurry. A delay of several hours to stabilise the mother is acceptable, assuming that there is no acute fetal concern such as a fetal bradycardia.

The mother's condition will always take priority over the fetal condition.

Treatment of seizures

- Magnesium sulphate is the therapy of choice; diazepam and phenytoin should no longer be used as a first-line treatment.
- The vast majority of initial seizures are self-limiting.
- The intravenous route is associated with fewer adverse effects than the intramuscular route.
- Dosage: see section above on seizure prophylaxis.
- Treatment is currently maintained for 24 hours after the last seizure, since commencing magnesium or 24 hours after delivery, whichever is longest.

- There is debate about whether drugs such as diazepam should be given to control the initial seizure. This is not usually necessary and would only be used in the case of a prolonged seizure or recurrent seizures not responding to magnesium sulphate. The risk of respiratory arrest is significantly increased by the use of multiple drugs.

Management of recurrent seizures

In the Collaborative Eclampsia Trial, a further bolus of 2 g or 4 g of magnesium sulphate was administered, depending on maternal weight.[4] The larger dose is appropriate for women over 70 kg. An alternative is to increase the rate of infusion of magnesium sulphate to 1.5 g/hour or 2 g/hour.

If there are repeated seizures, then alternative agents such as diazepam or thiopental may be used, the latter by an anaesthetist in conjunction with intubation. If convulsions persist, intubation will in any case be necessary to protect the airway and maintain oxygenation. Transfer to intensive care facilities with intermittent positive pressure ventilation is appropriate in these circumstances.

Women with recurrent seizures may have had an additional cerebral event and neuro-imaging may be helpful in excluding other pathology.

Eclampsia box

It has been recommended that each maternity unit should have an 'emergency box' for eclampsia, based on the treatment packs that were available for the Collaborative Eclampsia Trial. This will ensure that appropriate drugs are readily available. Equipment to secure the airway and venous access are dealt with in other chapters. The box should be regularly checked to keep drugs in date (Table 24.4).

Table 24.4 Contents of emergency box for eclampsia (agents included will depend on local protocols)

Drugs/fluids	Presentation	Quantity
Magnesium sulphate (ampoules of either 10, 20 or 50%)		10 ampoules
Normal saline injection if 20 or 50% magnesium sulphate being used	10 ml ampoules	20 ampoules
Calcium gluconate 10%	8.4 mg/ml 10 ml ampoules	2 ampoules
Labetalol	200 mg in 20 ml ampoule	2 ampoules
Nifedipine tabs	10 mg tabs	20 tabs
Hydralazine for injection	20 mg powder in ampoule	5 ampoules
Normal saline injection	250 ml	5 bags

HELLP syndrome

HELLP is a syndrome comprising **h**aemolysis, **e**levated **l**iver enzymes and **l**ow **p**latelets. It occurs in 4–12% of women with severe pre-eclampsia. Severe hypertension is not always a feature, and the degree of hypertension rarely reflects overall disease severity. It is more common in multiparous women and is associated with a high perinatal mortality rate.

HELLP can present with vague symptoms including nausea, vomiting and epigastric/right upper-quadrant pain, and there is often a delay in diagnosis. Severe epigastric pain not relieved by antacids should raise the index of suspicion. One unique (if somewhat late) feature of HELLP syndrome is 'Coca Cola urine', where small amounts of dark brown/black urine are produced caused by intravascular haemolysis.

The management of HELLP, as for severe pre-eclampsia, involves evaluating severity, stabilising the mother and delivery. The postnatal course for these women is often complicated by oliguria and slow recovery of biochemical parameters. High-dose corticosteroids may promote biochemical recovery, rather than preventing morbidity and are no longer recommended. The risk of recurrence of the HELLP syndrome is approximately 20%.

Postpartum care and follow-up

Up to 44% of cases of eclampsia have been reported to occur postnatally. Women delivered with severe pre-eclampsia (and/or eclampsia) should have continued close observation postnatally. As eclampsia has been reported up to 4 weeks postnatally, the optimum length of inpatient postnatal stay is unclear, but the incidence of eclampsia and severe pre-eclampsia falls after the fourth postpartum day. Women should stay in hospital until their general condition has improved, hypertension is controlled and proteinuria and any other biochemical abnormalities are improving.

Antihypertensive therapy should be continued after delivery. Although initially the blood pressure may fall, it usually rises again at around 24 hours postpartum. Antihypertensive therapy should be reduced in a stepwise fashion. There is no reason why the woman cannot go home on treatment, to be weaned off therapy as an outpatient. The blood pressure can take up to three months to return to normal. During this time, levels should not be allowed to exceed 160/110 mmHg.

Summary

The best ways to keep morbidity and mortality to a minimum in this common, but sometimes life-threatening condition, include making a timely diagnosis and effecting timely delivery involving senior personnel, accompanied by:

- seizure prophylaxis
- control of hypertension
- fluid restriction and attention to fluid balance

- close monitoring
- respect that the condition can deteriorate in the post-partum period before it gets better.

References and further reading

1 Milne F, Redman C, Walker J, *et al.* The pre-eclampsia community guideline (PRECOG): how to screen for and detect onset of pre-eclampsia in the community. *BMJ* 2005;330: 576–80.
2 CMACE Saving Mother's Lives 2006–2008 *BJOG* 2011;118(Suppl. 1).
3 Altman D, Carroli G, Duley L, *et al.* Do women with pre-eclampsia, and their babies, benefit from magnesium sulphate? The Magpie Trial: a randomised placebo-controlled trial. *Lancet* 2002;359:1877–90.
4 Eclampsia Trial Collaborative Group. Which anticonvulsant for women with eclampsia? Evidence from the Collaborative Eclampsia Trial. *Lancet* 1995:345:1455–63.
5 Douglas KA, Redman CW. Eclampsia in the United Kingdom. *BMJ* 1994;309:1395–400.
6 Duley L. Magnesium sulphate regimes for women with eclampsia: messages from the Collaborative Eclampsia trial. *BJOG* 1996:103:103–5.
7 Knight M. Eclampsia in the United Kingdom 2005 *BJOG* 2007;114:1072–8.
8 Magee LA, Cham C, Waterman EJ, *et al.* Hydralazine for treatment of severe hypertension in pregnancy: meta-analysis. *BMJ* 2003;327:955–60.
9 NICE guidelines. *Hypertension in pregnancy. The management of hypertensive disorders during pregnancy* August 2010.
10 Royal College of Obstetricians and Gynaecologists. *The Management of Severe Pre-eclampsia/Eclampsia.* Guideline No. 10(A). London: RCOG 2006.
11 Tuffnell DJ, Jankowicz, D, Lindow SW, *et al.* Outcomes of severe pre-eclampsia/eclampsia in Yorkshire 1999/2003. *BJOG* 2005;112:875–80.

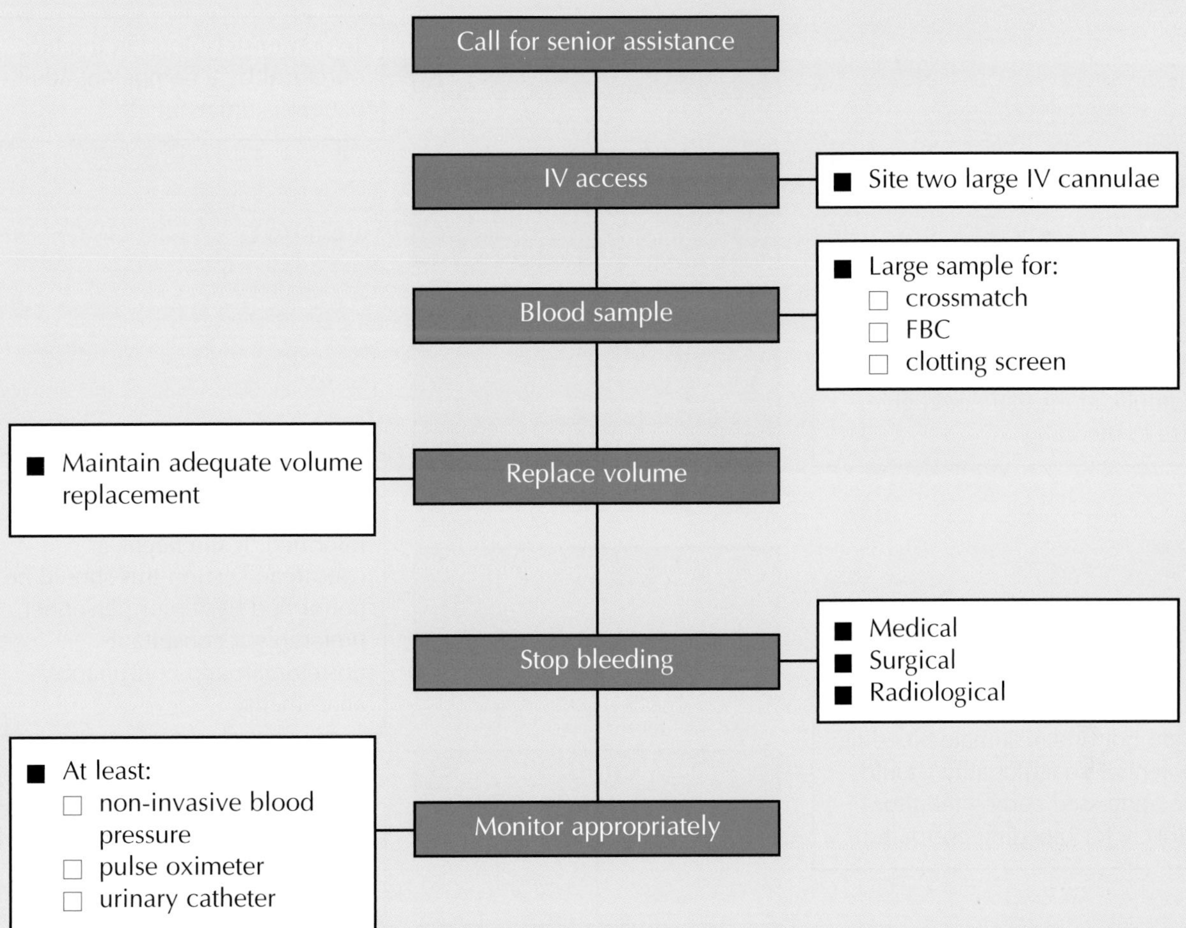
Call for senior assistance
IV access
■ Site two large IV cannulae
Blood sample
■ Large sample for:
□ crossmatch
□ FBC
□ clotting screen
Replace volume
■ Maintain adequate volume replacement
Stop bleeding
■ Medical
■ Surgical
■ Radiological
Monitor appropriately
■ At least:
□ non-invasive blood pressure
□ pulse oximeter
□ urinary catheter

ALGORITHM 25.2 Patients declining blood and blood products

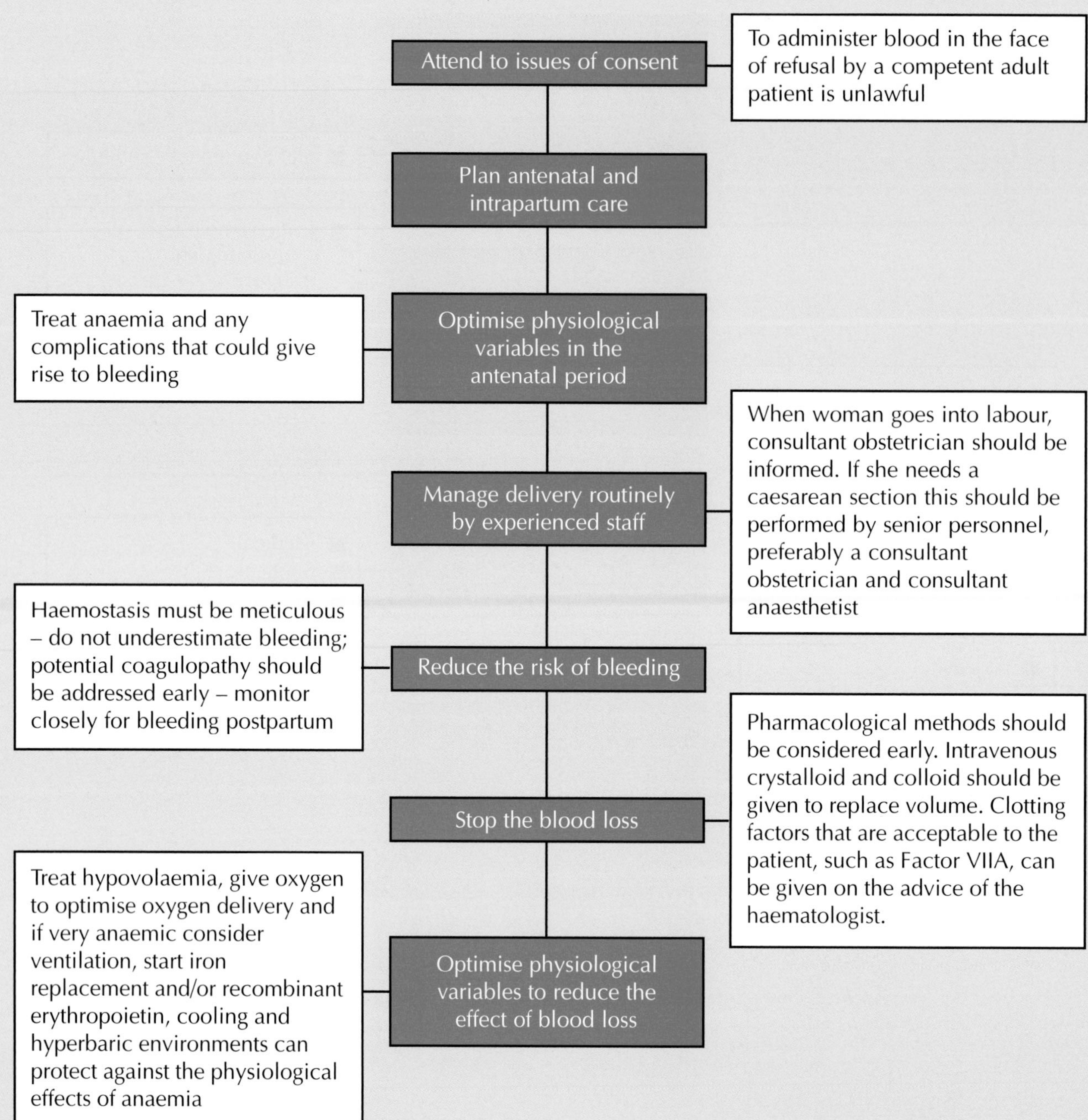

CHAPTER 25

Major obstetric haemorrhage

Objectives

On successfully completing this topic, you will be able to:

- understand the definition and causes of major obstetric haemorrhage
- recognise and manage maternal collapse caused by obstetric haemorrhage
- understand the pharmacological and surgical options for the treatment of major obstetric haemorrhage
- make a plan to facilitate optimum management in your environment
- understand the concerns to be discussed with a woman declining blood and blood products during pregnancy.

Introduction

Major haemorrhage remains a leading cause of maternal mortality despite modern improvements in obstetric practice and transfusion services. In addition, all 'near miss' audits, in developed as well as developing countries, show major haemorrhage to be one of the leading causes of severe maternal morbidity.

Complications of haemorrhage associated with first-trimester bleeding due to miscarriage or ectopic pregnancy are not within the remit of the MOET course, although most general principles will apply.

Maternal mortality and incidence of major haemorrhage

The CMACE Confidential Enquiry into maternal deaths 2006 to 2008 showed a welcome reduction in deaths due to postpartum haemorrhage.[1] However, despite a halving in the number of such deaths since the previous triennial report, obstetric haemorrhage remains a source of concern in the UK, with evidence of substandard care in three out of the five cases. In particular, a lack of routine observations in the postpartum period and failure to appreciate that significant (concealed) bleeding was occurring led to a lack of appropriate action including no early senior involvement. The report restates previous comments that all units should have procedures in place for the identification and management of major obstetric haemorrhage, and that regular skills training sessions should take place. It also draws attention to the importance of the use of MEOWS charts for 24 hours after CS, with immediate action if abnormalities are detected. A further comment is the importance of detecting and treating anaemia antenatally, thereby mitigating the effects of major obstetric haemorrhage should it occur.

Mortality statistics give no data on the incidence of major haemorrhage or on the maternal and fetal morbidity associated with haemorrhage and transfusion. Specific complications include: transfusion-related reactions and infections; genital tract trauma; loss of fertility following hysterectomy; and the rare Sheehan's syndrome (hypopituitarism).

Definition and epidemiology

Major obstetric haemorrhage is defined as the loss of more than 1000 ml blood as either antepartum or postpartum loss. Antepartum haemorrhage is often followed by postpartum haemorrhage.

Considerable problems are recognised in the accurate measurement of blood loss, and a definition based on volume alone has some shortcomings. Both visual and measured loss can be highly inaccurate, and loss from placental abruption, uterine rupture or post-CS may be partially or completely concealed. Underestimation of blood loss may delay active steps being taken to prepare for or prevent further bleeding.

Major causes of obstetric haemorrhage (primary or secondary)

Resulting initially in hypovolaemia:

- uterine atony (multiple causes)
- placenta praevia
- retained or adherent placenta or placental fragments
- genital tract injury including broad ligament haematoma
- uterine rupture
- uterine inversion
- uterine anatomical abnormalities, e.g. multiple fibroids.

Associated with coagulation failure:

- placental abruption
- pre-eclampsia
- septicaemia/intrauterine sepsis
- retained dead fetus

- amniotic fluid embolus
- incompatible blood transfusion
- existing coagulation abnormalities.

Guidelines for the management of major haemorrhage

The recommendations of the Royal College of Obstetricians and Gynaecologists (RCOG) Greentop Guideline 52, *Prevention and Management of Postpartum Haemorrhage*, updated in 2011, form the basis of this chapter.[2]

Most obstetric units in the UK now have a 'Major Obstetric Haemorrhage' procedure, as recommended by CMACE and endorsed by the RCOG. This now forms part of the requirements of the Clinical Negligence Scheme for Trusts (CNST). This protocol should be readily available on the delivery suite, including details of senior staff to be contacted in obstetrics, anaesthetics and haematology. Its use should also be subject to local audit. Blood loss of greater than 1000 ml or the recognition of maternal signs of shock in the absence of large *visible* loss should prompt the initiation of the protocol set out in the major haemorrhage guideline.

Practical management

The cornerstones in the management of major obstetric haemorrhage are early recognition, the restoration of the circulating blood volume and oxygen-carrying capacity, and the prevention of further loss. Failure to maintain adequate tissue perfusion leads to loss of vital organ function, and care becomes increasingly more complex.

Recognition of haemorrhage

Not all haemorrhage is revealed and large volumes of blood can be lost from the circulation while remaining concealed in the peritoneal cavity, the uterus, the retroperitoneal space or the ischiorectal fossa. A high index of suspicion should be maintained while assessing patients with abdominal pain, unusual levels of perineal discomfort post delivery, fainting and any signs of shock as listed below. The classes of increasing severity of blood loss are described in detail in Chapter 5 on shock.

Maternal signs of shock

These include (see also Chapter 5):

- tachycardia (on occasions a normal pulse rate or bradycardia can be seen – beware the patient on beta-blockers)
- tachypnoea
- poor peripheral perfusion

- confusion or unresponsiveness
- oliguria
- hypotension
- requiring more than 2 units of colloid to maintain blood pressure
- unexplained metabolic acidosis.

Management

Management involves various elements, all of which need to be undertaken simultaneously:

- communication and documentation
- resuscitation
- fluid replacement
- arresting the bleeding and obstetric intervention
- monitoring and investigation
- anaesthetic management.

Communication ('call for help') and documentation

Institute the following:

- call senior midwife, obstetric and anaesthetic registrars
- inform consultant obstetrician and anaesthetist
- inform blood bank technician and consultant haematologist (most units will have an agreed form of words, e.g. 'Major obstetric haemorrhage' to which the laboratory will respond)
- call porter for delivery of specimens and blood products
- allocate one member of resuscitation team as team leader and one to record events, fluids, drugs and vital signs.

Ongoing written and verbal communication between senior staff is essential. This may involve the assistance of other specialists, such as intensive care specialists, vascular surgeons or radiologists.

Resuscitation

Assess airway and breathing (see Chapter 8 for details). Conscious level and airway control usually improve rapidly once the circulating volume is restored. If the mother is shocked and there is no means of measuring saturations (or if saturations are reduced ≤95%), then administer high-flow oxygen.

Evaluate the circulation (see Chapters 5 [Shock] and 7 [Intravenous access and fluid administration] for details).

Correction of circulation within primary survey:

- establish two 14-gauge intravenous lines
- take 20 ml blood for diagnostic tests
- commence 2 litres of warmed crystalloid intravenously
- left lateral position should be adopted, to minimise the effects of aortocaval compression in an undelivered woman
- lateral tilt with a wedge (or manual displacement of the uterus by an assistant) should continue to be used when obstetric procedures are in progress
- stop any epidural infusion pending review by an anaesthetist; compensatory lower-limb vasoconstriction will be limited, so the effects of positioning may be more marked
- head-down tilt can be used as a short-term measure to improve venous return, but this may compromise respiration.

Fluid, blood product, cell salvage and clotting factor replacement is all described in detail in Chapters 5 and 7 and is not repeated here.

Diagnostic tests

These include:

- full blood count
- coagulation screen including fibrinogen
- cross match 4–6 units group specific if urgent
- baseline renal function
- blood gas.

Regular checks of the haematocrit, clotting studies and blood gases will help guide resuscitation.

Immediate bedside testing of haematocrit

This may guide the need for red blood cells, but if haemodilution has not yet occurred (as is the case with acute haemorrhage) then the result can be falsely reassuring. In addition, the Serious Hazards of Transfusion Scheme (SHOTS) report states that, 'Blood gas machines must not be used for haemoglobin estimations on which to base a transfusion request. All point of care testing devices for haemoglobin estimation must be fully validated and both internal quality control and participation in external quality assurance schemes must be ensured.' It is possible to overenthusiastically transfuse red blood cells, forgetting that these are concentrated red cells, not whole blood, and cannot be used as full replacement for loss on a volume-for-volume basis.

Monitoring – evaluation of response

A MEOWS early warning score chart should be used. This will record the following:

- pulse
- blood pressure
- respiratory rate
- SaO_2
- temperature
- urinary output via a urinary catheter
- record a detailed fluid balance
- fetal heart rate should be monitored as appropriate.

NB: Healthy women can maintain a normal or even high blood pressure while large volumes of blood are lost intra-abdominally. Most, but not all, women will demonstrate a tachycardia if bleeding significantly, but paradoxical bradycardia has also been observed (peritoneal irritation). This tachycardic response is unlikely to be present in women who have been given labetalol to treat high blood pressure. Additional monitoring by means of arterial lines and central venous monitoring may be indicated. Again, the reader is referred to Chapters 5 and 7.

Management of haemorrhage

'The four Ts' acts as an effective *aide memoire* regarding causes of postpartum haemorrhage:

- *tone* (poor uterine contraction)
- *tissue* (retained placenta or placental fragment)
- *trauma* (of the genital tract)
- *thrombin* (as a means of remembering coagulation abnormalities).

Tone

Major obstetric haemorrhage is very commonly due to uterine atony. In this situation, the following mechanical and pharmacological measures should be instituted, in turn, until the bleeding stops.

Mechanical

- Bimanual uterine compression ('rubbing up the uterus'), to stimulate contractions.
- Ensuring bladder is empty by inserting indwelling Foley catheter.

Pharmacological

- Syntocinon 5 units by slow IV injection, which may be repeated.
- Ergometrine 0.5 mg by slow IV or IM injection (c*ontraindicated in hypertension).*
- Syntocinon infusion (40 units in 500 ml Hartmann's solution at 125 ml per hour) unless fluid restriction is necessary when a more concentrated solution should be used.
- Carboprost® 0.25 mg by deep IM injection, repeated at intervals of not less than 15 minutes, to a maximum of 8 doses. This drug is contraindicated in asthma. Intramyo - metrial injection of carboprost is unlicensed and its manufacturer has recently circulated a warning against its use in this way. The hypervascular and atonic uterus certainly carries a high risk of intravascular drug administration with any direct myometrial injection.
- Misoprostol 600 microgrammes oral or per rectum is no more effective than oxytocin, but may be of use particularly in home deliveries, or in asthmatics where carboprost is contraindicated.

Advanced techniques

If the above measures fail to control the haemorrhage, invasive advanced haemostatic techniques must be initiated. This will invariably require an examination with some form of anaesthesia in an operating theatre.

Intrauterine tamponade

Tamponade should be supplemented with some adjustment to uterine tone (e.g. uterotonics).

- Intrauterine balloon tamponade (e.g. Rusch balloon) is an appropriate first-line 'surgical' intervention for most women where uterine atony is the only or the main cause of haemorrhage. The balloon should be inflated until bleeding is controlled and then left in place for 6–12 hours. (Condom catheters have been used successfully in developing countries to provide haemostasis.) This technique can also be used to manage an atonic uterus at CS.
- Uterine packing may be undertaken if a hydrostatic balloon is not available. A ribbon gauze (bandage rolls securely tied to each other) is inserted into the uterus and snugly packed in a zigzag fashion. This technique can also be used to manage an atonic uterus at CS. The pack should be removed by the vaginal route after 24 hours under the cover of intravenous antibiotics and a Syntocinon infusion.

If tamponade fails to stop the bleeding, the following conservative surgical interventions may be attempted, depending on clinical circumstances and available expertise:

Haemostatic brace suturing (B-Lynch or Modified B-Lynch)

The B-Lynch suture was devised for use at CS. It should only be used if the bleeding is controlled by bimanual pressure. A rapidly absorbable stitch is passed through the anterior wall of the uterus at the level of the uterine incision, over the right cornu, horizontally through the lower posterior wall, over the left cornu, back through the anterior wall at the left side of the uterine incision and tied in front (Figure 25.1). An assistant compresses the uterus manually as the suture is tightened. Various modifications not requiring opening of the uterus have been described.

It is recommended that a laminated diagram of the brace technique be kept in theatre

Stepwise uterine artery ligation

Bilateral ligation of iliac arteries

This procedure is rarely indicated and makes subsequent interventional radiology with embolisation extremely difficult. If needed it is best carried out by a vascular surgeon or one with equivalent experience as it is a hazardous procedure.

Selective arterial embolisation by an interventional radiologist

This may not be possible during an acute bleed as the patient may need to be transported to an imaging suite for insertion of catheters. Successful use may avert the need for hysterectomy and allow future fertility.

The UK Obstetric Surveillance System (UKOSS) reported on 272 women who required second-line therapy for management of postpartum haemorrhage. Compression sutures were used in 161 women, and were successful in 121 (75%); interventional radiology was used in 14 women with success in 12 (86%). Overall 71 (26%) women required a hysterectomy.

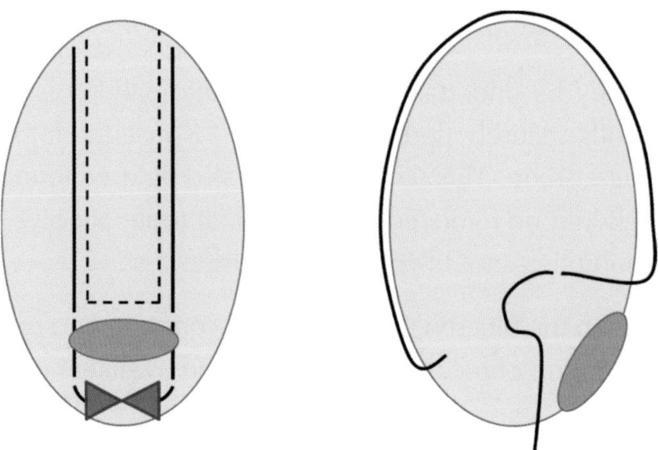

Figure 25.1 B-Lynch brace suture

Tissue and trauma

When bleeding persists despite a contracted uterus, or when a uterus fails to contract in response to oxytocic agents, or contracts but then keeps relaxing again, there may be retained tissue, or trauma to the genital tract. Once initial resuscitation is effective, the vagina, cervix and uterine cavity need to be explored urgently. Further interventions will depend on the cause found, if any. Interventional radiology techniques may be appropriate.

Hysterectomy should be undertaken sooner rather than later when haemostasis cannot be secured.

Manual compression of the aorta may allow catch-up resuscitation.

Specific situations leading to obstetric haemorrhage

These include the following:

- bleeding associated with CS (see Chapter 26)
- placenta praevia and accreta (see Chapter 27)
- placental abruption.

Placental abruption

An abruption results from the separation of the placenta from the uterine wall. Blood is driven into the myometrium ('Couvelairing'), which interferes with uterine contractility, causing postpartum haemorrhage. The associated release of thromboplastins can cause DIC.

Classic features of abruption are sudden onset of severe abdominal pain, associated with shock and a tender, hard uterus. However, with abruption of a posterior placenta, the abdomen may be soft.

Fetal heart sounds may be muffled or absent; abdominal ultrasound is often necessary to establish fetal viability but is not useful for diagnosis of the abruption itself unless the retroplacental clot is large (and this should already be obvious clinically).

If there is fetal death in association with abruption, then the abruption is major, and represents significant maternal blood loss. The blood loss may be without any vaginal loss (concealed) and may be compensated for in the maternal circulation by the shutting down of the blood supply to the fetoplacental unit. It is therefore frequently underestimated. As a rule of thumb, an abruption resulting in fetal death requires maternal transfusion.

Initial management is:

- A B C
- send blood samples for tests, including Kleihauer
- deliver the fetus
- treat coagulopathy.

If significant haemorrhage has occurred and the fetus is viable, immediate delivery by CS should be considered. However, labour may progress rapidly in the presence of an abruption; if the CTG is satisfactory, it may be prudent to aim for a vaginal delivery. If the fetus is dead, induction with a view to a vaginal delivery is usually advisable.

Expect massive postpartum haemorrhage. The combination of antepartum and postpartum haemorrhage may result in cardiovascular compromise.

Consider CVP monitoring, involve senior staff and arrange for high-dependency care postoperatively.

There is a possibility of caesarean hysterectomy. Senior staff should be involved.

Anaesthetic management for obstetric haemorrhage

The general approach should be the same regardless of the aetiology of the haemorrhage. The anaesthetist needs to be able to assess the patient quickly, to initiate or continue to resuscitate to restore the intravascular volume and provide safe anaesthesia.

Important points in the assessment will include:

- previous medical, obstetric and anaesthetic history
- a working diagnosis
- current vital signs and laboratory results
- an examination of the cardiovascular and respiratory systems
- an assessment of the upper airway as regards ease of intubation for rapid sequence induction of anaesthesia.

Prophylaxis against acid aspiration is recommended for all patients.

Regional or general anaesthesia

The presence of cardiovascular instability is a relative contraindication to regional blockade. The accompanying sympathetic blockade has the potential to worsen hypotension due to haemorrhage. There are no controlled data comparing techniques in the context of haemorrhage for either maternal or fetal outcomes. Choice for each patient will involve discussion with both the mother and surgeon together with the anaesthetist.

If cardiovascular stability has been achieved and there is no evidence of coagulation failure, regional anaesthesia can be used. This may be particularly appropriate where a working epidural has been in place during labour. Continuous epidural block may be preferred to a single-injection spinal technique, to allow better control of blood pressure and for prolonged surgery. Adequate quantities of blood, equipment, intravenous lines and monitoring must be available to cope with further bleeding. The height of the block needs to be well maintained to allow intra-abdominal handling of viscera without discomfort.

When bleeding is torrential and cardiovascular stability cannot be achieved, rapid sequence induction of general anaesthesia is more appropriate. Induction agents with minimal peripheral vasodilator action, such as ketamine 1–2 mg/kg (Ketalar®, Parke-Davis) or etomidate 100–300 microgram/kg (Hypnomidate®, Janssen-Cilag) should be considered and in extreme circumstances adrenaline and atropine should be ready in case of cardiovascular collapse on induction. Ventilation with high concentrations of oxygen may be needed until bleeding is controlled.

Volatile agents have been associated with increased blood loss due to their relaxant effects on uterine muscle. Anaesthesia should be maintained with intravenous agents if uterine atony is a problem.

Patients declining blood and blood products

Establishing wishes

Patients may decline blood and blood products because of their religious commitment or other personal belief. Many Jehovah's Witnesses believe that blood transfusion is forbidden and wish to be treated with effective nonblood alternatives. For all patients, doctors are obliged to deliver the best care in keeping with the patient's wishes. The legal position is that any adult patient (i.e. 16 years of age and over) who has the necessary mental capacity to do so is entitled to refuse treatment, even if it is likely that refusal will result in the patient's death. No other person is legally able to consent to treatment for that adult or to refuse treatment on that person's behalf and the patient should be seen alone at some point in her pregnancy to clarify their exact wishes and ensure they are not being coerced in any way. Having a witness at these discussions is helpful and should be clearly documented.

Generally speaking, Jehovah's Witnesses decline the transfusion of whole blood, packed red blood cells, white blood cells, plasma (FFP) and platelets. However, when it comes to derivatives of blood components (for example, albumin, freeze-dried synthetic coagulation factors, immunoglobulins, etc.) the use of these products is variably acceptable and all products must be discussed and a note made of anything acceptable. There is also variation as to which blood-saving techniques are acceptable, but cell salvaging with leucocyte depletion filters is usually acceptable. This should come with a caveat that it will not return essential clotting factors (see Chapter 7 on intravenous fluids).

Obtaining consent

Document content of discussions clearly, including persons present. Obtain from the patient a clear statement of what products and techniques she understands and will accept and what she refuses. Complete a 'no blood' consent form (featured as an appendix in the Royal College of Surgeons Code of Practice for The Surgical Management of Jehovah's Witnesses: www.rcseng.ac.uk).

Explain the risk of refusal of allogenic blood frankly but not dramatically. Discuss earlier surgical intervention, including the possibility of an earlier decision to proceed to CS for antepartum haemorrhage or hysterectomy in uncontrolled postpartum haemorrhage.

Most Jehovah's Witnesses will carry with them a clear Advance Directive prohibiting blood transfusions and including information relating to the patient's view of blood products and autologous transfusion procedures. The Advance Directive should be lodged with the patient's GP, as well as with family and friends. If the patient is not in a condition to give or withhold consent but has expressed a wish at an earlier date (Advanced Directive or Healthcare Advance Directive), respect the patient's instructions in the Advance Directive or Healthcare Advance Directive.

If such instructions do not specifically apply to the patient's current condition, if the patient's instructions are vague and open to interpretation or if there is good reason to believe that the patient has had a change of mind since making the declaration, the doctor's duty is to exercise good medical judgement and treat the patient in her best interests as determined by a responsible body of medical opinion.

Allow the patient the opportunity to speak with the Hospital Liaison Committee for Jehovah's Witnesses and, if requested, join their discussion.

A verbally expressed change of mind should be honoured. Again, it should be given in the presence of a witness and recorded in the notes. It is relevant to ensure that women are given an opportunity to change their minds at any stage, but they will eventually become unconscious as they lose blood and will be unable to affect the decision-making process from this point.

Plan antenatal and intrapartum care

Massive obstetric haemorrhage is often unpredictable and can become life threatening in a short time. Delivery should be planned in a unit that has the facilities to cope with massive obstetric haemorrhage to include appropriate surgical expertise, interventional radiology and the option of cell salvage. Management should be geared to anticipating, preventing or stopping bleeding early. If any complications are noted during the antenatal period, the consultant obstetrician must be informed.

Optimise physiological variables in the antenatal period. The woman's blood group and antibody status should be checked in the usual way and the haemoglobin and serum ferritin should be checked regularly. Haematinics should be given throughout pregnancy to maximise iron stores. Treat any complications that could give rise to bleeding.

Manage delivery routinely by experienced staff. The consultant obstetrician should be informed when a woman who will refuse blood transfusion is admitted in labour. Consultants in other specialties need not be alerted unless complications occur. The labour should be managed routinely by experienced staff and prolonged labour should be avoided. If an operative delivery is needed it should be conducted by a senior obstetrician. Oxytocics should be given when the baby is delivered. The woman should not be left alone for at least an hour after delivery and there should be early intervention to stem any postpartum bleeding.

When the mother is discharged from hospital, she should be advised to report promptly if she has any concerns about bleeding during the puerperium.

If unusual bleeding occurs at any time during pregnancy, labour or the puerperium, the consultant obstetrician (and possibly anaesthetist and haematologist) should be informed and the standard management should be commenced promptly. The principle of management of haemorrhage in these cases is to avoid delay. Rapid decision-making may be necessary, particularly with regard to surgical intervention and the threshold for such intervention should be lower than in other patients. Extra vigilance should be exercised to quantify any abnormal bleeding and to detect complications, such as clotting abnormalities, as promptly as possible.

Optimise physiological variables to reduce the effect of blood loss. Treat hypovolaemia with nonblood products and use vasopressors to maintain blood pressure if necessary. Give oxygen to optimise oxygen delivery and, if very anaemic, consider ventilation to deliver oxygen maximally. Start iron replacement and/or recombinant erythropoietin. Cooling and hyperbaric environments can protect against the physiological effects of anaemia, but in the latter case are rarely available.

Summary

Major obstetric haemorrhage is common and all units must have clear guidance and protocols for its management:

- early recognition
- prompt resuscitation (ABC) and volume replacement
- turn off the tap (four Ts)
- close monitoring
- plan for care of women refusing blood products.

References and further reading

1 Centre for Maternal and Child Enquiries (CMACE). *Saving Mothers' Lives*: reviewing maternal deaths to make motherhood safer: 2006–08. The Eighth Report on Confidential Enquiries into Maternal Deaths in the United Kingdom. *BJOG* 2011;118(Suppl. 1):1–203.

2 Royal College of Obstetricians and Gynaecologists Greentop Guideline No. 52 *Postpartum Haemorrhage. Prevention and Management.* London: RCOG 2011.

3 Royal College of Obstetricians Greentop Guideline No. 63 *Antepartum Haemorrhage.* London: RCOG 2011.

4 B-Lynch C, Keith LG, Lalonde AB, Karoshi M (editors). A textbook of postpartum haemorrhage. Duncow, Dumfriesshire: Sapiens Publishing 2006.

5 Intraoperative cell salvage survey (www.transfusionguidelines.org.uk/docs/pdfs/bbt_UKCSAG_ICS_Survey_2010.pdf).

6 Kayem G, Kurinczuk J, Alfirevic Z, *et al.* Specific second-line therapies for postpartum haemorrhage: a national cohort study. *BJOG* 2011;118:856–64.

ALGORITHM 26.1 Prerequisites for caesarean section

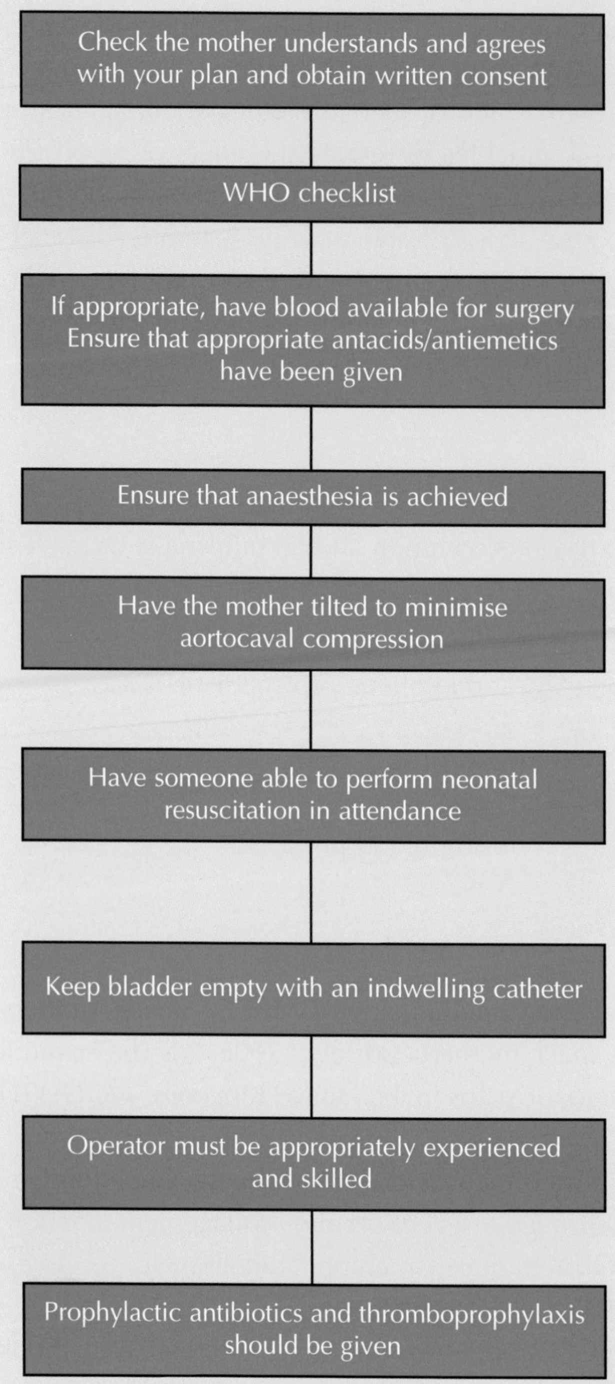

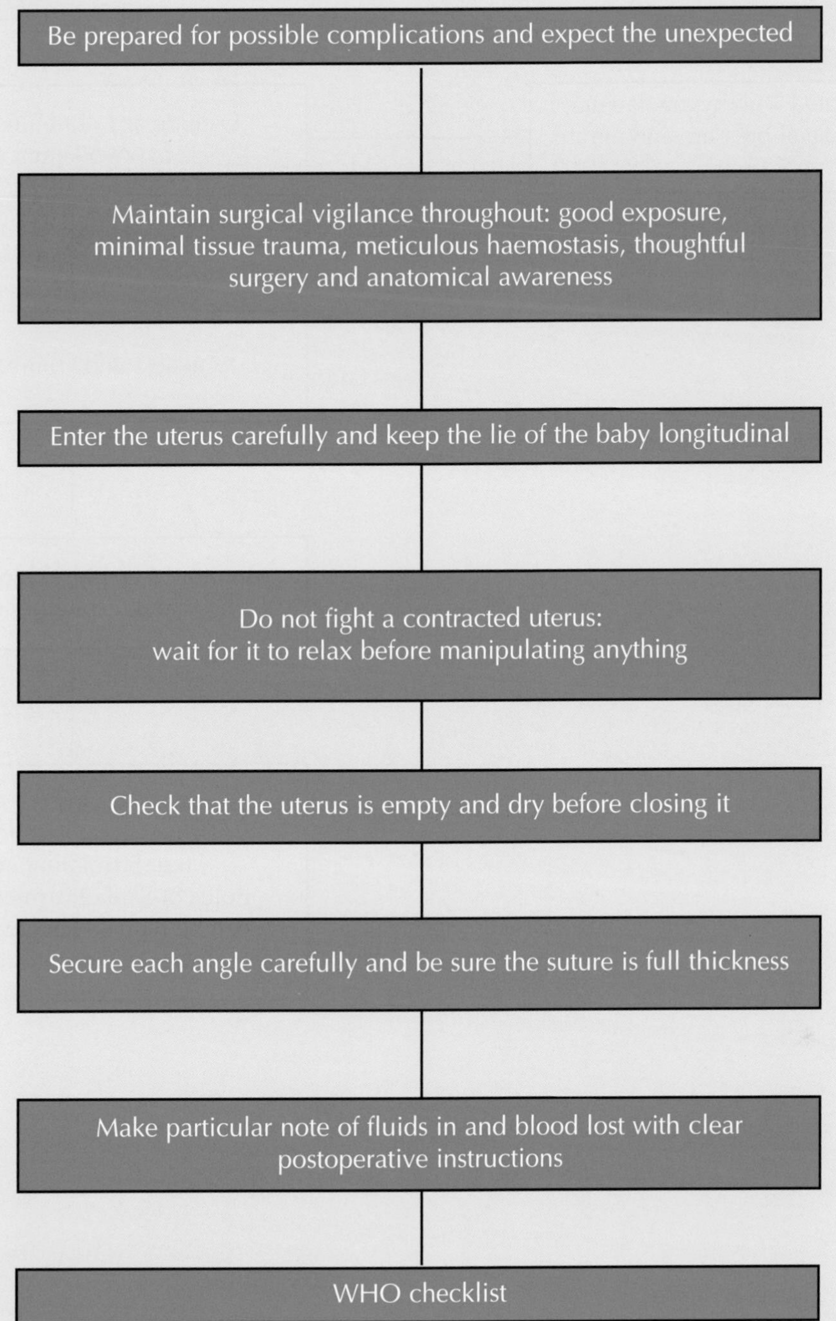
Be prepared for possible complications and expect the unexpected
Maintain surgical vigilance throughout: good exposure, minimal tissue trauma, meticulous haemostasis, thoughtful surgery and anatomical awareness
Enter the uterus carefully and keep the lie of the baby longitudinal
Do not fight a contracted uterus: wait for it to relax before manipulating anything
Check that the uterus is empty and dry before closing it
Secure each angle carefully and be sure the suture is full thickness
Make particular note of fluids in and blood lost with clear postoperative instructions
WHO checklist

ALGORITHM 26.3 Rules for the safe use of intravenous GTN

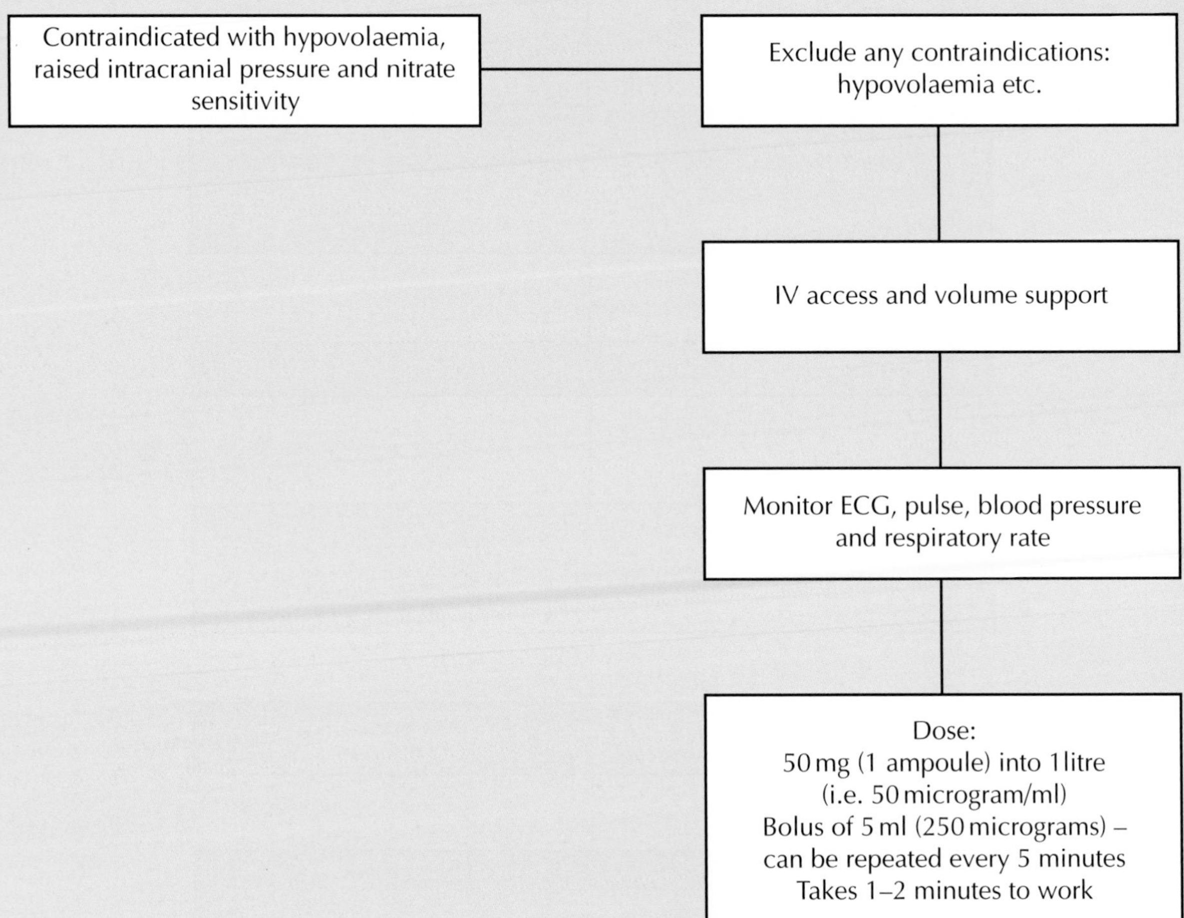

CHAPTER 26

Caesarean section

Objectives

On successfully completing this topic, you will be able to:

- understand how to anticipate and, to some extent, avoid difficulties encountered at CS
- appreciate the techniques that can help you cope with such difficulties.

Introduction

CS is the process of delivering a baby abdominally. It may be required on fetal grounds or on maternal grounds. Rates vary enormously, not only between countries but also between hospitals, but trends are generally increasing worldwide. In the UK, the CS rate for 2011–12 was 25%, according to the NHS maternity statistics report. This reflects the fact that, in most developed countries, around one in four women will deliver by CS. The caesarean rate continues to rise in developing countries as well, and has now reached 50% in China. CS has become one of the most (if not *the* most) commonly performed operations in the world.

The decision to perform a CS can be obvious in some circumstances, while in others it can be extremely difficult. This decision-making skill in terms of timing and mode of delivery is acquired over many years, with experience and clinical judgement. CS should never be seen as the easy option. All risks of CS, as opposed to those of proceeding with an attempt at labour and vaginal delivery, should be considered and balanced in each individual circumstance, taking into account both maternal and fetal interests.

This chapter is not designed to list the indications or arguments for CS, nor to give intricate detail into surgical technique, but rather to highlight the difficulties that can be encountered (both anticipated and unexpected) and to suggest ways in which they can be predicted, recognised and dealt with in the acute situation.

Prerequisites for CS

- The woman should understand the indications for the procedure and agree to it, giving written informed consent.

- Anaesthesia should be achieved (either regional or general).
- The patient or operating table should be tilted laterally 30°, to minimise aortocaval compression during the procedure.
- The bladder should be kept empty with a urethral catheter.
- Someone should be in attendance that is capable of performing neonatal resuscitation.
- The operator must have appropriate experience and competence.
- Prophylactic antibiotics and appropriate thromboprophylaxis should be used.
- Blood may need to be grouped and saved or crossmatched, depending on the clinical situation at hand and local arrangements.

Anticipating problems in specific circumstances

Before embarking on any surgery, rehearse the principles of good and safe surgical technique:

- maintain a sterile operative field
- achieve good exposure with an appropriate incision
- keep tissue handling to a minimum and avoid unnecessary dissection and trauma
- treat the tissues with respect
- achieve meticulous haemostasis
- while operating, positively consider and avoid the common problems that could turn a straightforward procedure into a complex one.

Skin incision

A low transverse skin incision is usually adequate for all uterine incisions except the true high classic incision extending up to the fundus. Make sure that the incision used affords adequate access.

Entry

Entry to the peritoneal cavity should be careful and safe. Special care is needed if there has been previous surgery (bowel can be tethered or bladder can be high).

The operator and the assistant should avoid hooking fingers under the rectus muscle (between the rectus muscle and the peritoneum), as this can seriously threaten the inferior epigastric vascular bundle.

Before extending the peritoneal incision, check there are no adhesions hidden from view; the tearing that is done at this stage of surgery can be frighteningly vicious – be gentle.

Assess the lower uterine segment

The uterovesical peritoneal reflexion identifies the upper limit of the lower uterine segment, and is invaluable in planning the uterine incision in difficult circumstances, such as CS at full dilatation, preterm delivery or abnormal lie situations.

Always check the degree of uterine rotation, and correct it, or allow for it, prior to making the uterine incision to reduce the likelihood of angle extension into the broad ligament.

Exposure

Make sure the peritoneum is reflected well clear of the proposed angles of the uterine incision, as failure to do this can compromise access, haemostasis and closure of the angles if they have extended during delivery.

Uterine incision

Do not do this until you have either checked and confirmed that there is a presenting part in the pelvis, or you have felt for the fetal lie and made a plan with your assistant regarding how to conduct the delivery.

In making the uterine incision, always try to leave membranes intact, as this will make it less likely that you will cut the baby (the membranes can then be carefully nicked just prior to delivery).

Remember that the thicker the uterine segment (preterm, placenta praevia, a high presenting part or an abnormal lie) the less space it affords you in terms of access to the baby – make sure the incision is big enough.

Be careful during this stage of the surgery to get your assistant to keep the lie of the baby longitudinal – this is especially important if the lower segment is poorly formed or full of fibroid or placenta – the last thing you need in this difficult situation with compromised space is for the baby to drift off into an oblique or transverse lie.

Delivery

At CS, the baby's head delivers into the wound in the occipitotransverse position by lateral flexion. This procedure should be conducted gently and slowly to avoid trauma to and extension of the uterine angles.

Fundal pressure during the delivery should be sustained and should follow the distal end of the fetus on its way out (like squeezing toothpaste from a tube).

Placenta

While the placenta is attached, the placental site will not bleed and there is no need to hurry this process. Wait for separation to occur rather than precipitating a problem. If there is bleeding then Green-Armytage clamps can be placed on the bleeding sinuses or angles as needed.

Check that all placenta and membranes have been removed.

Check the patency of the internal cervical os and that it is not covered with membrane.

Closure of uterus

Both uterine angles need to be secured carefully and accurately, with each stitch passing full thickness into the uterine cavity; failure to achieve this full thickness can leave a bleeding vessel within the cavity, which will remain hidden from the surgeon's view and produce vaginal bleeding later.

If there are placental bed bleeders (commonly seen with placenta praevia), then attention should be given to these before closing the uterus, as once closed such bleeding is hidden from the surgeon's view. These can be dealt with by systemic uterotonics but may also need an under-running suture or a local injection of uterotonics (e.g. a solution of Syntocinon 10units diluted in 20 ml physiological saline). Persistent placental bed bleeding can also be dealt with using tamponade with a balloon catheter, such as a Rusch or Cook-Bakri balloon, once the uterus is closed.

The uterus should routinely be closed in a double layer suture (a single layer has a higher rate of future dehiscence and rupture). Occasionally, the lower segment is so thin that a single layer is all that is possible.

Haemostasis

Once the uterus is closed, the suture line and both angles should be checked for haemostasis while exposed without tension.

Great care should then be taken checking the peritoneal edges, the subrectus space and, if exposed, the inferior epigastric bundles for haemostasis before the sheath is closed. Where the visceral peritoneum is not closed, this process of haemostasis is even more vital than previously as there is no tamponade effect on bleeding vessels in this layer, and massive obstetric haemorrhage occurring due to bleeding from this site has been reported.

Drains

Anyone who claims never to need drains because they 'never close if everything isn't perfectly dry' paints an enviable but rather naïve picture. While haemostasis should always be the aim, occasionally drains can be useful if there has been extremely difficult surgery with extensive dissection and raw surfaces, or if there is likely to be a postpartum clotting problem (fulminating pre-eclampsia, HELLP, DIC, sepsis).

Any drain placed within the peritoneal cavity should be soft and large bore (such as the Robinson drain) and not suctioned. If a suctioned drain is placed in the rectus space then the peritoneum should be closed (otherwise the drain is effectively intra-abdominal).

Closure

Close the sheath, then check for haemostasis before closing the fat layer and skin.

Postoperatively

If the baby is delivered in good condition it should be handed to the mother as soon as possible to encourage skin–skin contact – the midwife can facilitate this during surgery.

After surgery, the uterus should be palpated and the vagina should be swabbed out to check that the uterus has contracted well, and there is no continued bleeding. If there is concern at this stage, the mother should not leave theatre until the uterus is contracted and the bleeding has stopped.

The swabs and instruments should be counted.

Every aspect of the delivery should be documented but, most particularly, the findings, including the position of the baby's head, should be clearly described, as should any problems that were encountered.

Prior to leaving theatre, the estimated blood loss, the urine output (and colour) and the amount and type of fluids the anaesthetist has given should all be clearly noted. They can be summarised on a fluid/recovery chart, and discrepancies noted and managed.

Supervising a CS

The supervisor is responsible for the quality and safety of the surgery. They must be comfortable that the procedure is within the scope of the trainee, and they must be able to stop unsafe hands quickly, effectively and subtly if indicated. Conversation needs to maintain calm and demonstrate control, and frank feedback may have to wait until after the procedure is over.

During the delivery of the head, there needs to be communication as to whether progress is being made or not. This is usually what trainees find most difficult and talking them through the process of rotation and flexion of the fetal head, followed by lateral flexion into the wound, can be helpful.

Specific difficulties encountered at CS

Difficulty delivering the head in advanced labour

CS in the second stage of labour is associated with high maternal morbidity and can be extremely difficult. In the UK, there have been some instances of severe fetal trauma caused by difficulty in delivering an impacted fetal head at CS. There is some work that suggests that this is due to decreasing skill in effecting instrumental vaginal delivery, making CS necessary when forceps or ventouse would have been more appropriate and successful previously. CS at full dilatation is not straightforward and should be decided upon in conjunction with a senior obstetrician, and conducted or supervised by the same (i.e. Year 6/7 registrar or consultant).

Do not fight the uterus: if the head is deeply impacted in the pelvis in advanced labour, then once the uterus is opened at CS and the hand inserted into the pelvis a uterine contraction will follow. This can be felt as huge pressure on the operator's hand. Struggling to manipulate the fetal head against uterine activity in this situation should be avoided – it will prolong the uterine contraction and is highly likely to fail or will cause extension of the uterine angles. Wait with the hand unmoving until the contraction eases off, and the hand no longer feels so squashed. Then proceed with disimpaction, flexion with or without rotation (depending on the position) lateral flexion and delivery, which can usually be achieved gently without force.

Pushing the head up from below, or pushing up on the fetal shoulder is common practice, but if the uterus is contracting, this can also be unhelpful and patiently awaiting uterine relaxation is the key. Equally, trying to apply one blade of the forceps to try to scoop the head up is illogical and potentially dangerous.

In the rare circumstances when, despite doing the above, the head still cannot be disimpacted, then the uterus can be further relaxed by the anaesthetist administering a tocolytic (for example, an intravenous tocolytic of either 250 microgram terbutaline or 250 microgram glyceryl trinitrate – with circulatory support and intensive monitoring – see Algorithm 26.3).

The uterine incision can be extended (either in an inverted T or a J) to improve access if it is inadequate although this is rarely needed. Patwardhan's procedure can also be used (see below).

Access to the uterine cavity

When performing a CS in the second stage of labour, the lower segment will have stretched and its upper limit can extend much higher than initially thought. The danger in this situation is to enter the 'lower segment' too low and inadvertently go straight into the vagina. Such inadvertent laparoelytrotomies have been reported and, to avoid this, the uterovesical fold should be positively identified and then the uterine incision should be made approximately 3cm below it.

Fibroids can seriously hamper access to the uterine cavity and antenatal ultrasound scans, however descriptive of the fibroids, are not conducted with surgical access in mind. For this reason, an ultrasound scan performed immediately before surgery, by the surgeon, can check the thickness of the anterior wall over the proposed incision site and the relative positions of the fibroids to this and to the fetal lie. This can be of enormous benefit in planning the most accessible route of entry and how best to conduct the delivery. Another problem regarding fibroids relates to the degree of uterine rotation that they can cause, so checking the position of the fibroids in early pregnancy can help anticipate potential problems.

Access to the baby

Babies with an unstable or abnormal lie can cause problems with delivery at CS. The question 'why is this baby lying abnormally' should be asked and answered prior to surgery. An experienced surgeon should be present in all such 'unexplained' cases in nulliparous women, as the technical problems encountered, if they are due to amniotic bands or uterine anomaly, can be demanding.

Placenta praevia

Access to the uterine cavity and the baby is hampered by a thick vascular lower segment as well as by the placenta itself. The assistant should maintain the longitudinal lie of the baby while the uterus is being incised and not get distracted by the bleeding. Interrupting the continuous pressure on the abdomen should be avoided as it can allow the baby to drift away from a longitudinal lie if the placenta is filling the lower segment.

Anterior placenta

Depending on where the placenta is lying, it may be possible to incise the uterus down to the placenta and then separate it from uterine wall to expose membranes without dividing the placenta itself. Planning this preoperatively is aided by an ultrasound scan by the surgeon just prior to surgery (to decide which direction to work towards). Sometimes it is necessary to go through the placenta, and, in such cases, avoiding the cord insertion site (again helped with pre-op scan) is important and then the cord should be clamped as soon as possible on delivering the baby to minimise any fetal blood loss from the torn placenta. The neonatologist in attendance should also be warned that this is what is expected so they are prepared in case the baby does show signs of acute haemorrhage.

Breech

Many obstetricians believe the breech is much more at risk of being cut by the scalpel at uterine incision than with a cephalic baby, but studies have shown no difference with a rate of around 1% and this reiterates the previous advice – always take care and try to leave the membranes intact until the uterine incision is complete.

Make the incision big enough and all the principles of vaginal breech delivery hold true at CS. Pressure from above (do not pull) and do not lift the body till the nape of the neck is visible. In most cases, manipulation can be kept to a minimum if the initial incision is adequate.

A trapped fetal head during a breech delivery at CS is particularly stressful for the obstetrician, and it can be helpful if the anaesthetist administers a uterine relaxant.

In anticipation of an entrapment, always ensure that both abdominal and uterine incisions are adequate. If problems are still encountered and tocolysis does not resolve the problem, consider converting the incision to a 'J' incision by extending upwards from the angle of the incision.

Wrigley's forceps can be applied to assist in the delivery of the breech head at CS, but care still needs to be taken in avoiding hyperextension of the neck during the application of the blades and then the direction of traction must flex the neck.

Shoulder presentation

If a fetal arm is prolapsed through the vagina, consider ***Patwardhan's procedure***, which involves delivering the fetal breech first: usually, a transverse incision in the uterus is adequate, although the incision can be extended by converting it to a 'J' shape. The operator's hand is passed upwards until a leg is reached and either the leg or the breech is delivered. The rest of the delivery is as for a caesarean breech delivery. This technique can also be used if the head is deeply engaged and disimpaction is unsuccessful.

Premature infant

A very premature infant in the transverse or breech position with absent liquor may best be managed with a vertical incision in the uterus.

Uterine trauma

The uterine incision may extend into the broad ligament, tearing uterine vessels and leading to brisk bleeding. After consultation with the anaesthetist, if the woman is awake, it may be helpful to exteriorise the uterus, so that the posterior aspect of the uterus and broad ligament can be examined. In addition, traction to elevate the uterus may slow the blood loss and help to identify the bleeding areas requiring attention. The proximity of the ureter must be borne in mind and an effort made to sweep the bladder down and with it the ureter. This will enable better access to the uterine vessels. If bleeding is heavy it may be very difficult to identify the ureter. The first priority is to control haemorrhage and subsequent expert urological help should always be requested, if damage is suspected.

Troublesome haemorrhage from the angle of the uterine incision may be controlled by the insertion of a suture to control the uterine artery. Again, every effort should be made to identify the ureter.

Thromboprophylaxis

The need for thromboprophylaxis should be considered in all women undergoing CS. The widespread application of thromboprophylaxis protocols following CS is likely to be the cause of the significant reduction in the rate of maternal death from venous thromboembolism in the latest CMACE Reports. It should be remembered that risk factors are multiplicative, including advanced maternal age, caesarean in labour, pre-eclampsia, sepsis or other inflammatory conditions, haemorrhage and maternal obesity.

Audit standards

The following should be audited routinely (RCOG 2005):

- rates of CS, especially in different groups of women (e.g. Robson groups)
- incidence of massive blood loss associated with CS
- returns to theatre
- wound infections
- standard of documentation (including operative findings).

Summary

- CS is common and attention to detail is essential to minimise morbidity.
- Anticipation of problems and an awareness of the techniques described in this chapter, together with senior experienced help when appropriate are most likely to lead to the best outcomes.

References and further reading

1 Althabe F, Belizan JM, Villar J, *et al.* Mandatory second opinion to reduce rates of unnecessary caesarean sections in Latin America: a cluster randomised controlled trial. *Lancet* 2004;363:1934–40.

2 Bujold E, Bujold C, Hamilton EF, *et al.* The impact of a single-layer or double-layer closure on the uterine rupture. *Am J Obstet Gynecol* 2002;186:1326–30.

3 Centre for Maternal and Child Enquiries (CMACE). Saving Mothers' Lives: reviewing maternal deaths to make motherhood safer: 2006–08. The Eighth Report on Confidential Enquiries into Maternal Deaths in the United Kingdom. *Br J Obstet Gynaecol* 2011;118(Suppl. 1):1–203.

4 Cetin A. Superficial wound disruption after cesarean delivery: effect of the depth and closure of subcutaneous tissue. *Int J Gynecol Obstet* 1997;57:17–21.

5 Clark AS. Nonclosure of peritoneum at surgery. *Br J Obstet Gynaecol* 1997;104: 1099–1200.

6 Department of Health. *NHS Maternity Statistics, England – 2009/10.* (www.ic.nhs.uk/ pubs/maternity0910).

7 Haaz DM, Ayres AW. Laceration injury at cesarean section. *J Matern Fetal Neonatal Med* 2002;11:196–8.

8 Murphy DJ, Liebling RE, Patel R, *et al.* Cohort study of operative delivery in the second stage of labour and standard of obstetric care. *BJOG* 2003;110:610–15.

9 Murphy DJ, Liebling RE, Verity L, *et al.* Early maternal and neonaatal morbidity associated with operative delivery in second stage of labour: a cohort study. *Lancet* 2001;358:1203–8.

10 Murphy DJ, Pope C, Frost J, Liebling RE. Women's views on the impact of operative delivery in the second stage of labour: qualitative interview study. *BMJ* 2003;327: 1132–5.

11 National Collaborating Centre for Women's and Children's Health. *Caesarean Section. Clinical Guideline.* London: RCOG Press 2004.

12 Olah KS. Reversal of the decision for casesarean section in the second stage of labour on the basis of consultant vaginal assessment. *J Obstet Gynaecol* 2005;25:115–16.

13 Peleg D, Perlitz Y, Pansky S, *et al.* Accidental delivery through a vaginal incision (laparoelytrotomy) during caesarean section in the second stage of labour. *BJOG* 2001;108: 659–60.

14 Porter S, Paterson-Brown S. Avoiding inadvertent laparoelytrotomy. *BJOG* 2003;110: 91–2.

15 Royal College of Obstetricians and Gynaecologists Clinical Effectiveness Support Unit. *The National Sentinel Caesarean Section Audit Report.* London: RCOG Press 2001.

16 Wiener JJ, Westwood J. Fetal lacerations at caesarean section. *J Obstet Gynaecol* 2002;22:23–4.

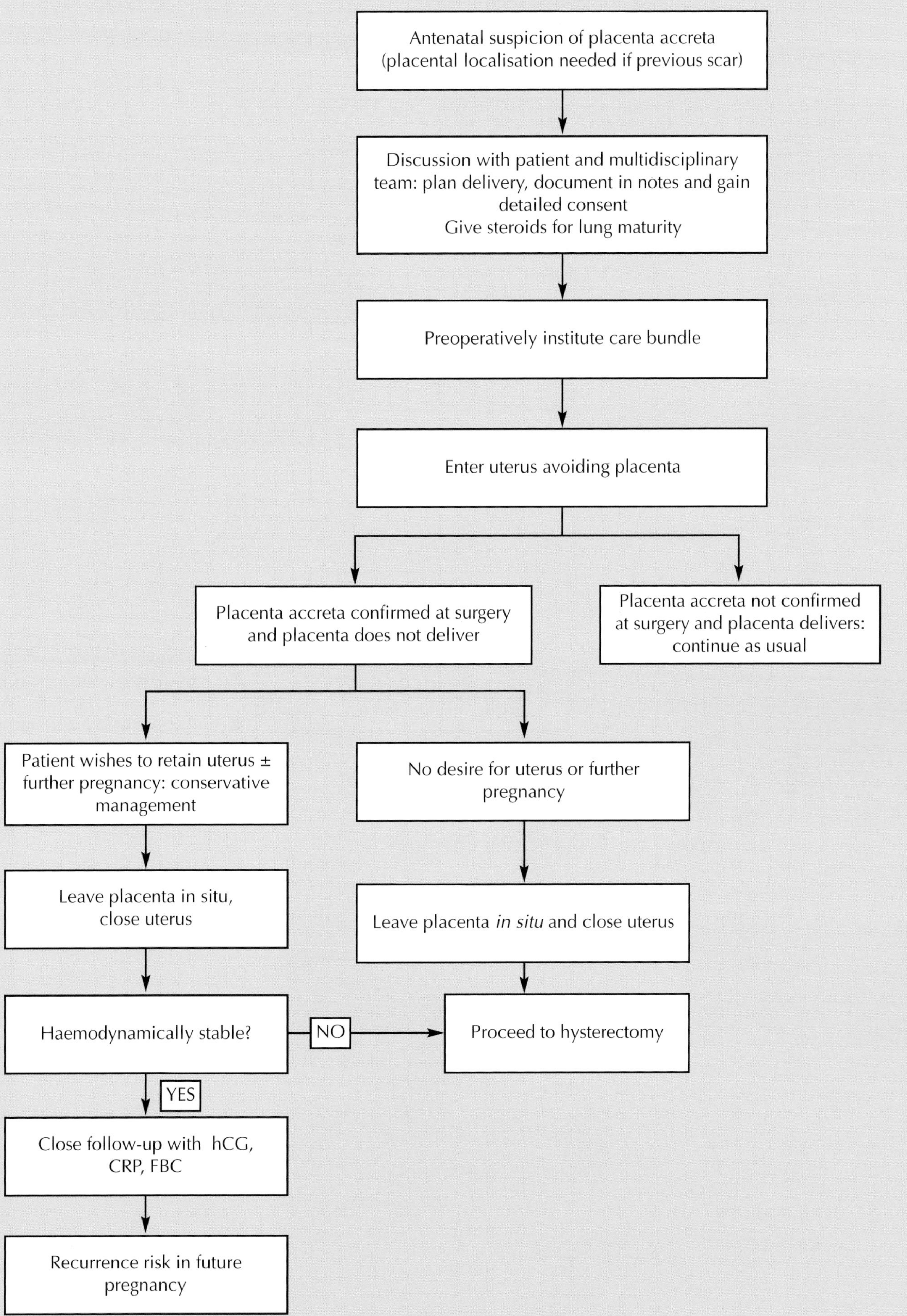
Antenatal suspicion of placenta accreta (placental localisation needed if previous scar)
Discussion with patient and multidisciplinary team: plan delivery, document in notes and gain detailed consent
Give steroids for lung maturity
Preoperatively institute care bundle
Enter uterus avoiding placenta
Placenta accreta confirmed at surgery and placenta does not deliver
Placenta accreta not confirmed at surgery and placenta delivers: continue as usual
Patient wishes to retain uterus ± further pregnancy: conservative management
No desire for uterus or further pregnancy
Leave placenta in situ, close uterus
Leave placenta in situ and close uterus
Haemodynamically stable?
NO
Proceed to hysterectomy
YES
Close follow-up with hCG, CRP, FBC
Recurrence risk in future pregnancy

ALGORITHM 27.2 Retained placenta

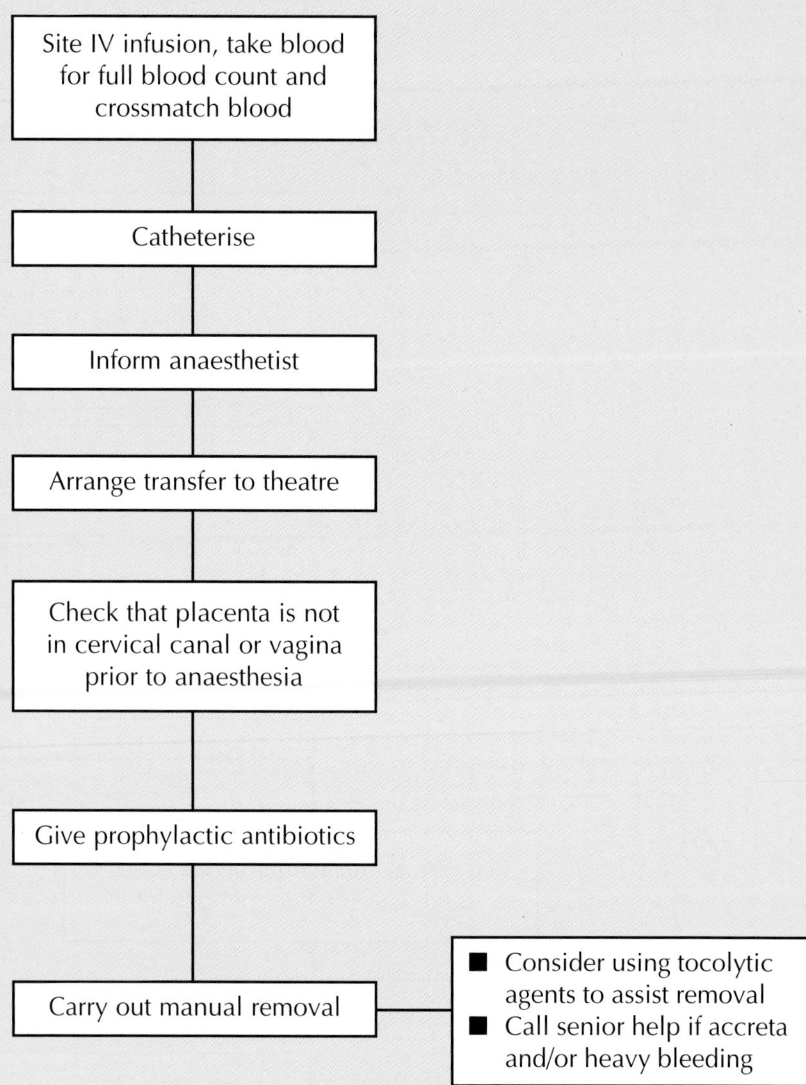

CHAPTER 27

Placenta accreta and retained placenta

Objectives

On successfully completing this topic, you will be able to:

- recognise risk factors for a morbidly adherent placenta
- understand the need for a multidisciplinary plan of management where accreta is suspected
- understand the technique of manual removal of the placenta.

Introduction

Postpartum haemorrhage is a major cause of maternal morbidity and mortality. Chapter 25 has covered the management of major obstetric haemorrhage; this chapter will look at the management of problems associated with an adherent placenta, where separation does not occur and manual removal is required or where the placenta is morbidly adherent.

Placenta accreta

Definition and incidence

Normally, the placenta does not penetrate deeper than the decidua basalis. If it invades further it will be morbidly attached, and heavy bleeding is likely if separation is attempted. The terms placenta accreta, increta and percreta refer to deeper penetration of the chorionic villi into, and ultimately through, the myometrium and possibly into adjacent organs, such as the bladder. In this chapter, placenta accreta will be used to refer to all grades of abnormal penetration.

The incidence is rising and is currently 2 per 1000 deliveries. It is usually associated with previous surgery to the uterus – most commonly a CS. The risk of accreta rises with the number of previous caesarean sections, and is greatest when associated with placenta praevia. If a woman having her third CS has a placenta praevia, she has a 40% chance of a placenta accreta. In the 2005–06 UK Obstetric Surveillance System study of peripartum hysterectomy, 39% of women having this operation had a morbidly adherent placenta, and the main risk factor was a previous CS.

The 2006–08 Confidential Enquiry into Maternal Mortality reported two deaths associated with placenta accreta.

Diagnosis

All women who have had a previous CS should undergo ultrasound assessment of the placental site, even if they decline an anomaly scan. If the placenta is anterior and appears to cover the scar (i.e. reaches the internal cervical os), the scan should be repeated at 32 weeks. Sonographic features that suggest accreta are:

- a loss of the hypoechoic retroplacental zone
- multiple vascular lacunae in the placenta giving a 'Swiss cheese' appearance
- blood vessels or placental tissue bridging uterine–placental margin, myometrial–bladder interface or crossing uterine serosa
- retroplacental myometrial thickness of <1mm
- numerous coherent vessels visualised with 3D power Doppler in basal view.

Studies suggest that colour Doppler has the highest sensitivity and moderate specificity.

MRI is recommended in cases where the scan is inconclusive, or where there is suspicion that the placenta has invaded adjacent organs. The features which suggest accreta are:

- uterine bulging
- heterogenous signal density within the placenta
- dark intraplacental bands on T2-weighted imaging.

Measurement of cell-free placental messenger RNA (mRNA) in the maternal plasma has been described as a means of improving the accuracy of the diagnosis, but is not clinically available. Elevated levels of alpha fetoprotein, free beta-human chorionic gonadotrophin and creatine kinase have also been associated with accreta, but are not advocated as screening or diagnostic tests.

Despite these investigations, it is not possible to diagnose or exclude placenta accreta with certainty in the antenatal period, and if the placenta still appears to overlie the scar at 32 weeks the management plan for a woman with a previous CS should assume that there is a risk of accreta.

Management

Any pregnant woman with a low anterior placenta or a placenta praevia and a previous CS is at risk of major haemorrhage and should have a regular assessment of full blood count (give iron supplements where appropriate). Care should be consultant based and follow the

Placenta Praevia after Caesarean Section care bundle:

- consultant obstetrician planned and directly supervising the delivery
- consultant anaesthetist planned and directly supervising anaesthesia at delivery
- blood and blood products available on site
- multidisciplinary involvement in preoperative planning
- discussion and consent including possible interventions (such as hysterectomy, leaving the placenta in situ, cell salvage and interventional radiology)
- local availability of level 2 critical care bed.

The optimal timing of delivery depends on the clinical features but is generally advocated around 37 weeks to reduce the risks of an emergency procedure should labour start spontaneously or heavy antepartum haemorrhage occur. It is advisable to administer steroids to improve fetal lung maturity.

Multidisciplinary discussion should involve:

- theatre staff to plan equipment required, such as cell salvage and additional instruments for hysterectomy and balloon tamponade
- interventional radiologists to decide if preoperative placement of femoral balloons is required, advise on imaging modalities required in theatre or to be on standby should the need arise
- anaesthetists to plan anaesthesia technique and equipment required, to liaise with critical care
- haematologist to alert laboratory staff to possible need for large amounts of blood and clotting factors
- consideration of the need for other surgical support: gynaecologist, vascular surgeon, urologist
- neonatal team, especially if surgery has to take place away from the normal theatre to allow access for interventional radiology.

It is advisable to draw up a checklist with the names and contact details of all involved in the case. This should be in the patient's notes in case labour starts prior to the planned date.

The consultant obstetrician should discuss plans with the woman and her partner, and document these in the notes. If their family is complete and the placenta does not readily separate, then immediate hysterectomy leaving the placenta in place is the best course of action. If the woman wishes to preserve her fertility, then it may be possible to leave the placenta in situ, and close the uterus. She must understand that hysterectomy may still be required, and she will have to attend for prolonged follow up; there is also a risk of infection to consider.

A retrospective, multicentre study in France from 1993–2007 reviewed 167 cases of accreta treated conservatively. Management was successful in 78%, spontaneous placental resorption occurred in 75% of these women – taking a median of 13.5 weeks (range 4–60 weeks). One woman died of complications related to administration of methotrexate. There were 21 successful subsequent pregnancies, but placenta accreta recurred in six pregnancies.

Surgical considerations

Ideally, the uterus should be opened avoiding the placenta; a vertical skin incision may be required. It is good practice to confirm the placental position by ultrasound scan immediately prior to the operation. If necessary, a scan probe can be covered with a sterile sleeve and used directly on the uterus intraoperatively. Exteriorisation of the uterus and a posterior uterine wall incision has been performed in cases where the placenta covers the entire anterior uterine wall.

If the placenta does not separate following administration of Syntocinon, the cord should be unclamped and drained of blood, and the cord ligated close to the placenta and cut short, and the uterine incision should be closed. Depending on the patient's wishes and clinical needs, hysterectomy or conservative treatment follows as appropriate. Prophylactic antibiotics are needed for a few days if the placenta is left in situ. Serum beta human chorionic gonadotropin (hCG) levels should be checked twice weekly, together with full blood count and C-reactive protein levels to look for signs of infection, and the woman kept under close review. Methotrexate has been used with varying degrees of success. As it precludes breastfeeding it should not be routinely used, but may be considered if the beta hCG levels do not fall.

In the situation where accreta was not anticipated, surgical entry has failed to avoid the placenta, or the placenta partially separates and bleeding ensues, the situation is more hazardous and associated with heavy bleeding. In these situations, it is advisable to remove the placenta as best possible, small portions of myometrium can be removed/sutured to reduce bleeding and local infiltration of uterotonics or balloon tamponade may be helpful. Hysterectomy is, however, likely to be needed in up to 50% of such cases and recognising this and performing it in a timely fashion, before the patient is in extremis, can be lifesaving. See Algorithm 27.1 for a diagrammatic representation of the management of placenta accreta.

Anaesthetic considerations

The operation is likely to be prolonged; if regional techniques are used it may be necessary to convert to general anaesthesia. Large-bore intravenous access and haemodynamic monitoring will be required, anticipating a large blood loss. Particular attention should be paid to positioning the patient to avoid nerve compression, and measures taken to reduce thromboembolism and hypothermia. If blood loss is excessive, cell salvage and reinfusion may reduce the need for blood transfusion, but it is important to monitor blood coagulation, as proportionally more platelets and cryoprecipitate may be required. If embolisation is required, it may be necessary to transport the patient from theatre to an imaging department.

Retained placenta

NICE intrapartum care guidelines define a placenta as retained if it is not delivered within 30 minutes of birth when the third stage is actively managed, or longer than an hour when physiologically managed, without signs of postpartum haemorrhage or maternal collapse. The longer the placenta remains undelivered, the greater the risk of haemorrhage. The common risk factors for retained placenta are:

- previous retained placenta
- multiparity
- preterm labour
- induced labour
- uterine fibroids and uterine anomaly, such as a bicornuate uterus
- uterine scar.

The placenta may be retained due to ordinary adherence, in which case there is not usually much bleeding until separation occurs, or due to abnormal adherence with accreta as discussed above. It may also be retained due to a contraction ring in the uterine body or corneal region; in these cases bleeding is heavier as the placenta has partially separated, but the uterus cannot contract down fully.

Management

Large-bore intravenous access should be secured, and blood taken for matching as there is a risk of major haemorrhage. It is likely that the midwife will have already catheterised the patient, but if not an indwelling catheter should be inserted.

A number of medical treatments have been advocated, but manual removal of the placenta is likely to be required. Nitroglycerin may be beneficial if the problem is due to a constriction ring. The drug is given sublingually, as a spray in a dose of 800 microgram, or intravenously (see below). There is no evidence to support the use of intravenous infusion or umbilical injection of oxytocin. The NICE guidelines did advocate the use of umbilical injection of oxytocin, but the subsequently published Release trial did not show any benefit, so this should no longer delay treatment. The patient should be moved to theatre, and a check made prior to anaesthesia that the placenta has not separated.

Anaesthesia for manual removal of placenta

If the patient is haemodynamically stable, regional anaesthesia is safer for the mother, although it may be necessary to give a uterine relaxant to enable the surgeon to get past the constriction ring. This is best achieved by intravenous nitroglycerin:

- add contents of one 5 mg ampoule to 100 ml normal saline: 1 ml of this solution will give 50 microgram; a dose of 50–250 microgram will be required. The drug acts within 90 seconds and, as it is rapidly metabolised with a half-life of 2 minutes, the effect soon wears off, thus minimising the risk of bleeding due to uterine atony following delivery of the placenta.

If there is significant bleeding, general anaesthesia will be necessary. This also provides an opportunity to use inhalational agents to relax the uterus. Prophylactic antibiotics should be given, and an oxytocin infusion will be commenced after the placenta has been removed.

Technique of manual removal

Full aseptic precautions are used in theatre. It is advisable to wear gauntlet length gloves and a nonpermeable gown as the operator's arm will usually need to go high into the uterus.

- If the cord is still attached, the operator's well-lubricated, dominant hand should follow this through the cervix with the fingers held in a cone shape. The other hand is placed on the patient's abdomen to steady the fundus and push it downwards. If there is a constriction ring, steady pressure should allow the hand to pass, but if not uterine relaxation may be required.
- The fingers and thumb should be kept together and the edge of the placenta identified, the placenta can then be steadily detached by sweeping movements. Clawing should be avoided as it may lead to rupture of the uterus and retention of placental cotyledons.
- The abdominal hand maintains pressure on the fundus and pushes it down onto the internal hand to facilitate the detachment of the placenta.
- Once the placenta is separated, it is grasped in the hand and removed slowly to prevent inversion, which may occur if there is still some placenta attached to the uterus. If the cord is still attached, the abdominal hand moves to the cord to apply traction, or grasps the edge of the placenta as it emerges in the vagina.
- The hand in the uterus should remain there after the placenta is removed to check the cavity to ensure there are no remaining pieces of placenta and the uterine wall is intact.
- Bimanual compression may be necessary to reduce blood loss until the uterus contracts in response to oxytocin.

Summary

- Retained placenta is relatively common and can be managed with little difficulty on most cases, although preparation for significant blood loss must be made.
- Placenta accreta is much less common, although incidence is rising. The condition carries significant risks for morbidity, mortality and subsequent fertility. Management requires senior multidisciplinary preparation and involvement. The available comprehensive guidelines (see Further reading) should be used.

References and further reading

1 RCOG. Greentop Guideline No 27. Placenta praevia, placenta praevia accreta and vasapraevia; diagnosis and management. London: RCOG, 2011.

2 Society for Maternal-Fetal Medicine. Clinical opinion: placenta accreta *Am J Obstet Gynecol* 2010;430–39.

3 NPSA. *Placenta praevia after CS care bundle: background information for healthcare professionals.* National Patient Safety Agency 2010. (www.nrls.npsa.nhs.uk/resources/?EntryId45=66359, accessed 10 March 2012).

4 Weeks AD, Alia G, Vernon G, *et al.*, Umbilical vein oxytocin for the treatment of retained placenta (Release Study): a double-blind, randomised controlled trial. *Lancet* 2010;375:141–7.

5 NICE. Clinical guideline 55. *Intrapartum care* 2007 (www.nice.org.uk/CG055, accessed 12 March 2012).

ALGORITHM 28.1 Uterine inversion

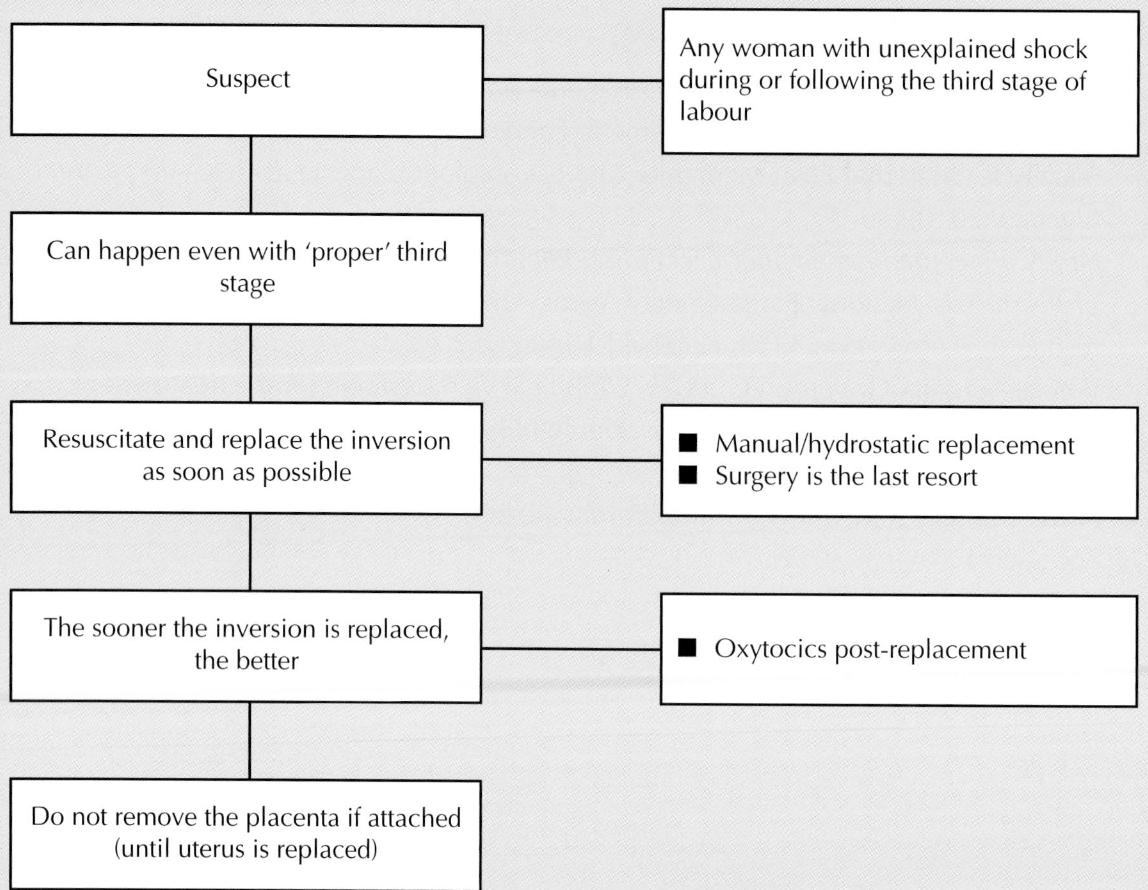

CHAPTER 28

Uterine inversion

Objectives

On successfully completing this topic, you will be able to:

- recognise and manage uterine inversion.

Introduction

Reported incidence ranges from 1/2000 to 1/6400. Although it has often been thought to be related to mismanagement of the third stage, uterine inversion was found even in an institution that did not use the Crede's manoeuvre, where they strongly discourage vigorous cord traction and where oxytocin was not given until after placental separation. Brar *et al.* found a fundal placenta in the majority of women.[1] Other associated obstetric conditions include a short cord, a morbidly adherent placenta and uterine anomalies.

Inversion of the uterus can be puerperal and nonpuerperal. However, chronic nonpuerperal uterine inversions are rare. In a study by Mwinyoglee *et al.*, only 77 cases were reported; 75 (97.4%) were tumour-produced and 20% of these tumours were malignant.[2]

Puerperal uterine inversions can follow vaginal delivery or occur at CS. Usual causes are cord traction before the uterus has contracted, but especially when there is a short umbilical cord, fundal insertion of placenta or an adherent placenta. Prompt understanding and repositioning by manual replacement will prevent further complications.

Immediate, nonsurgical measures are successful in the vast majority of cases of uterine inversion. The pooled experience of Brar *et al.*[1] and Watson[3] demonstrated only three laparotomies requiring surgical reposition out of a total of 102 uterine inversions.

Recognition

Early recognition of uterine inversion is vital to enable prompt treatment and to reduce morbidity and mortality.

Symptoms and signs

These include:

- severe lower abdominal pain in the third stage
- shock that is out of proportion to the blood loss, owing to parasympathetic stimulation
- haemorrhage (present in 94% of cases)
- placenta may or may not be attached
- uterine fundus not palpable per abdomen (in milder degrees there may be a dimple in the fundal area)
- pelvic examination showing a mass in the vagina (in milder degrees) or at/outside the introitus; if the placenta is still attached then it is palpable / visible as above.

Prevention

Mismanagement of the third stage should be avoided, and cord traction should not be applied until the signs of placental separation are apparent.

Management

1. Call for help (experienced obstetrician/anaesthetist/midwives).
2. Arrange replacement of uterus concurrently with antishock measures, as resuscitation may not be successful until the inversion is corrected. Sometimes the delivering attendant may be successful at immediate replacement, within seconds of the inversion.
3. Insert two wide-bore intravenous cannulae.
4. Collect blood for full blood count, coagulation studies and group and crossmatch (4–6 units).
5. Start fluid replacement immediately (colloids and crystalloids).
6. Continuously monitor blood pressure, pulse, respiratory rate, urine output, O_2 saturation.
7. If the bradycardia is pronounced, atropine can be administered.
8. Arrange appropriate analgesia.
9. Transfer to theatre.
10. If oxytocin has been running it should be stopped, as replacement requires the uterus to be relaxed.
11. If the placenta is still attached, it should be left as such until after repositioning. Attempts to remove the placenta may result in major bleeding, as there will be no uterine muscular contraction to constrict blood vessels in the placental bed.
12. Attempt to reposition the uterus; the earlier the restoration, the more likely the success.

Replace the uterus using one of the following techniques:

- manual replacement (the Johnson manoeuvre)
- hydrostatic repositioning (O'Sullivan's technique)
- medical approach
- surgery (laparotomy and Haultain's procedure or Huntingdon's operation).

Manual replacement

Manual replacement should be performed preferably under general anaesthesia. The uterus may require relaxation for manual replacement to succeed, and the aim should be to reduce the uterus in the order of 'last out first back in', gradually progressing such that the first bit out (the fundus) is replaced last. Once the replacement is complete the hand should be left inside the uterus while a uterotonic is administered and only when the uterus has contracted should a manual removal of the placenta ensue, with precautions for and treatment of post-partum haemorrhage.

Hydrostatic repositioning (O'Sullivan's technique)

Uterine rupture must be excluded first. Warm saline is infused into the posterior fornix of the vagina under gravity, from a height of about 2metres while the vaginal orifice is closed. The water distends the vagina gradually so that it stretches, the cervical constriction relaxes and the uterus gradually returns to its correct position. The process takes about 10–15 minutes and up to 2 litres of warm saline may be needed.

The fluid is best given by attaching the intravenous giving set to a silicone ventouse cup inserted into the vagina; this tends to produce a good seal facilitated by holding the vulva closed over the intravaginal cup.

A hard, black, rubber anaesthetic facemask can be used, which may fit over the vulva. The oxygen inlet allows access for fluid input.

Medical approach

Drugs are used to relax the cervical ring to facilitate replacement. Agents include:

- magnesium sulphate 2 g infused intravenously over 5 minutes
- ritodrine 0.15 mg intravenous bolus slowly
- terbutaline 0.25 mg intravenously
- nitroglycerin 100 microgrammes intravenously.

Surgery

Surgery is only used if all other attempts fail. In Huntingdon's procedure, Allis forceps are placed within the dimple of the inverted uterus and gentle upward traction is exerted on the clamps, with a further placement of forceps on the advancing fundus.

Haultain's technique involves incising the cervical ring posteriorly (where the incision is least likely to involve the bladder or uterine vessels) with a longitudinal incision and facilitates uterine placement by Huntingdon's method. After replacement has been completed the hysterotomy site is repaired.

Oxytocics should be administered after repositioning to keep the uterus contracted and prevent recurrence. The attendant's hand should remain in the uterine cavity until a firm contraction occurs.

Summary

- Prompt replacement of the inverted uterus has the best chance of success; shock must be treated concurrently and, once in place, the uterus must be allowed to, or stimulated to, contract before active placental delivery.

References and further reading

1 Brar HS, Greenspoon JS, Platt LD, Paul RH. Acute puerperal uterine inversion. New approaches to management. *J Reprod Med* 1989;34:173–7.

2 Mwinyoglee J, Simelela N, Marivate M. Non-puerperal uterine inversions. A two case report and review of the literature. *Cent Afr J Med* 1997;43:268–72.

3 Watson P, Besch N, Bowes WA Jr. Management of acute and subacute puerperal inversion of the uterus. *Obstet Gynecol* 1980;55:12–16.

4 Abouleish E, Ali V, Joumaa B, *et al.* Anaesthetic management of acute puerperal uterine inversion. *Br J Anaesth* 1995;75:486–7.

5 Clark S. Use of ritodrine in uterine inversion. *Am J Obstet Gynecol* 1984;151:705.

6 Dayan SS, Schwalbe SS. The use of small dose nitroglycerine in a case of uterine inversion. *Anesth Analg* 1996;82:1091–3.

7 Grossman R. Magnesium sulphate for uterine inversion. *J Reprod Med* 1980;20:161–2.

8 Huntington JL, Irving FC, Kellog FS. Abdominal reposition in acute inversion of the puerperal uterus. *Am J Obstet Gynecol* 1928;15:34–40.

9 Kriplani A, Relan S, Kumar R, *et al.* Complete inversion of the uterus during caesarean section: a case report. *Aust N Z Obstet Gynaecol* 1996;36:17–19.

10 Loeffler F. Postpartum haemorrhage and abnormalities of the third stage of labour. In: Chamberlain G (editor). *Turnbull's Obstetrics.* 2nd edn. Edinburgh: Churchill Livingstone 1995.

11 Manassiev N, Shaw G. Uterine inversion. *Modern Midwife* 1996;6(5):32–4.

12 Mohanty AK, Trehan AK. Puerperal uterine inversion: analysis of three cases managed by repositioning, and literature review. *J Obstet Gynecol* 1998;18:353–4.

13 Ogueh O, Ayida G. Acute uterine inversion: a new technique of hydrostatic replacement. *Br J Obstet Gynaecol* 1997;104:951–2.

14 O'Sullivan J. Acute inversion of the uterus. *Br Med J* 1945;2:282–3.

15 Shah-Hosseini R, Evrard JR. Puerperal uterine inversion. *Obstet Gynecol* 1989;73: 567–70.

16 Thomson AJ, Greer IA. Non-haemorrhagic obstetric shock. *Baillieres Best Pract Res Clin Obstet Gynaecol* 2000;14(1):19–41.

17 World Health Organization, UNFPA, UNICEG, World Bank. *Managing Complications in Pregnancy and Childbirth. A guide for midwives and doctors.* Geneva: WHO 2001.

ALGORITHM 29.1 Ruptured uterus

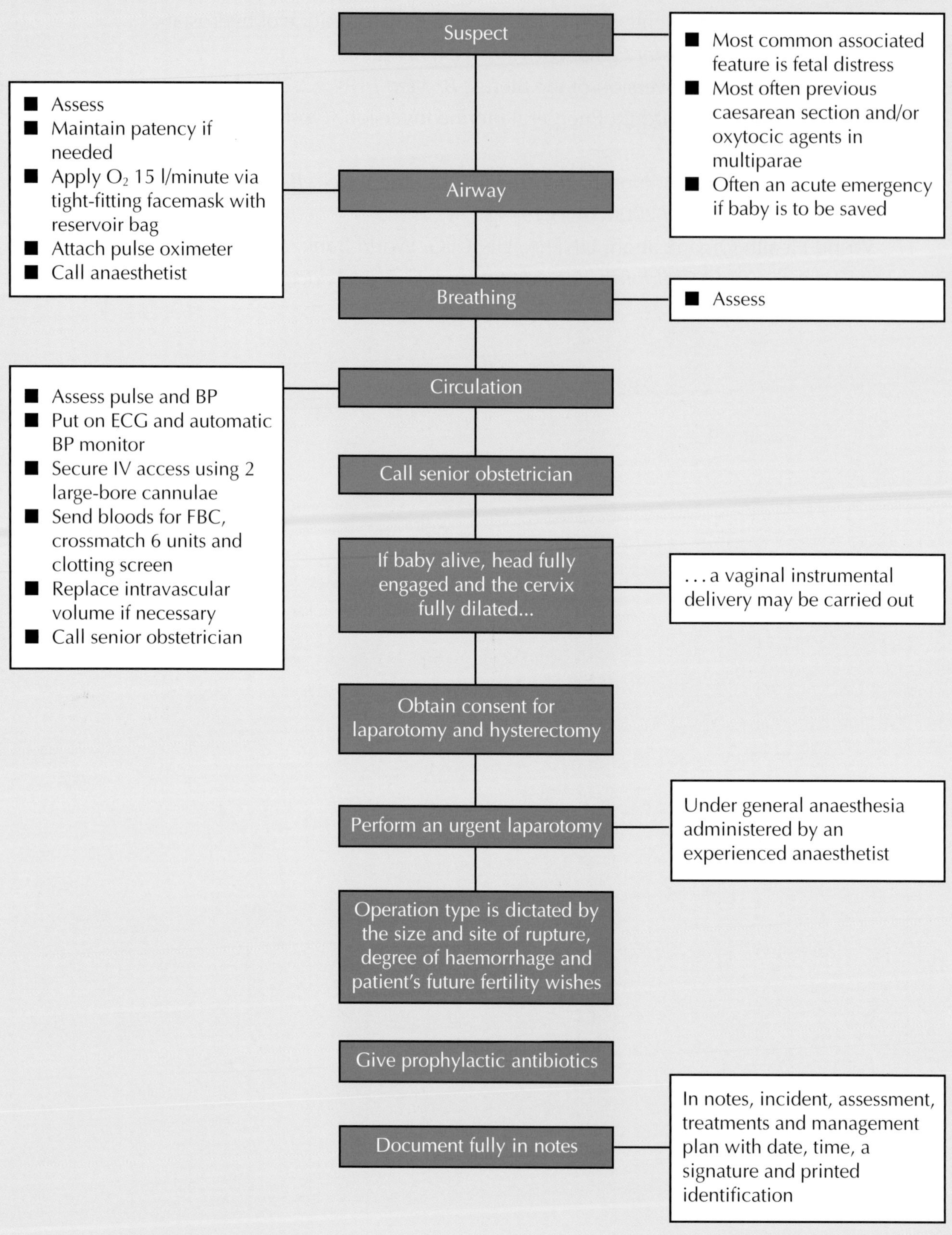

CHAPTER 29

Ruptured uterus

Objectives

On successfully completing this topic, you will be able to:

- discuss the risk factors for uterine rupture
- recognise a ruptured uterus early
- plan and manage a ruptured uterus.

Introduction

Complete rupture of the uterus can be a life-threatening emergency. Fortunately, however, the condition is rare in modern obstetrics, despite the increase in CS rates, and serious sequelae are even more rare.

Incidence and predisposing factors

Population studies, including large numbers (>50 000) of patients over the last few decades, give a low overall incidence of uterine rupture at approximately 0.3/1000 deliveries. Rupture is more likely in multigravid women, especially those who have undergone previous CS, but spontaneous rupture of the unscarred uterus does occur. Risk factors for rupture of an unscarred uterus include:

- grand multiparity
- undiagnosed cephalopelvic disproportion or malpresentation
- oxytocin administration
- macrosomic fetus
- placenta percreta
- prior uterine surgery
- version
- uterine abnormalities (e.g. rudimentary horn).

Previous CS

Smith *et al.* looked at 35 854 women who laboured with a previous CS: 74.2% had a vaginal delivery and the incidence of uterine rupture was 0.35%.[1] The risk was higher among women who had not previously given birth vaginally and those whose labour was induced with prostaglandin. Al Zirqi *et al.* reviewed 18 794 women who gave birth after a CS in Norway from 1999 to 2005.[2] Compared with elective prelabour CS, the odds ratio for rupture with spontaneous labour was 6.65, and for induced labour 12.6. Induction, using prostaglandins, increased the odds for rupture by 2.72 compared with spontaneous labour.

NICE recommendation

The NICE induction of labour guideline recommends that the induction of women with a previous CS is reasonable, and that prostin is appropriate, but that it should not occur on antenatal wards.

Hospital units need to provide:

- local guidelines regarding the augmentation of labour and induction of labour
- local guidelines regarding intrapartum fetal and maternal surveillance in women with a uterine scar.

Perinatal morbidity and mortality from uterine rupture

Leung *et al.* undertook a retrospective review of 106 cases of uterine rupture.[3,4] They found perinatal mortality and morbidity to be associated with complete fetal extrusion and more than 18 minutes delay between the onset of prolonged decelerations and delivery.

CESDI data

In the 1995 CESDI report of intrapartum deaths, there were 12 cases of ruptured uterus.[5] The two clinical features that stood out were:

- delay in making the diagnosis – fetal distress was invariably present but no action was taken
- the use of prostaglandins to induce labour.

Following this, a focus group was set up to review cases of ruptured uterus that were reported in the fifth CESDI report (1998).[6] Forty-two cases of ruptured uterus with fetal death were found, 75% of which were considered to have had significantly substandard care and 18 were only diagnosed at laparotomy.

Factors identified in the CESDI report

- Obesity (46% BMI greater than 30 compared with 14% of the female population in this age group).
- Uterine scar (30/42); of the 12 women without a scar, only one was nulliparous.

- Antenatal issues: absence of a recorded plan (five cases), failure to involve seniors (four cases) and inappropriate decision about induction (four cases).
- Induction (60%) and augmentation (25%): all 12 women without scars had oxytocics; 23/30 of women with previous CS had oxytocics.
- Fifty percent of ruptures occurred at or close to full dilatation.
- Failure to involve senior staff was common.
- Delay in transfer to theatre (five cases).

Maternal morbidity and mortality

Thankfully, while there is significant maternal morbidity, mortality from uterine rupture is extremely rare. Nine of the 42 women in the CESDI report required hysterectomy, but all lived.

Confidential maternal UK death data

Deaths from uterine rupture in the confidential maternal UK death reports has steadily fallen over the last two decades from five in 1994–96 to only one in 2006–08: this most recent death was in a woman who had placenta accreta.

Practice and training issues

All involved in intrapartum care of women must be aware of the factors that may lead to uterine rupture. In particular, they must recognise that women with a uterine scar are 'high risk' and should be managed appropriately.

- Antenatal management needs to include plans for delivery and induction, with a documented discussion with senior obstetrician (ideally a consultant but at least ST6 or higher).
- Attentive intrapartum fetal and maternal surveillance in a setting where CS can be performed within 30 minutes.
- No more than one dose of prostaglandin, unless great vigilance is exercised.
- Raise awareness of the warning signs:
  - fetal heart rate anomalies
  - fetal bradycardia
  - scar pain and/or tenderness
  - vaginal bleeding
  - concealed bleeding (shoulder tip pain)
  - poor progress in labour.

Findings at the time of laparotomy

Lower uterine segment dehiscence is the most common finding. The rupture of the lower segment may extend anteriorly into the back of the bladder or laterally towards the region of the uterine artery, or even into the broad ligament plexus of veins, causing extensive haemorrhage and damage. Posterior rupture of the uterus is uncommon and would usually be seen in relation to previous uterine surgery or intrauterine manipulation, but can occur spontaneously.

Management

Three options exist in terms of managing uterine rupture. Two experienced obstetricians should be present.

Simple repair

This depends on the extent of the injury and on the wishes of the mother. In one series of 23 cases of ruptured uterus, hysterectomy was undertaken in 15 (65%) cases and repair in the other eight. Five successful further pregnancies were reported without repeat rupture (all delivered by CS).

Subtotal hysterectomy

The choice of subtotal hysterectomy may be dictated by the individual situation, the anatomy and the extent of the trauma.

Total hysterectomy

There should be particular concern about the ureters when the rupture has extended laterally into the broad ligament or inferolaterally towards the vagina (and there may be value in obtaining postnatal imaging to check).

Summary

- Constant vigilance, antenatal, as well as intrapartum is required to diagnose and manage uterine rupture.
- Listen to the woman.
- Anticipate complications.
- Monitor carefully.
- Respond quickly.
- Follow national recommendations.

References and further reading

1 Smith GC, Pell JP, Pasupathy D, Dobbie R. Factors predisposing to perinatal death related to uterine rupture during attempted vaginal birth after caesarean section: retrospective cohort study. *BMJ* 2004;329:375.

2 Al-Zirqi, Stray-Pedersen B, Forsen L, Vangen S. Uterine rupture after previous caesarean section. *BJOG* 2010; 117:809–20.

3 Leung AS, Farmer RM, Leung EK, *et al.* Risk factors associated with uterine rupture during trial of labor after cesarean delivery: a case control study. *Am J Obstet Gynecol* 1993;168:1358–63.

4 Leung AS, Leung EK, Paul RH. Uterine rupture after previous cesarean delivery: maternal and fetal consequences. *Am J Obstet Gynecol* 1993;169:945–50.

5 Maternal and Child Health Research Consortium. *Confidential Enquiry into Stillbirths and Deaths in Infancy. Annual Report 1 January to 31 December 1993.* London: Maternal and Child Health Research Consortium 1995.

6 Maternal and Child Health Research Consortium. *Confidential Enquiry into Stillbirths and Deaths in Infancy. Annual Report 1 January to 31 December 1996.* London: Maternal and Child Health Research Consortium 1998.

7 Enkin M. Labour and delivery following previous caesarean section. In: Chalmers I, Enkin M, Keirse MJNC (eds). *Effective Care in Pregnancy and Childbirth.* Oxford: Oxford University Press 1989;1196–215.

8 Fedorkow DM, Nimrod CA, Taylor PJ. Ruptured uterus in pregnancy: a Canadian hospital's experience. *CMAJ* 1987;137:27–9.

9 Phelan JP, Korst LM, Settles DK. Uterine activity patterns in uterine rupture: a case–control study. *Obstet Gynecol* 1998;92:394–7.

ALGORITHM 30.1 Prerequisites for instrumental vaginal delivery

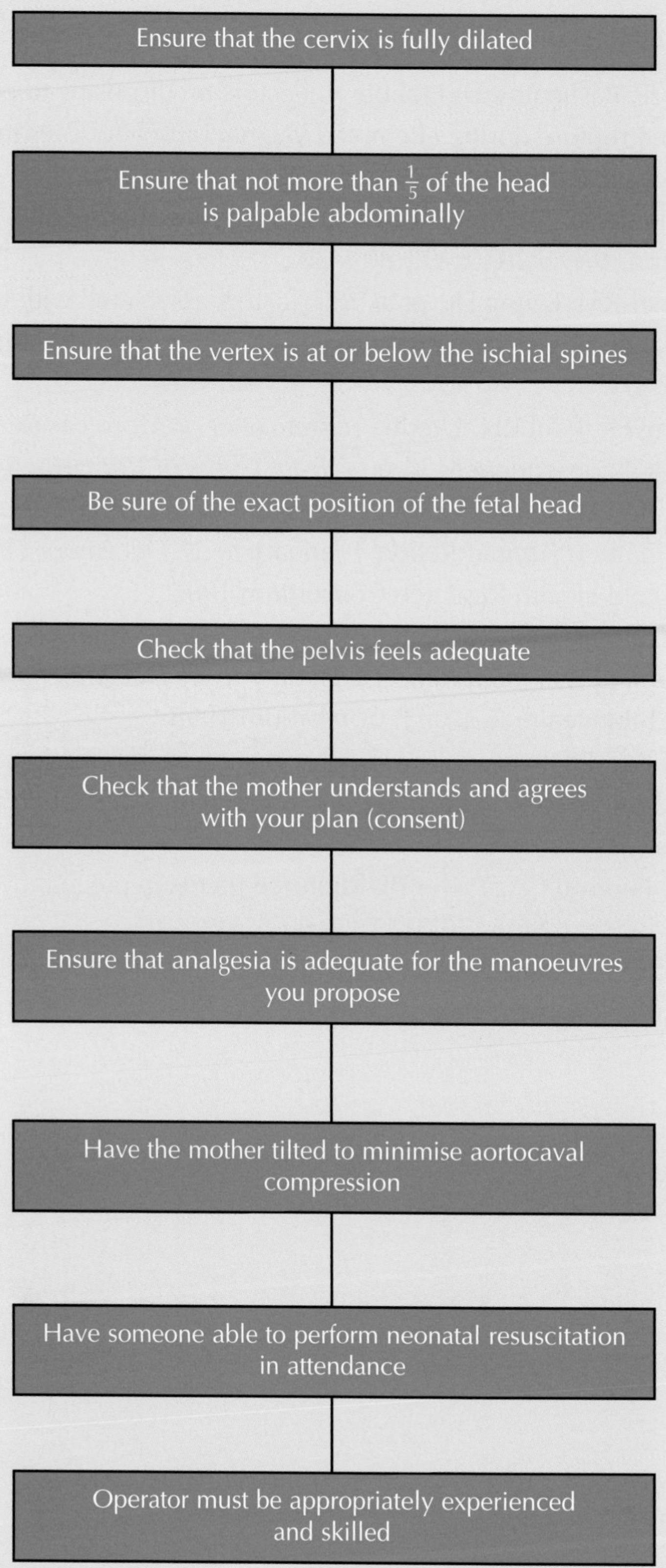

ALGORITHM 30.2 Rules for safety when conducting ventouse delivery

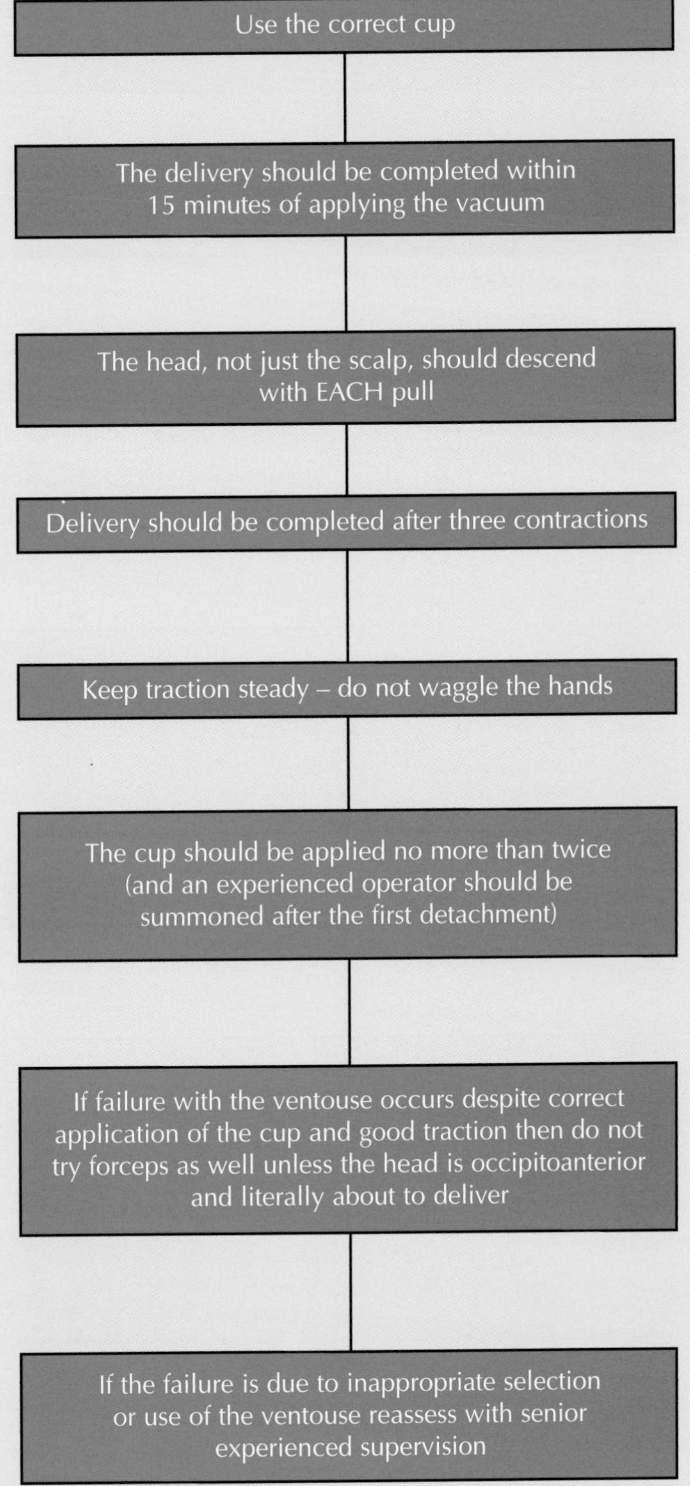

ALGORITHM 30.3 Rules for safety when conducting forceps delivery

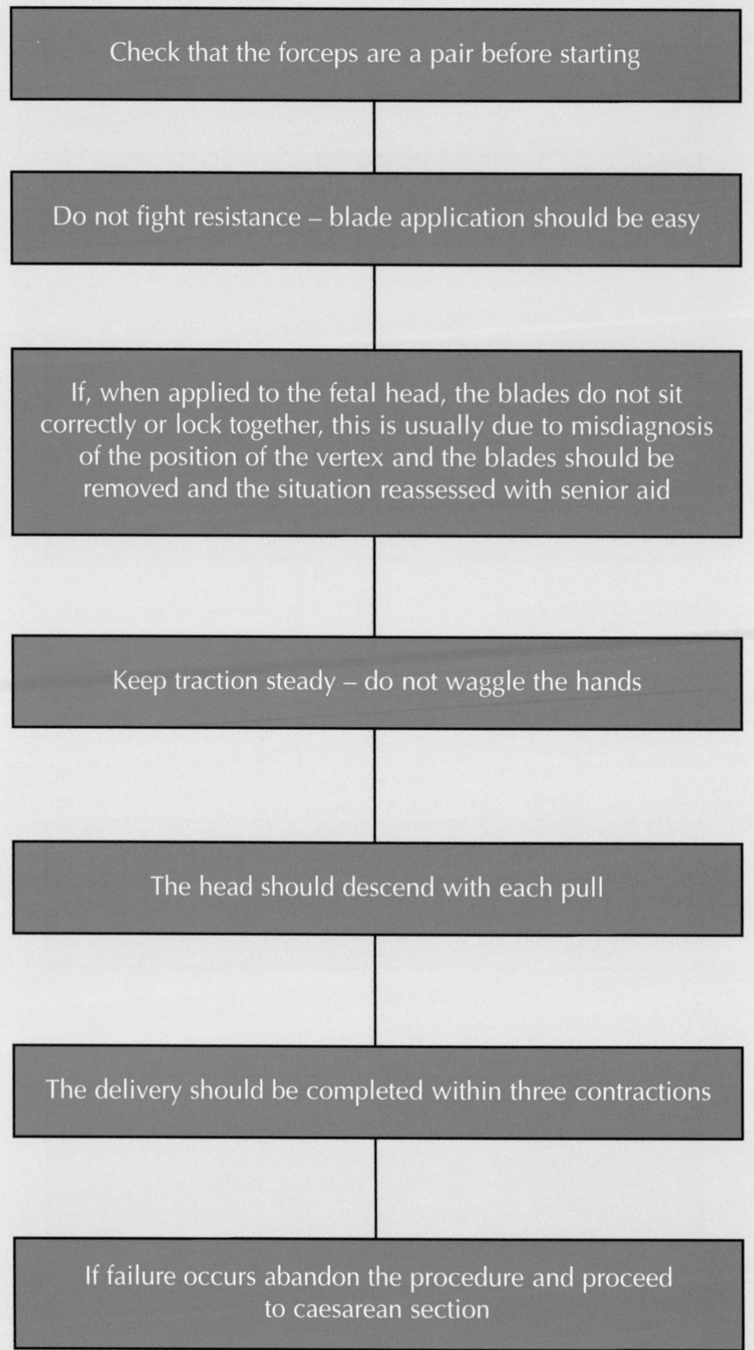

CHAPTER 30

Ventouse and forceps delivery

Objectives

On successfully completing this topic, you will be able to:

- decide when an instrumental delivery is appropriate
- decide which instrument is most appropriate in a specific circumstance
- appreciate the techniques required for vacuum and forceps delivery
- recognise and appreciate the causes of failure to deliver with the instrument selected
- know what to do when the instrumental delivery has failed.

Introduction

Operative vaginal delivery (OVD) aims to expedite the delivery of a baby who is believed to be at risk of compromise or when the mother is unable to push it out herself. Worldwide, assisted vaginal delivery remains an integral part of the obstetrician's duties. Rates vary from 1.5% of deliveries (Czech Republic) to 15% (Australia and Canada) and from 9% to 13% regionally in the UK. These varying rates reflect not only different clinical practices but also different attitudes. Low OVD rates may reflect high CS rates, including those performed at full dilatation, because of a reluctance to perform instrumental deliveries. There is evidence of an increasing trend towards using emergency CS directly for delay in the second stage, without resort to a trial of instrumental delivery. This is particularly with occipito-posterior positions at midcavity. Although instrumental vaginal delivery can be hazardous and should be undertaken with care, the difficulty of CS at full dilatation should not be underestimated; it can be extremely difficult and is associated with high maternal morbidity. There is emerging evidence to support the direct supervision of trainees in this situation in order to maximise the appropriate number of operative vaginal deliveries both attempted and achieved.

Women who labour are, by definition, aiming for vaginal delivery and therefore efforts should be focused on helping them to achieve this normally and safely. Various techniques may help in achieving high spontaneous vaginal delivery rates, such as the use of a partogram, companionship in labour, delaying pushing in women who have had epidural anaesthesia, upright posture and active management of the second stage of labour using oxytocin in nulliparae with epidurals.

Training and simulation in obstetrics

Simulation has an increasing role in developing appropriate skills for OVD. Use of 'high fidelity' manikins such as the PROMPT pelvic simulator, can allow objective assessment of traction force. Dupuis *et al.* have shown that sophisticated simulators can accelerate gaining competence in accurate forceps application (using computer-aided tracking technology).[1]

Importance of nontechnical skills in OVD

Bahl *et al.*[2] initially described the 'technical skills' required to undertake an operative vacuum delivery and described three 'skills' covering the areas of:

- assessment and preparation
- cup application
- traction with the cup.

These are particularly useful in teaching trainees, both on simulators and in early patient contact. In their subsequent paper, they outline the vital importance of 'nontechnical skills' which include:

- situation awareness
- decision-making
- task management
- teamwork/communication
- appropriate professional behaviour
- crossmonitoring of performance.

It is often errors in these areas that compromise patient safety – one example being loss of situational awareness with an inappropriate number of pulls to try and achieve vaginal delivery. The experienced operator should consider how they teach these skills to their trainees.

Indications for OVD

Indications are:

- delay in the second stage of labour
- fetal compromise in the second stage of labour
- maternal conditions that require either a short second stage or avoidance of Valsalva.

Prerequisites for OVD

Clinical examination should include both abdominal palpation and vaginal examination:

- preferably, the fetal head should not be palpable abdominally (i.e. 0/5 palpable); an experienced clinician can consider OVD if the head is no more than 1/5 palpable (this is usually associated with midcavity arrest and malposition)
- the cervix should be fully dilated
- the vertex (bone, not caput) should be at or below the ischial spines
- the exact position of the fetal head should be established
- the pelvis should feel adequate clinically.

Informed consent is needed: check that the mother understands and agrees with your plan. The RCOG (2010) has produced advice on consent for OVD.[3] The guideline paper outlines which risks should ideally be discussed (within the constraints of the individual clinical situation). A model consent form is provided in the guideline.

Adequate analgesia is needed but this will vary according to the type of delivery proposed, as discussed below.

Make sure the woman is sitting up and tilted as far as practicable to minimise aortocaval compression during the procedure – ideally this should be towards her left side (this is best achieved by placing a wedge underneath her right hip).

Someone should be in attendance that is capable of performing neonatal resuscitation. The operator must be appropriately experienced and skilled.

Safety matters and choice of instrument

When an assisted vaginal delivery is contemplated, careful clinical assessment is vital in order to confirm whether it is appropriate to proceed and to select the most suitable instrument. The different types of ventouse and forceps instruments both have their advantages and disadvantages. Promoting one type over another is inappropriate, as the instrument most suited for the situation at hand, with which the operator is experienced and skilled, is what matters to each individual mother and baby. The advantage of the ventouse cup over forceps relates to its being associated with significantly less maternal trauma and requiring less analgesia, but it is more likely to cause fetal cephalohaematoma and retinal haemorrhage. In addition, ventouse deliveries are significantly more likely to fail than forceps deliveries. Both forceps and vacuum deliveries are associated with an increased risk of shoulder dystocia, but the risk is highest with vacuum (3.5% versus 1.5%). Using a combination of instruments is associated with increased complications. It is best to choose one likely to achieve success.

Different types of ventouse and forceps instruments are available to deal with lift out and rotational deliveries, but the rotational deliveries require particular skills, especially when using forceps. Use of Kjelland's forceps has declined because of concerns about the risks of increased neonatal and maternal morbidity. However, in skilled hands and following appropriate training and supervision, the overall rates of morbidity are low and can avoid the trauma associated with CS at full dilatation. Recent observational data suggests that the risk of third/fourth degree is no higher with Kjelland's forceps than with nonrotational forceps (although both have a higher risk than vacuum delivery). Whichever instrument is selected, the operator must be experienced and skilled in its use (or be supervised directly by someone who is). In all cases, as mentioned above, the exact position of the baby's head must be established before proceeding. There have been many publications over the past 5 years confirming that ultrasound assessment in the second stage of labour allows more accurate confirmation of fetal position. This technique is particularly useful when there is marked caput and can be used as an adjunct (rather than as a replacement) to careful abdominal and vaginal assessment. The operator should place the ultrasound probe suprapubically and seek to delineate the prominent orbital ridges. Ultrasound has also been used in labour to measure degree of asynclitism and descent, as well as predicting the likelihood of achieving a vaginal delivery. It is universally acknowledged that the tendency to put a ventouse on a baby because the position is not clear is totally unacceptable and dangerous. One study demonstrated that 17 of 64 (27%) fetal head positions diagnosed clinically on digital vaginal examination were incorrect when checked with ultrasound and continued vigilance, training and supervision in this area is urgently needed.

Conditions where ventouse should be preferred to forceps

1 Urgent delivery required with no previous analgesia when a low lift out, easy delivery is anticipated.
2 Low lift out delivery, especially if there has been no prior analgesia.
3 Rotational delivery, if operator has inadequate experience with Kjelland's forceps.
4 Operator or maternal preference, when either instrument would be suitable.

Conditions where forceps should be preferred to ventouse

1 Face presentation (an absolute contraindication to ventouse).
2 Aftercoming head of the breech.
3 Marked active bleeding from a fetal blood-sampling site.
4 Gestation of less than 34 weeks (between 34 and 36 weeks the ventouse is 'relatively' contraindicated).
5 Large amount of caput.
6 Certain fetal or maternal haematological conditions (e.g. autoimmune thrombocytopenia [AITP], haemophilia).
7 Mother who is unable or unwilling to push.
8 Operator or maternal preference when either instrument would be suitable.

Ventouse/vacuum

There are a number of soft cups in common use which are smoothly applied to the contour of the baby's head and do not develop a 'chignon'. The vacuum achieved is particularly poor when soft cups are applied to moderate or severe caput (as adhesion to folds of oedematous skin is poor). In addition, they have limited manoeuvrability and cannot be correctly placed when the head is deflexed. Consequently, soft cups have a poorer success rate than metal cups, but are less likely to be associated with scalp trauma. Being soft, they are easy to apply and unlikely to injure the mother. As they are cleaned and sterilised as one item, they present no problems with assembly or leakage.

The hard cups are traditionally metal, the most widely used being the 'Bird-modification' cups. These have a central traction chain and a separate vacuum pipe. The anterior cups come in 4, 5 and 6cm sizes. The posterior cup is 5cm in diameter and has either the standard chain or the new cord for traction. The posterior cup is designed to be inserted higher up in the vagina than the anterior cups, to allow correct placement when the head is deflexed. Many units will use the 'Kiwi' omnicup cup (a light, disposable, hard plastic cup with integrated vacuum mechanism). A variant has an additional display which allows semi-objective estimation of traction force applied. These cups are useful for both rotational and nonrotational deliveries, but operators should be aware that two studies have suggested a higher failure rate compared with standard metal cup ventouse. Experienced operators usually recommend use of the largest metal cup available when trying to achieve delivery from transverse or posterior positions at pelvic mid-cavity level (i.e. from '0' to '+2cm' below the ischial spines).

It has been shown that successful delivery is most likely with the ventouse when the cup is applied over the flexion point, which lies in the midline just in front of the posterior fontanelle. A cup is ideally positioned when it covers the posterior fontanelle with the sagittal suture pointing to the centre of the cup. A well-placed cup will result in a well-flexed head (Figure 30.1), while failure to put the cup far enough back will result in deflexion and a higher chance of detachment and failure.

Safe delivery with the ventouse

To minimise the chances of any fetal damage, the basic rules for delivery with the ventouse should be followed. Overall, the risks of perinatal trauma using the vacuum extractor correlate with the duration of application, the station of the fetal head at the commencement of the delivery, the degree of difficulty of the delivery and the condition of the baby at the time of commencement of the procedure. When contemplating using the ventouse, in addition to the factors mentioned above, it is particularly important that there are good uterine contractions and that the mother is fully cooperative and able and willing to push. The increasing tendency to perform operative deliveries in theatre as 'trials' (which are conducted under dense regional blockade with associated significant compromise to maternal efforts) may be increasing the likelihood of failures with these instruments.

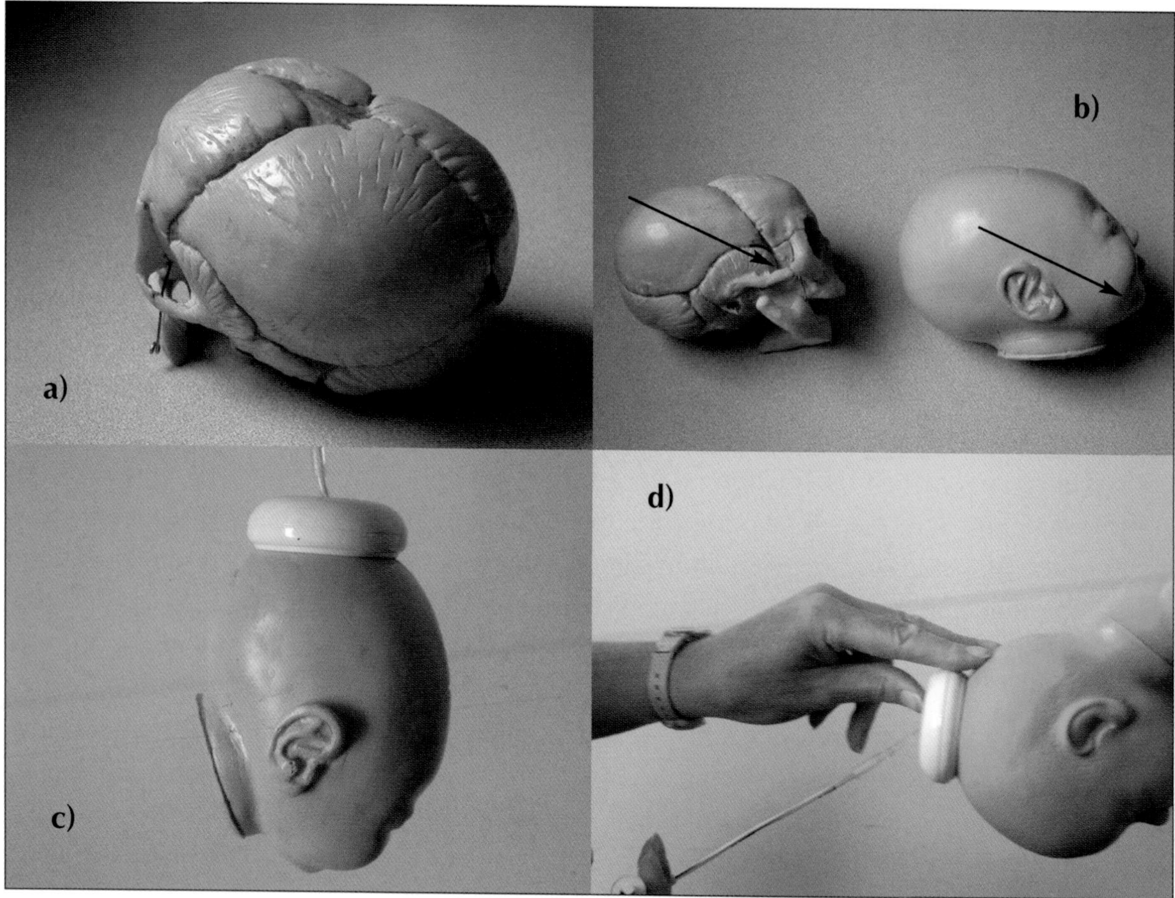

Figure 30.1 Ventouse: (a) Note how far back the posterior fontanelle is; (b) Note the axis through the flexion point, which results in the smallest presenting diameter; (c) The ventouse cup applied over the flexion point; (d) traction (along the pelvic axis) and the three-fingered grip of the ventouse cup with the second hand.

Basic rules for safe use of the ventouse

1. The delivery should be completed within 15 minutes of application of the vacuum (15 minutes is given as the maximum time allowed for application but the average time from insertion of the cup to delivery in over 400 deliveries was 6 minutes).
2. The head, not just the scalp, should descend with each pull.
3. Delivery should be complete within three pulls (if the head is crowning a fourth pull is allowed).
4. Keep the hands steady during traction – do not waggle, as this increases scalp trauma.
5. The cup should be reapplied no more than twice (and after one detachment an experienced operator should be summoned).
6. If failure with the ventouse occurs despite good cup placement and good traction, do not try the forceps as well.

Method

There is no need to catheterise the woman (unless there is another indication, such as epidural anaesthesia). No additional anaesthesia is required (perineal infiltration will suffice if an episiotomy is needed). Lithotomy is the most common position used (and should be used with lateral tilt) but delivery may be possible in dorsal, lateral or squatting positions.

Examine the woman carefully. Estimate the size of the baby by abdominal examination and ensure that the head is fully engaged (less than one-fifth of the head should be palpable). Confirm vertex presentation, position and the amount of caput through vaginal examination. Describe the attitude of the presenting part as 'flexed' or 'deflexed' (any situation where the anterior fontanelle can be felt easily) and take note of any asynclitisim.

The appropriate cup should be chosen

1 The silicone rubber cup can be used with any well-flexed vertex presentation, as long as the mother is cooperative, the baby is average-sized and there is minimal caput (i.e. by pressing firmly all details of the cranium should be felt, the skin will not be deep and will feel only slightly spongy). This cup is rarely suitable for occipitolateral positions, as the asynclitism associated with them tends to make placement of this cup over the posterior fontanelle difficult.

2 The anterior metal cup should be chosen if the baby is big, if the second stage is prolonged and if there is a moderate degree or more of caput (the skin may feel deep, may be folded and will definitely be spongy). It may also be used if the head is only slightly deflexed or slightly rotated, provided correct cup placement can be achieved. The 6 cm cup is preferable to the 5 cm cup because it allows greater traction without increasing the risk of scalp trauma. Only where the vagina is narrow should the 5 cm cup be used. The small 4 cm cup is reserved for use with the second twin, particularly if the cervix is no longer fully dilated.

3 The most valuable posterior metal cup, as its name indicates, is used for occipito-posterior positions, but also for occipito-lateral positions. It is particularly useful in situations with significant asynclitism and/or deflexion.

Once the correct cup has been chosen and connected to its pump as required (electric or hand) a check should be made for leakages prior to commencing the delivery. Common problems include suction bottles not tightly screwed in or tubing loosely attached to the metal cups (not locked with the small plastic ring). The metal cups should have a meshed bottom plate, which functions to maintain a clear space between the scalp and the cup so that an effective vacuum can be applied.

Silicone rubber cup

The silicone rubber cup is used in the following manner: it is folded and gently inserted into the vagina with one hand from above downwards, while the other hand parts the labia. A gentle twist may help it to unfold into place in the vagina and thereafter it is essentially not manoeuvrable, being larger in diameter than the metal cup and having a relatively inflexible handle.

Take the pressure up to 0.2 kg/cm^2, check that no maternal tissue is caught under the cup and then continue directly to 0.8 kg/cm^2, beginning traction with the next contraction after this pressure has been achieved. In a recent randomised controlled trial (RCT), there was no significant difference in successful vaginal delivery rates where this method was used (as opposed to sequential pressure increases of 0.2 kg/cm^2).[4] There were significant reductions in the mean application-maximum negative pressure time (–4.6 95% CI [–4.4 to –4.8]) minutes and in mean application-delivery time (–4.4 95% CI [–4.8 to –4.0]) minutes. Where gentle to moderate traction is required, it is reasonable to take the pressure to 0.6kg/cm^2 and in those rare situations where deliveries are undertaken between 34 and 36 weeks, it may suffice to stop at 0.4 kg/cm^2.

Traction should be along the pelvic axis for the duration of the contraction. One hand should rest on the bell of the cup (Figure 30.1) while the other applies traction. Malmstrom said: 'Vacuum extraction is a matter of cooperation between the traction hand and the backward-pressing hand'[5]. The hand on the cup detects any early detachment and also indicates whether the head moves downwards with each pull. The fingers on the head can promote flexion and can help to guide the head under the arch of the pubis by using the space in front of the sacrum. As the head crowns, the angle of traction changes through an arc of over 90°, but the fetal head should guide the hands, not the other way around: raising the hands too early causes extension of the fetal head, increasing the diameter of the presenting part. This, in turn, increases the risk of trauma to the perineum and can cause cup detachment.

At this point, if necessary, an episiotomy can be cut but if the perineum is stretching as normal, it is simply supported with the hand that was on the bell. Occasionally, an edge of the cup might lift off at the introitus (this is more likely to happen if there is caput present or if the hands have been raised too early). If this occurs, you must be careful not to catch maternal tissue under the cup as it reattaches, and thus this should be rechecked before final delivery of the head.

Anterior metal cup

The metal cup is lightly lubricated and then inserted sideways into the vagina. To orientate the cup, make sure the chain and vacuum pipe lie centrally over the posterior fontanelle. Check that no maternal tissue is included at low pressure then traction can commence once a negative pressure of 0.8kg/cm^2 has been achieved. Otherwise, the controlled two-handed manner of delivery is similar to that described for the soft cup above, classically using the 'three-finger grip' for the fingers on the cup and head (Figure 30.1). This not only helps to confirm that the fetal head and not just the scalp is descending but also that the fingers apply a force which opposes the lifting tendency of the upper edge of the rigid cup when pulling downwards earlier in the delivery and which oppose the lifting tendency of the lower edge when pulling upwards at the end of the delivery.

Posterior metal cup

When confronted with a deflexed head in an occipitoposterior position, the 'OP' cup should be used. It is applied as far back on the head as possible, again aiming to lie in the midline over the posterior fontanelle. To allow good placement of the cup, it sometimes helps to try to flex the head, with two fingers of the left hand pressing on the sinciput, while the right hand inserts the cup behind the head. Once correctly placed, the vacuum can be started and taken directly to the required level (because the cup lies parallel to the vagina it is unlikely to catch any maternal tissue).

The first pull will be in the direction required to flex the head and with this flexion the presenting diameter immediately becomes smaller. Thereafter, traction should be along the pelvic axis. The delivery may be completed simply by a standard spontaneous rotation with maternal effort and gentle assistance. It is important not to try to twist the cup to rotate the baby as this can increase scalp injuries.

Difficulty is sometimes encountered once the head flexes, as the suction pipe can tend to kink, making it more likely to detach. If the cup detaches at this point (after flexion and rotation) it may be simplest to change to an anterior cup or, if speed is essential, to perform a lift-out forceps.

Avoiding failure with the ventouse

Failure rates reported in the literature vary enormously but studies report rates from 6% to as much as 20–30%. There is increasing concern that failure rates are rising and with the evidence that caesarean sections in second stage are associated with significant morbidity attention to technique is vital. The following factors contribute to ventouse failure:

1 Inadequate initial assessment of the case: the head is too high. A classic mistake is to assume that because caput can be felt below the ischial spines the head must be engaged: always palpate the abdomen carefully.

2 Misdiagnosis of the position and attitude of the head: attention to simple detail will minimise the occurrence of this problem.

3 Incorrect instrument selected: failures with the silicone rubber cup will be common if it is used inappropriately when there is deflexion of the head, excess caput, a big baby, a prolonged second stage of labour or an uncooperative mother.

4 Either anterior or lateral placements of the cup will increase the failure rate: anterior placements are also more likely to be associated with fetal injury. In this respect, preterm infants are more vulnerable (even greater care should be taken to check position before application in these cases). If the cup placement is found to be incorrect, it may be appropriate to begin again with correct placement: midline over the posterior fontanelle or change to forceps.

5 Failures due to traction in the wrong direction; these may be amenable simply to a change in angle of traction.

6 Excessive caput, rarely, even with the metal cups, adequate traction is not possible because of excessive caput and forceps may be more appropriate.
7 Poor maternal effort, there is no doubt that maternal effort can contribute substantially to the success of the delivery. Adequate encouragement and instruction should be given to the mother.

The incidence of cephalopelvic disproportion (true failure) is low.

Special indications for ventouse delivery

The use of the ventouse in the first stage of labour has lost favour since two maternal deaths were reported on and reviewed in a recent Confidential Enquiry. If it is ever to be contemplated, all other prerequisites for ventouse delivery should be fulfilled. Use before full dilatation should be reserved for acute fetal distress (e.g. abruption), where a straightforward normal delivery would have been expected within the next half hour. Nevertheless, this is a potentially dangerous practice and should only be undertaken by an experienced operator.

In the hands of an experienced operator, the ventouse can also be used to expedite delivery complicated by a prolapsed cord at full dilatation and for delivery of the second twin with fetal distress (thereby avoiding a CS).

Forceps

There are over 700 makes of forceps. Most authors subscribe to a classification system that divides forceps into classic and specialised subtypes. Classic subtypes that are traction in design include Simpson, Anderson and Neville-Barnes forceps, while specialised forceps include Kjelland (for rotation) and Piper (for the aftercoming head of the breech). Variations in cephalic curvature, fenestration and design of shank allow selection to be made on the basis of individual circumstances. There have been no RCTs comparing different types of forceps and it is recognised that the choice is often subjective. One RCT was identified; in this study decreased facial marking was found when soft blade pads were used.

Safe delivery with forceps

It is important that the practitioner is comfortable with and skilled in the use of the instrument selected and that adequate supervision is available as required. To minimise morbidity, the prerequisites for any instrumental delivery should be followed and particular points of safety for forceps delivery should be respected.

Basic rules for safe use of the forceps

1 Check the forceps are a pair before starting. This is done by locking them together and checking that they produce a symmetrical neat fit. It is also useful to check the maximum diameter between the two blades (a pair that is not true will have maximum diameter as little as 7cm or 7.5cm. The maximum diameter should be at least 9cm).
2 If there is resistance when trying to apply the blades or if, when applied to the fetal head, the blades do not sit correctly or lock together, this is usually due to misdiagnosis of the position of the vertex and the blades should be removed and the situation reassessed with senior aid.
3 The head should descend with each pull.
4 Traction should be steady and the hands should not waggle, as this risks fetal injury.
5 The delivery should be completed within three contractions.
6 If failure occurs, abandon the procedure and proceed to CS.

Method of delivery with traction forceps

The woman is placed in lithotomy and tilted by means of a wedge under the right hip.

An in–out catheterisation is required to empty the bladder prior to forceps delivery.

Checks that the forceps are a pair.

The blades should be applied in turn when the uterus is relaxed between contractions with one hand guiding the blade in (while following in from the line of the contralateral femur) while the other protects the maternal soft tissues. If the blades do not insert easily then they should be removed and the situation reassessed with senior aid: there is no place for forcing the blades.

Once applied the blades should lock together easily (no force should be needed to achieve this) and their position should be checked relative to the fetal landmarks (Figure 30.2).

Traction during a contraction attempts to follow the pelvic curve by using Pajot's manoeuvre, which involves two separate components: the dominant hand applies traction while the other hand gently presses downwards on the shank of the forceps (Figure 30.3). The strength of the left hand is crucial to successful and safe delivery: too strong a left hand increases perineal trauma and too weak a left hand means the traction is transmitted too anteriorly – i.e. up against the bladder – causing inefficiency, possible failure and possible bladder trauma. This latter effect is also produced if the direction of traction is too vertical.

The timing of the episiotomy should be when the perineum has thinned out and once the operator is totally confident the delivery is going to be completed successfully.

As the head crowns, the hands will need to rise up but, as for ventouse delivery, they should follow the head, not lead it, to minimise perineal trauma.

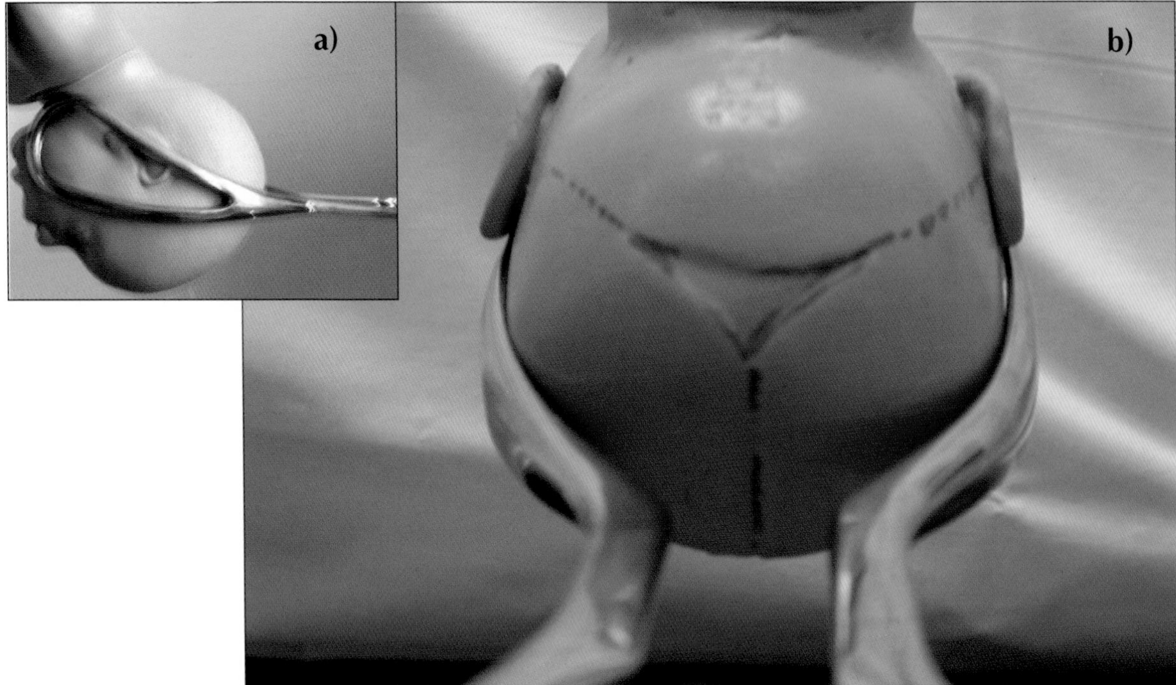

Figure 30.2 (a) Forceps blades correctly applied – lying along mento-vertical axis. (b) The forceps blades should lie *parallel* to the sagittal suture and *equidistant* from the lambdoidal suture on each side – always check these bony landmarks after forceps application *before* traction is applied.

Special indications for forceps delivery

Rotation

Rotational delivery for occipito-transverse or occipito-posterior positions can be effected following manual rotation or using a suitable ventouse cup as described above. However, Kjelland's forceps still have an important place in operative obstetrics for rotational deliveries, but they do require special expertise.

Be especially careful in the abdominal palpation to identify which side of the mother the baby's back is lying, as this will define which direction (clockwise or anticlockwise) that the baby's head should be rotated. When occiput and fetal back are on the same side, the direction of rotation is obvious, but when they lie on opposite sides (sometimes seen with occipitoposterior positions), the occiput should be rotated towards the fetal back to avoid traction on the fetal neck (e.g. left occipitoposterior and fetal back on maternal right then rotation should occur clockwise i.e. the long way round).

Check that the blades are a pair. The blades are applied ensuring that the nipple on the shank is facing towards the occiput.

Blade application is achieved during uterine relaxation between contractions:

- with occipito-posterior positions the blades are usually applied directly
- with occipito-transverse positions, the blade destined to lie anteriorly is applied first and usually wandered over from the lateral position across the brow. It should not be inserted

far enough such that it ends up wandering over the face. Particular attention to this point should be made in training and supervising this technique. (In some cases, it may be possible to insert the anterior blade 'directly' by careful insertion under the pubic bone. This may not be possible when the head is lower in the pelvis). The posterior blade is then applied directly and negotiating the coccyx is usually the technically demanding part of this step.

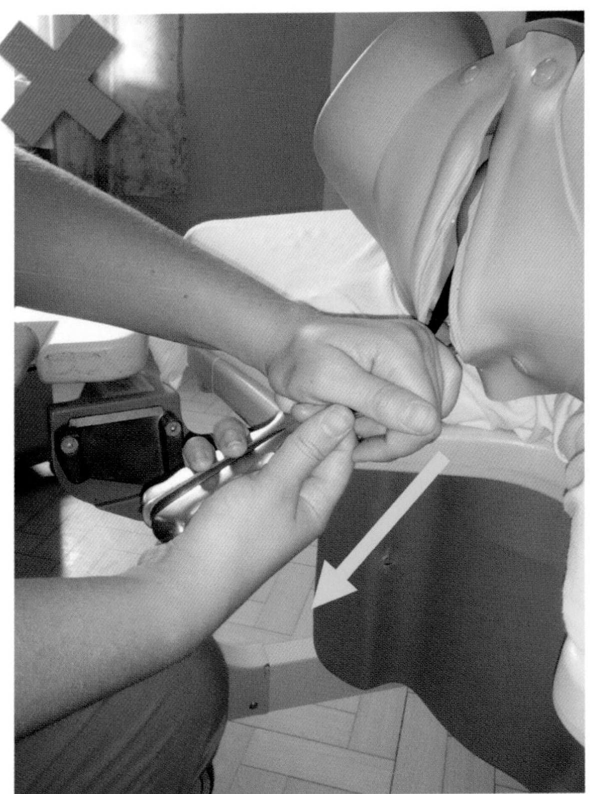

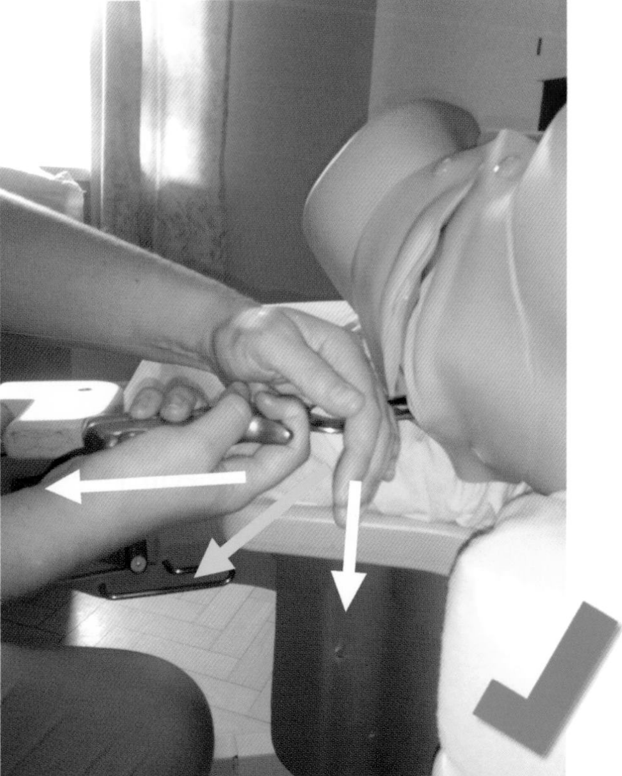

Figure 30.3 Left image – incorrect interpretation of Pajot's manoeuvre – the forceps handles have been dropped to about 45° below the horizontal. Right image – correct application of Pajot's manoeuvre: the dominant hand applies traction along the long axis of the forceps horizontally, while the other hand applies downward pressure on the shanks. This produces a resultant vector (yellow arrow) with direction of traction in line with the pelvic axis until the head is passing under the symphysis pubis.

Once the blades are applied they should be gently approximated and the lock engaged but rather than clasping the handles together as with other types of forceps (which compresses the Kjelland blades) they should be held with the thumb between the handles, which serves to fix the blades together without squashing them (Figure 30.4). Their position relative to the fetal landmarks should be confirmed.

Once locked together, the handles are very likely to lie slightly removed from each other (enabled by the sliding lock on Kjelland) due to asynclitism. This is normal and attempts should not be made to force them to correct, as this should occur naturally as rotation is completed and asynclitism resolved.

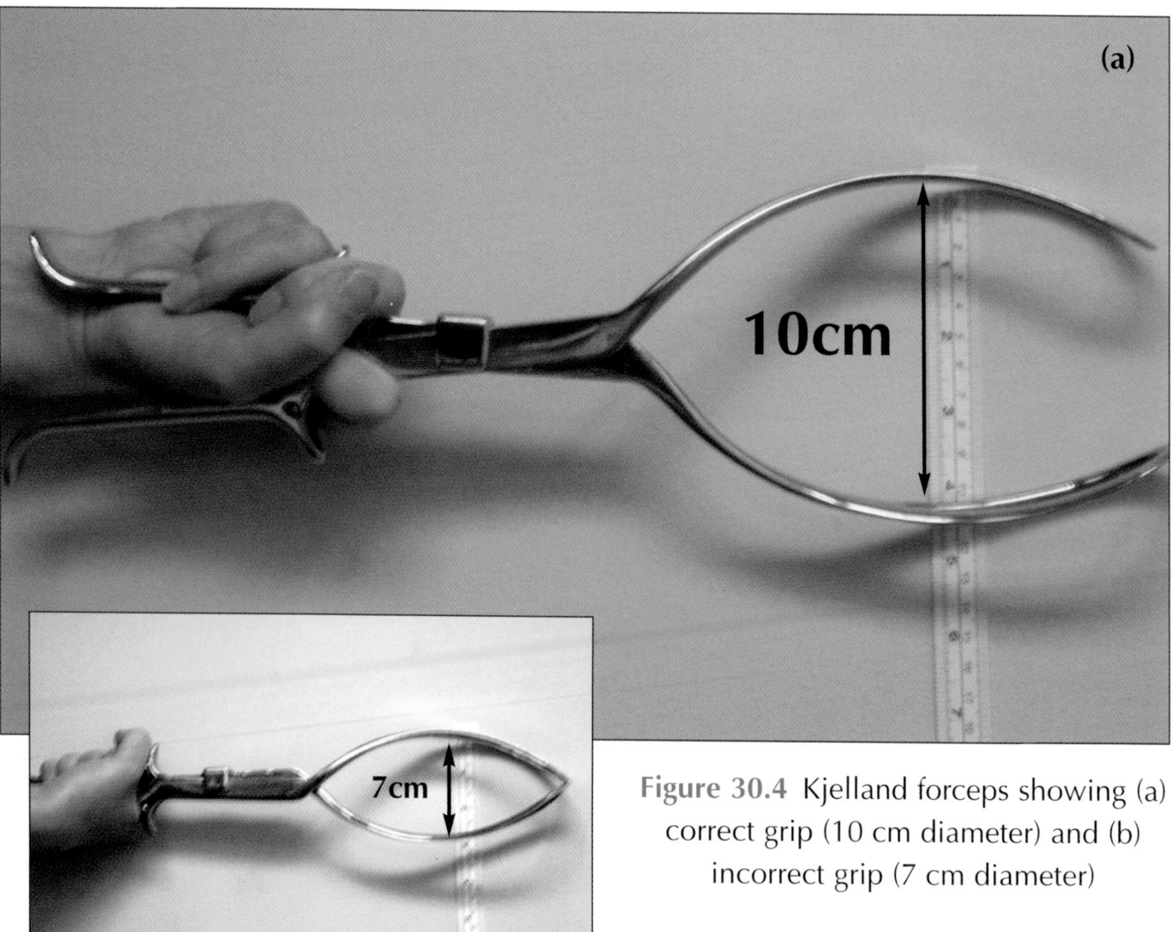

Figure 30.4 Kjelland forceps showing (a) correct grip (10 cm diameter) and (b) incorrect grip (7 cm diameter)

Rotation should be attempted between contractions when the uterus is relaxed and the force required should be minimal. This is a 'feeling' technique and it should never be forced. It is vitally important, at this point, that the operator lowers the handles by lowering the hands. The aim is to angle the forceps to lie in the true axis of the pelvis and to encourage flexion of the head at the same time. The commonest reason for unsuccessful rotation (in terms of technique) is the failure to have the handles moved low enough to allow the forceps blades to lie in the line of the true pelvic axis. This can be facilitated by the operator kneeling down between the patient's legs.

Rotation should only be attempted between contractions. Rotation can first be attempted at the level at which the blades are lying after application. If an initial attempt at rotation is unsuccessful, first re-check that the handles have been pushed downwards adequately. If so, the operator can gently try and move the fetal head either marginally upwards (by no more than 1cm) or marginally downwards (again by no more than 1cm). Rotation may be easier at the slightly higher or lower levels. *Attempts should never be made to 'disimpact' the head back into the upper pelvis.* If a contraction develops during rotation, further movement should cease until it relaxes again but keep gentle hold of the handles of the forceps otherwise they tend to drift.

Once rotation is complete, it is imperative that the fetal head is palpated to check its position and to confirm it is now occipito-anterior. The blades can slip round the fetal head and traction must not be applied until the operator is confident that this has not occurred.

Traction with Kjelland's forceps requires the handles to be kept in a low position as there is no pelvic curve (as in standard nonrotational forceps). Traction is then applied in the line of the true pelvic axis and therefore Pajot's manoeuvre is not required. The operator should take care to maintain the safe Kjelland grip during traction. An episiotomy will be required (in nearly all cases) as the lack of pelvic curve means that the Kjelland shafts do cause additional perineal stretch. As the fetal head crowns, delivery is completed by raising the handles as in a standard forceps delivery. However, because of the absence of a pelvic curve, the Kjelland's handles will not end up as high over the symphysis pubis as occurs with standard forceps.

Face presentation

Face presentation is covered in Chapter 33, but it is noteworthy to reiterate that it is essential to judge the station of the head prior to embarking on a forceps-assisted mentoanterior delivery. The head in these circumstances is always higher than one thinks and not only is careful abdominal palpation crucial, but a careful vaginal examination is mandatory. If vaginal examination reveals a hollow sacrum then the head is not fully engaged and vaginal delivery is not appropriate.

The aftercoming head of the breech

The Piper forceps were designed for this manoeuvre but any traction forceps can be used. If the operator is familiar with Kjelland's forceps, these may be used. The absence of a pelvic curve has the advantage that the forceps are easier to apply because they lie away from the baby's body. The breech delivery is covered in Chapter 34 and, as mentioned, forceps may not be needed but, if required, their principle of application and direction of traction is similar to that described above.

The place of trial of instrumental delivery

If there is uncertainty about whether an instrumental delivery is appropriate because the operator is uncertain about the position or degree of engagement of the head, good analgesia should be achieved to allow adequate examination. If uncertainty remains, someone of greater experience should be called to assess and assist prior to attempting delivery. There is no place for a 'try-it-and-see' approach in these situations and the suggestion that 'the indications for the use of the vacuum extractor as an alternative to forceps delivery include uncertainty with regard to the position of the sagittal suture and situations where the fetal head is assumed to be too high for application of forceps' is quite clearly both untrue and dangerous. Any trial-of-instrument in theatre must be sanctioned and/or supervised by a consultant or experienced registrar. There is an ongoing debate about the need for senior staff to be present for every trial of forceps undertaken in theatre. In a recent small study,

Safety points for forceps delivery of aftercoming head of a breech baby:

1. Forceps are not appropriate for delivery of the head of a breech that has not entered the pelvis. The nape of the neck/base of occiput must be seen before the baby's body is lifted up.
2. When conducting forceps delivery for the aftercoming head of the breech, an assistant is needed and coordination between operator and assistant must be maintained, as one is in control of the baby's body, the other the baby's head.
3. The baby should be lifted into the horizontal position but, as the arms tend to fall into the way, interfering with the forceps application, the assistant is advised to wrap the baby, including its arms, into a towel to keep things clear.
4. Hyperextension of the neck should be avoided at all times and the operator should keep strict control of the elevation of the baby provided by the assistant.
5. An episiotomy is required for delivery in this circumstance and, if not already cut when the breech distended the perineum, it should be cut after the application of the forceps.

Lewis confirmed that consultant presence resulted in a 70% (7/10) vaginal delivery rate compared with 30% (12/40) ($P<0.05$) when the registrar was unsupervised.[5] Further support - ive evidence is awaited.

The place of forceps after failure to deliver with the ventouse

There is no place for an attempt at forceps delivery if:

- the position of the fetal head was correctly diagnosed
- the cup was applied correctly
- adequate traction was applied and there was no descent with the ventouse.

If these were not the case and there was a misdiagnosis, misapplication of a cup or traction was inadequate (due to caput, leaking equipment, no maternal assistance) it may be justified to change to forceps. Murphy *et al.* showed that use of sequential instruments is more commonly associated with fetal malpositions (OR 1.8, 95% CI 1.3–2.6).[6] It is associated with increased maternal and neonatal morbidity compared to 'single instrument use':

- anal sphincter tear – 17.4% versus 8.4% (OR 2.1, 95% CI 1.2–3.3)
- umbilical artery pH <7.10 – 13.8% versus 5.0% (OR 3.3 95% CI 1.7–6.2).

This decision must therefore be made at an experienced level and will require a formal clinical assessment to be made by the senior clinician.

The situation may also arise that after rotation of the head and good descent into the lower pelvis (i.e. more than 2cm below the ischial spines), the ventouse cup detaches: in such cases what might have been a difficult Kjelland's delivery has now become a potentially straightforward 'lift-out' forceps delivery. Double instrumentation in this last circumstance is acceptable after careful re-assessment by the operator.

Following on from any instrumental delivery

- If the baby is delivered in good condition it should be handed to the mother as soon as possible to encourage skin–skin contact.
- After delivery, perineal damage should be assessed carefully with particular attention given to check for anal sphincter and anal mucosa integrity.
- After repairing any tear or episiotomy, the swabs and instruments should be counted.
- A vaginal and rectal examination should be performed at the end of the procedure to confirm restoration of anatomy, exclude any stray sutures having entered the rectum and confirm no swabs have been retained.
- Every aspect of the delivery should be documented.
- Examine the baby's head, when you get a chance, to confirm the positioning of the instrument used relative to where you thought it was, and where it should have been. This is important in self-audit of your technique and in teaching and feedback for trainees.

Supervising an instrumental delivery

The supervising obstetrician must make a full clinical assessment, otherwise they have no way of knowing whether the operative delivery is appropriate or the instrument selected is suitable for the task.

During traction, the supervisor needs to be confident descent is occurring with each traction and, if in doubt, they should feel for themselves to confirm this fact. Leaving the trainee to pull for three contractions before assessing the situation leaves an almost impossible decision of whether and how to continue and risks inappropriate excessive attempts at delivery.

After delivery, a careful examination of the extent of perineal trauma should be conducted together. This is not only important in identifying third- or fourth-degree tears (which are often underdiagnosed clinically), but can also provide useful feedback on instrument technique: tears or episiotomies that have extended may have been due to lifting the hands too early on crowning, or too strong a left hand with forceps deliveries.

Documentation and debriefing

After completion of the delivery, the operator should complete a detailed and (ideally) contemporaneous delivery note for the clinical records. A model example is appended to the RCOG OVD Greentop Guideline.[7]

Despite the problem of continuity of care related to shift systems in obstetrics, it is mandatory (and good clinical practice) to ensure that the operator meets up with the patient to offer a formal debrief before they are discharged home. If that is not possible, the operator should specifically ask a colleague to undertake the debrief on their behalf. This does not usually require more than a few minutes, but should include positive psychological support by confirming with the woman that her own efforts helped the operator to complete the delivery. Confirmation that a normal delivery in the future is most likely can also be very reassuring for the patient.

Audit standards

The RCOG Greentop Guideline recommends that the following should be audited routinely:

- maternity unit
    - rate of OVD.
- maternity unit and individual operator
    - percentage of women with failed OVD
    - rate of sequential instrument use
    - case notes review to audit appropriate management of women with failed OVD or sequential instrument use, i.e. when to use a sequential instrument and when to abandon
    - percentage of women with third- and fourth-degree perineal tears
    - rate of neonatal morbidity, composite trauma (subgaleal haemorrhage/brachial plexus injury/fracture/facial nerve palsy/cerebral haemorrhage), low Apgar <7 at 5 minutes and cord arterial pH <7.1
    - documentation of written or verbal consent for OVD
    - documentation of written consent for trial of OVD in operating theatre
    - accuracy of documentation.

Online resources

There are several excellent online resources and these are listed below. The RCOG resource is open access.

Sullivan C. EaSi – e-learning and simulation for instrumental delivery. RCOG StratOG 2012 (www.rcog.org.uk/stratog/page/introduction)(RCOG free access online resource).

O'Grady JP, Taugher C, Chelmow D (Chief Editor). Vacuum extraction. (http://emedicine.medscape.com/article/271175-overview).

Ross MG, Beal MH, Chelmow D (Chief Editor). Forceps. (http://emedicine.medscape.com/article/263603-overview).

Ross MG, Beal MH. Forceps delivery procedures. (http://emedicine.medscape.com/article/1848372-overview).

References and further reading

1 Dupuis O, Decullier E, Clerc J, *et al.* Does forceps training in a birth simulator allow obstetricians to improve forceps blade placement? *Europ J Obstet Gynecol Reprod Biol* 2011;159:305–9.

2 Bahl R, Murphy DJ, Strachan B. Qualitative analysis by interviews and video recordings to establish the components of a skilled low-cavity non-rotational vacuum delivery. *BJOG* 2009;116:319–26.

3 Edozien LC. Royal College of Obstetricians and Gynaecologists. *Consent Advice No 11*. London: RCOG 2010.

4 Suwannachat B, Laopaiboon M, Tonmat S, *et al.* Rapid versus stepwise application of negative pressure in vacuum extraction-assisted vaginal delivery: a multicentre randomised controlled non-inferiority trial. *BJOG* 2011;118:1247–52.

5 Lewis EA, Barr C, Thomas K. The mode of delivery in women taken to theatre at full dilatation: does consultant presence make a difference? *J Obstet Gynaecol* 2011;31(3): 229–31.

6 Murphy DJ, Macleod M, Bahl R, Strachan B. A cohort study of maternal and neonatal morbidity in relation to use of sequential instruments at operative vaginal delivery. *Europ J Obstet Gynaecol Reprod Biol* 2011;156:41–5.

7 Bahl R, Strachan BK, Murphy DJ. Royal College of Obstetricians and Gynaecologists. *Operative Vaginal Delivery.* Greentop Guideline No. 26. London: RCOG 2011.

8 Akmal S, Kametas N, Tsoi E, *et al.* Comparison of transvaginal digital examination with intrapartum sonography to determine fetal head position before instrumental delivery. *Ultrasound Obstet Gynecol* 2003;21:437–40.

9 Attilakos G, Sibanda T, Winter C, *et al.* A randomised controlled trial of a new handheld vacuum extraction device. *BJOG* 2005;112:1510–15.

10 Bahl R, Murphy DJ, Strachan B. Non-technical skills for obstetricians conducting forceps and vacuum deliveries: qualitative analysis by interviews and video recordings. *Europ J Obstet Gynecol Reprod Biol* 2010;150:147–51.

11 Barata S, Cardoso E, Ferreira-Santo S, *et al.* Maternal and neonatal immediate effects of sequential delivery. *J Maternal Fetal Neonat Med* 2012;25(7):981–3.

12 Bird GC. The importance of flexion in vacuum extractor delivery. *Br J Obstet Gynaecol* 1976;83:194–200.

13 Cheng YW, Shaffer BL, Bianco K, Caughey AB. Timing of operative delivery and assoc-iated perinatal outcomes in nulliparous women. *J Maternal Fetal Neonat Med* 2011;24(5):692–7.

14 Johanson RB, Menon V. Soft versus rigid vacuum extractor cups for assisted vaginal delivery. *Cochrane Database Syst Rev* 2004;(2).

15 Johanson RB, Menon V. Vacuum extraction versus forceps for assisted vaginal delivery. *Cochrane Database Syst Rev* 2004;(2).

16 Malvasi A, Stark M, Ghi T, *et al.* Intrapartum sonography for fetal head asynclitism and transverse position: sonographic signs and comparison of diagnostic performance

between transvaginal and digital examination. *J Maternal-Fetal Neonat Med* 2012;25(5):508–12.

17 Murphy DJ, Liebling RE, Patel R, *et al.* Cohort study of operative delivery in the second stage of labour and standard of obstetric care. *BJOG* 2003;110:610–15.

18 Murphy DJ, Liebling RE, Verity L, *et al.* Early maternal and neonatal morbidity associated with operative delivery in second stage of labour: a cohort study. *Lancet* 2001;358:1203–8.

19 O'Mahony F, Settatree R, Platt C, Johnson R. Review of singleton fetal and neonatal deaths associated with cranial trauma and cephalic delivery during a national intrapartum-related confidential enquiry. *BJOG* 2005;112:619–26.

20 Patel RR, Murphy DJ. Forceps delivery in modern obstetric practice. *BMJ* 2004;328: 1302–5.

21 Roodt A, Nikodem VC. Pushing/bearing down methods used during the second stage of labour. *Cochrane Database Syst Rev* 2002;(1).

22 Saunders NJ, Spiby H, Gilbert L, *et al.* Oxytocin infusion during second stage of labour in primiparous women using epidural analgesia: a randomized double-blind placebo-controlled trial. *BMJ* 1989;299:1423–6.

23 Siassakos D, Clark J, Sibanda T *et al.* A simple tool to measure patient perceptions of operative birth. *BJOG* 2009;116(13):1755–61.

24 Touqmatchi D, Schwaiger N, Cotzias C. How good are obstetric and gynaecology trainees at reviewing and debriefing patients following operative deliveries? *J Obstet Gynecol* 2011;31(8):687–91.

25 Towner D, Castro MA, Eby-Wilkens E, Gilbert WM. Effect of mode of delivery in nulliparous women on neonatal intracranial injury. *N Engl J Med* 1999;341:1709–14.

26 Unterscheider J, McMenamin M, Cullinane F. Rising rates of caesarean deliveries at full dilatation: a concerning trend. *Europ J Obstet Gynecol Reprod Biol* 2011;157:141–4.

27 Vacca A. The place of the vacuum extractor in modern obstetric practice. *Fetal Medicine Review* 1990;2:103–22.

28 Yeo L, Romero R. Sonographic evaluation in the second stage of labor to improve the assessment of labor progress and its outcome (Editorial/Opinion). *Ultrasound Obstet Gynecol* 2009;33:253–8.

ALGORITHM 31.1 Management of shoulder dystocia

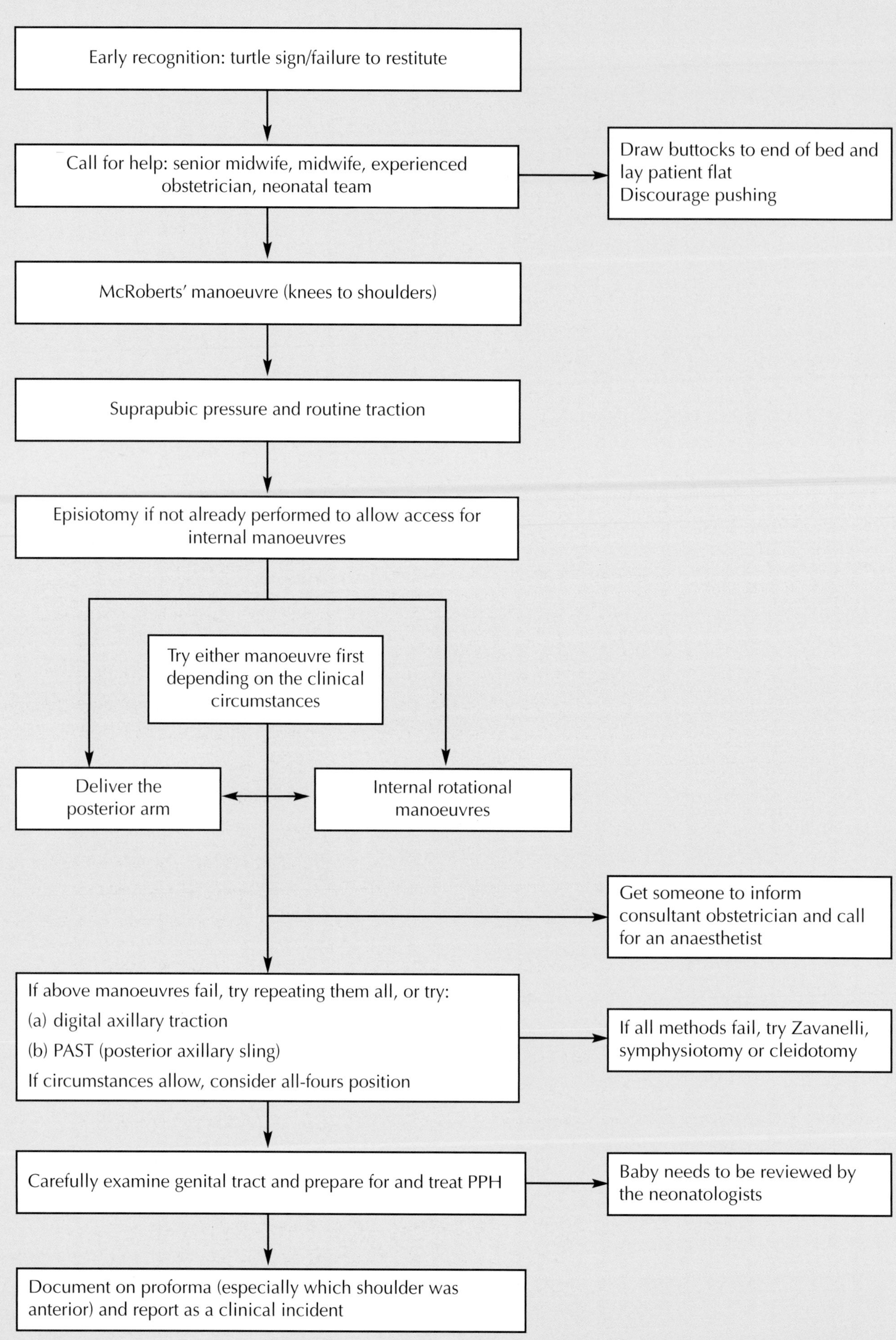

CHAPTER 31

Shoulder dystocia

Objectives

On successfully completing this topic, you will be able to:

- understand the aetiology and complications of shoulder dystocia
- understand the risk factors for shoulder dystocia
- be aware of strategies that can be tried to prevent shoulder dystocia
- be confident in understanding the variety of obstetric manoeuvres used to overcome shoulder dystocia
- appreciate the benefits of formal skills/drills training on maternal and fetal outcomes in cases of shoulder dystocia.

Introduction

Shoulder dystocia remains one of the most dreaded obstetric complications and one that is often unanticipated. It is associated with significant perinatal mortality and morbidity, maternal morbidity and is a costly source of litigation. In this chapter, a number of matters will be addressed.

Definition and incidence

Shoulder dystocia describes difficulties encountered with delivering the shoulders after the fetal head is born. Discrepancies in the definition have resulted in differences in the reported incidence of this obstetric emergency from 0.15% to 2% of all vaginal deliveries. MOET considers shoulder dystocia to be a condition requiring special manoeuvres to deliver the shoulders that have been arrested due to impaction of the anterior shoulder above the symphysis pubis.

Clinical risks and outcomes

Fetal mortality and morbidity

Shoulder dystocia is still a significant cause of term fetal mortality. In the CESDI annual report for 1993,[1] shoulder dystocia was responsible for 8% of all intrapartum fetal deaths. A later, focused report (1998) critically reviewed 56 cases of death associated with shoulder dystocia: 47% had died despite delivery within 5 minutes and, in 37 (66%) cases, the level of substandard care offered by professionals was graded at 'level 3' (i.e. a different management would have likely resulted in an improved outcome). The babies were delivered by both midwives and medical staff, emphasising the need for all professionals involved in delivery to be aware of appropriate drills.

Fetal morbidity:

- cerebral hypoxia
- cerebral palsy
- fracture clavicle and/or humerus
- brachial plexus injuries.

Following delivery of the head, the umbilical cord pH falls by 0.04 unit/minute, in addition, cranial venous congestion occurs, which exacerbates the fetal insult. As a result, delay in completing the delivery may result in asphyxia and, if the interval between head and trunk delivery is prolonged, permanent neurological deficit may occur. Delivery should occur within 5 minutes and permanent injury is progressively more likely with delays above 10 minutes.

Brachial plexus injuries can occur in shoulder dystocia due to downward traction with excessive lateral flexion of the neck, which stretches its soft tissues. Erb's palsy is the most common of these. A study in 2000 found 62 cases of brachial plexus injury in 13 366 deliveries (incidence 0.46%): 22 recovered completely within a month, while a further 23 had delayed but complete recovery.[2] Of 17 with residual paresis, 11 underwent surgery but only three had severe paresis. The most significant marker to predict the likelihood of 'nonrecovery' was birthweight greater than 4000 g (OR 51).

It has been suggested that intrauterine maladaptation may play a role in brachial plexus impairment, implying that brachial plexus impairment should not be taken as prima facie evidence of birth-process injury. The mechanism of damage may not always be clear, as brachial plexus injury has also been reported in the opposite arm to the trapped shoulder and also without any recorded dystocia. Furthermore, it has also been reported after delivery by CS, although clearly injudicious traction on the fetal head and neck can also occur during this delivery.

Bony injuries in the form of fractured clavicle or humerus can also occur. These fractures usually heal quickly and have a good prognosis.

Maternal morbidity

Postpartum haemorrhage and genital tract trauma are common following shoulder dystocia. Uterine rupture may also occur, especially if undue abdominal force is used.

Antenatal risk factors

Antenatal risk factors are so common that they lack sensitivity and specificity, and the majority of cases of shoulder dystocia occur without any risk factors. There is a strong correlation between fetal weight and shoulder dystocia. Increasing obesity, diabetes and gestational diabetes all increase the likelihood of macrosomia; however, shoulder dystocia occurs with a normal fetal weight therefore all professionals need to be prepared for unexpected shoulder dystocia at all deliveries.

Intrapartum risk factors

Secondary arrest and slow progress in the first stage of labour can be associated with increased incidence of shoulder dystocia, but many studies have shown labour abnormalities to be similar in both the shoulder dystocia and the control groups, making clinical predictors for subsequent development of shoulder dystocia imprecise.

Shoulder dystocia is more frequently encountered in assisted vaginal deliveries. Boekhuizen *et al.* analysed 256 vacuum extractions and 300 forceps deliveries.[3] They found an incidence of 4.6% of shoulder dystocia compared with 0.17% of all cephalic vaginal deliveries. This emphasises the importance of particularly careful abdominal and vaginal assessment before performing assisted deliveries for clinically macrosomic babies.

Risk factors for shoulder dystocia

Antepartum	Intrapartum
• Fetal macrosomia • Maternal obesity • Diabetes • Prolonged pregnancy • Advanced maternal age • Male gender • Excessive weight gain • Previous shoulder dystocia • Previous big baby	• Prolonged first stage • Prolonged second stage • Assisted delivery

How does shoulder dystocia happen?

The posterior shoulder usually enters the pelvic cavity, while the anterior shoulder remains hooked above the symphysis pubis. In the more severe forms of shoulder dystocia, both shoulders do not cross the pelvic brim.

Strategies suggested for prevention and management of shoulder dystocia

Identifying risk factors

Identify the risk of shoulder dystocia antenatally and recommend clearly in the mother's notes that an experienced obstetrician should be available for the second stage.

Training and teaching

In the CESDI report 1993 it is stated that: 'There should be regular rehearsals of emergency procedures and training sessions in the management of rare or troublesome complications for obstetricians and midwives involved in care.' Such complications include obstructed delivery... and shoulder dystocia.

There is now clear evidence of benefit from the work of the research team led by Draycott and Crofts. In a randomised trial of 450 clinicians, formal skills/drills training in SD resulted in an increase in successful delivery rate (72% prior to training versus 94% post-training), with a reduction in total force applied.[4] Of even greater importance is the improvement in neonatal outcomes following the introduction of training.[5] In an analysis of >29 000 births, the use of correct manoeuvres was significantly increased. This resulted in a significant reduction in neonatal injury at birth after shoulder dystocia: 30/324 (9.3%) to 6/262 (2.3%) (relative risk [RR] 0.25 [CI 0.11–0.57]).

Clinical approach

Prevention

Prevention by performing CS for macrosomic infants is not recommended from the evidence available.

Estimates of fetal weight antenatally are notoriously unreliable (especially at the extremes). Many cases of shoulder dystocia occur in babies of average weight, and most macrosomic fetuses delivered vaginally do not suffer from shoulder dystocia. Most cases of shoulder dystocia can be overcome without trauma to mother or baby if proper precautions are taken. Abdominal delivery is not 100% safe to the baby and causes morbidity to the mother. Thus, a policy of elective CS for all clinically big babies will not be effective in reducing the incidence of shoulder dystocia and subsequent brachial plexus injuries.

Prevention by induction of labour for suspected macrosomia

Induction of labour has been considered as an option for managing mothers with suspected macrosomic babies to try to reduce the incidence of shoulder dystocia and subsequent birth trauma. A 1995 study reviewed 186 mothers with suspected macrosomic fetuses at term.[6] Labour was induced in 46 cases, 23.9% of them needed CS while, with spontaneous onset of labour in 140 cases, the CS rate was 14%. This difference was statistically significant, regardless of parity or gestational age. The frequencies of shoulder dystocia, 1 minute Apgar score less than 7 and abnormal umbilical blood gas were not different. They concluded that spontaneous labour is associated with a lower chance of CS than induced labour when the birthweight is 4000g and above.

The situation in women with diabetes is different, for reasons mentioned earlier. Various authorities recommended CS for babies with estimated fetal weight 4000g or above. Induction of labour is also recommended for women with diabetes at 38 weeks, especially if their diabetic control has not been ideal, not only to avoid intrauterine death but also shoulder dystocia and birth trauma.

Documentation

Risk factors should be documented in the notes, especially if they are multiple. It is also recommended that an experienced clinician is present during the second stage. It is strongly recommended that events, manoeuvres and accurate times are documented in the notes. Using a proforma for this ensures all important facts are noted.

Early detection

- 'head bobbing' (the head coming down towards the introitus with pushing but retracting well back between contractions)
- 'turtle' sign at delivery (the delivered head becomes tightly pulled back against the perineum)
- failure of restitution.

Have a plan of action

As shoulder dystocia is infrequently predictable, every clinician should be armed with a plan of action; that is, a sequence of manoeuvres. All manoeuvres result from one (or a combination of) the following three mechanisms:

- increase in the available pelvic diameter
- narrowing of the transverse (bisacromial) diameter of the shoulders by adduction
- movement of the bisacromial diameter into a more favourable angle relative to the pelvic inlet (oblique diameter is larger than the anteroposterior pelvic diameter).

Plan of action

1 Call for help.
2 Draw buttocks to edge of bed.
3 Consider episiotomy.
4 McRoberts' manoeuvre + moderate traction.
5 Suprapubic pressure + moderate traction.
6 Episiotomy (if not already cut) to allow space to insert hand for internal manoeuvres.
7 Deliver posterior arm and shoulder or internal rotational manoeuvres (including Woods' screw manoeuvre).
8 Repeat manoeuvres or try:
   (a) Digital axillary traction
   (b) PAST (posterior axillary sling).
9 Change of position ('All fours' or 'Gaskin' manoeuvre).
10 If all the above fail, try symphysiotomy, cleidotomy or Zavanelli manoeuvre.
11 Ensure comprehensive and contemporaneous written records.

Call for help

This includes calling the most experienced obstetrician available, a paediatrician and an anaesthetist, and other nursing and ancillary staff as available.

Episiotomy

Episiotomy is recommended to allow more room for manoeuvres, such as delivering the posterior arm or internal rotation of the shoulders. Although it has been suggested that episiotomy does not affect the outcome of shoulder dystocia, there is strong evidence to suggest that the incidence of vaginal lacerations with shoulder dystocia is high and performing an episiotomy to reduce the chance of having severe lacerations is recommended. The main reason for recommending an episiotomy is to allow the operator more space to use the hollow of the sacrum to perform the different internal manoeuvres.

McRoberts' manoeuvre (with or without moderate traction)

Both thighs are sharply flexed, abducted and rotated outwards (knees to shoulders). The bed should be flat and legs should not be in lithotomy poles, as this would limit the amount of flexion obtained. This position serves to straighten the sacrum relative to the lumbar vertebrae and causes cephalic rotation of the pelvis to occur, which helps to free the impacted shoulder. One study tested McRoberts' position with laboratory maternal pelvic and fetal models. Their findings showed that this manoeuvre reduced the amount of traction needed and the likelihood of subsequent brachial plexus injuries or fractured clavicle. For this reason, patients should be put in McRoberts' before applying appropriate traction on the fetal neck. Lurie *et al.* reviewed 76 cases of shoulder dystocia and found that McRoberts' manoeuvre was sufficient to achieve delivery of the impacted shoulder in 67 cases (88%).[7] McRoberts' manoeuvre is associated with the least neonatal trauma.

The traction applied during delivery can be measured objectively using the PROMPT Trainer with studies showing a mean maximum applied traction force of 106Newtons, but a range varying from 6 to >250N. Computer modelling suggests that maximum traction force should not exceed 100N in order to reduce the risk of neonatal brachial plexus injury.

Suprapubic pressure (with moderate traction)

Suprapubic pressure is applied to adduct and internally rotate the anterior shoulder and thus reduce the bis-acromial diameter and push the anterior shoulder underneath the symphysis pubis into the pelvis. A 'cardiac massage' grip is used, with pressure applied to the posterior aspect of the shoulder with the heel of the hand. It is important to know where the fetal back lies so that pressure is applied in the right direction. If continuous pressure is not successful, a 'rocking' movement may be tried. This is also known as the 'Rubin I' manoeuvre. At this stage, only moderate traction is applied, strong traction, as well as fundal pressure, should always be avoided. Strong pushing may have similar effects to fundal pressure and maternal efforts should be discouraged until shoulder displacement is achieved, as these could increase the impaction of the shoulders and increase the neurological and orthopaedic complications.

Deliver posterior arm and shoulder

The hand of the operator should be passed up to the fetal axilla and the shoulder hooked down. There is always more room in the hollow of the sacrum. Traction on the posterior axilla usually enables the operator to bring the posterior arm within reach.

The posterior arm can then be delivered or, if the cubital fossa is within reach, backwards pressure on it will result in disengagement of the arm, which will then be brought down. This is achieved by getting hold of the hand and sweeping it across the chest and fetal face. This process is similar to the Pinard method for bringing down a leg in breech presentation. This procedure is usually successful.

Internal rotatory manoeuvres

Internal rotatory manoeuvres, such as Rubin II, Woods' screw and reverse Woods' screw, are often confused with each other and are often incorrectly described in the literature.

Rubin II

The operator inserts the fingers of one hand vaginally, positioning the fingertips behind the anterior shoulder. The shoulder is pushed towards the fetal chest (adducting the shoulders and rotating the bisacromial diameter into the oblique). If unsuccessful, this can then be combined with the Woods' screw manoeuvre.

Woods' screw

This manoeuvre was described by Woods in 1943. The fingers of the opposite hand are inserted vaginally to approach the posterior shoulder from the front of the fetus, aiming to rotate the shoulder towards the symphysis pubis. The Rubin II and Woods' screw can be combined to rotate the shoulders through 180° ('like a thread on a screw'). It is important not to twist the fetal head or neck.

Reverse Woods' screw

If the above fail, an attempt is made to rotate in the opposite direction to the original Woods' screw. If successful, the shoulders will rotate 180° in the opposite direction and deliver.

Hoffman *et al.* have confirmed that delivery of the posterior arm achieved the highest rate of delivery compared with other manoeuvres (84.4% versus 24.3–72.0% $P<0.005$ to $P<0.001$), but with no differences in rates of neonatal injury (8.4% versus 6.1–14.0% $P=0.23$ to $P=0.7$).[8] However, it was clear that the total number of manoeuvres performed correlated significantly with the rate of neonatal injury. Other papers have confirmed increased success rates with use of multiple manoeuvres (72% rising to 79% then 95% with two then three manoeuvres), but higher rates of neonatal injury with removal of the posterior arm relative to internal rotatory methods.

Overall, the literature supports the judicious use of multiple manoeuvres to achieve successful delivery and the accoucheur should be familiar with the different approaches. Which to use first will depend on training and familiarity. This is reflected in Algorithm 31.1 that shows use of internal rotatory manoeuvres and removal of the posterior arm at the same level.

Finally, using computer modelling, Grimm *et al.* confirmed that **all** manoeuvres *reduce the amount of force and resultant brachial plexus stretch required to achieve delivery.*[9] The greatest effect using the modelling technique, was with delivery of the posterior arm with a 71% decrease in nerve stretch and an 80% reduction in traction force.

All-fours position ('Gaskin' manoeuvre)

The maternal weight lies evenly on the four limbs and this increases the anteroposterior diameter of the inlet and facilitates other manoeuvres. The posterior shoulder (with respect to the maternal pelvis) may be delivered first in this position. Midwives will often use this manoeuvre early in the management of shoulder dystocia. In a series of 82 cases of shoulder dystocia among 4452 deliveries (incidence 1.8%), all babies were delivered successfully with this manoeuvre in a mean time of 2.3 (range 1–6) minutes. There were no cases of mortality and no cases of brachial plexus injury. One baby suffered a fractured humerus. Obstetricians should consider the merits of this alternative approach if it is practicable (i.e. no dense epidural blockade).

Other measures

'Sling' or posterior axillary traction

These techniques to deliver the posterior arm are described in two case series.[10,11] The approach may be particularly helpful when the posterior shoulder is held up on the sacral promontory, and other standard manoeuvres are unsuccessful. Menticoglou describes insertion of the clinician's hand along the sacral hollow and delivery of the *posterior shoulder* before delivering the posterior arm.[11] Cluver and Hofmeyr describes use of a soft silastic suction catheter that is looped around the posterior shoulder and under the axilla using the index fingertip.[10] The loop is retrieved with the opposite index finger and withdrawn to create a sling around the shoulder that can be used for downward traction (again aiming to deliver the *posterior shoulder* itself first). The techniques are associated with a high risk of humeral fracture.

Zavanelli manoeuvre (cephalic replacement)

This method has been named after the physician who first performed the manoeuvre in 1978. It describes reversal of the delivery process by rotating, flexing and reinserting the head into the vagina, followed by CS; that is, after failure of all manoeuvres to overcome shoulder dystocia, restitution and neck extension are reversed and the head recoils into the vagina. It may be of particular use when both shoulders remain in the abdomen (the double-shoulder dystocia) where cephalic replacement is relatively easier as the pelvis does not contain the posterior shoulder.

A study reported 59 women who underwent cephalic replacement. All but six were successfully replaced and delivered by CS without excessive maternal or fetal morbidity. The study described the need for a tocolytic and used 0.25 mg subcutaneous terbutaline, depressing the posterior wall and using firm and constant pressure on the head. Those who have had experience of applying this technique have reported very good outcomes.

Descriptions in the literature report an almost automatic ease in performance of the Zavanelli manoeuvre and a complication-free procedure. However, it has been reported how difficult the process can be. One author reported three cases of hysterectomies necessitated because of uterine rupture during the procedure. There have also been cases of severe perinatal hypoxia, which ultimately resulted in brain damage and/or death. It has been recommended that it should be used as a last resort.

Symphysiotomy

Symphysiotomy is described in Chapter 37. The procedure requires inserting a urethral catheter to move the urethra to one side, which is extremely difficult, if not impossible, to achieve when the head has been born. Two assistants support the legs after taking them out off the stirrups. An incomplete midline cut in the symphyseal joint is made. This, in addition to an episiotomy, will increase the space available and facilitate the delivery of the shoulders. Performance of this uncommon procedure, in an emergency situation, by an operator who has never performed it before must carry a considerable risk. However, the successful use of the technique has been described. The importance of supporting the woman's legs when the incision is made must be emphasised, in order to prevent sudden abduction.

Intentional fracture of the clavicle

The clavicle may fracture spontaneously with the above manoeuvres but to perform this deliberately is really a last resort.

Approaches advocated by other authors

Several authors have advocated the use of similar systematic approaches to the hands-on management of shoulder dystocia. They vary in the order in which manoeuvres may be recommended, but the more important principle of having an orderly, logical and calm approach is advocated by all. The ALSO approach uses the mnemonic 'HELPERR' (the order of manoeuvres is not mandatory):

H Help (call for plenty)

E Evaluate for episiotomy

L Legs (McRoberts' manoeuvre)

P Pressure (suprapubic)

E Enter (rotational manoeuvres)

R Remove the posterior arm

R Roll (Gaskin manoeuvre).

Guidelines may differ at the point where internal manoeuvres are required. Should one 'enter and rotate (the shoulders)' first or 'enter and remove' (the posterior arm) first? There is no scientific evidence on which to base this choice. Therefore, it should be left to the attending professional to use the manoeuvre with which they are most familiar and most comfortable. In a survey of obstetricians, it was found that 56% would attempt delivery of the posterior arm first and 36% would attempt the internal rotatory manoeuvres first. MOET instructs in both techniques as each may be invaluable in any specific case.

Medico-legal aspects

Courts have found in favour of the professionals involved, when the allegations have been that shoulder dystocia 'should have been predicted' and CS offered in order to avoid the complication. It is accepted that the majority of cases are unpredictable and that professionals cannot be expected to predict this catastrophe antenatally. However, in many cases, there were no departmental guidelines available for the management of shoulder dystocia once it had occurred. Inappropriate manoeuvres, such as excessive lateral traction and fundal pressure, would not be acceptable and, indeed, would be difficult to defend in present-day practice.

Units should continually review and revise their management guidelines with reference to changing evidence-based practice. It is accepted that it is not possible to produce Grade A (randomised controlled trial) evidence in this field. Therefore, the manoeuvres recommended by 'expert' opinion will be the basis of best practice.

Summary

- Although shoulder dystocia is usually an unpredictable obstetric emergency, having guidelines and a plan of action and being vigilant to the possibility of shoulder dystocia should minimise the fetal and maternal trauma. There is now Grade A evidence that simulation with skills/drills training can result in improved operator technique and a reduced incidence of brachial plexus injury.
- It is important that every institution has a guideline and documentation proforma, with which all staff are familiar and comfortable.
- Run mock 'fire drills'.
- Confidence with this rare emergency can be enhanced with the use of 'fire drills' and by completing structured skills-training courses.

References and further reading

1. *Confidential Enquiry into Stillbirths and Deaths in Infancy. Annual Report 1 January to 31 December 1993.* London: Maternal and Child Health Research Consortium 1995.
2. Wolf H, Hoeksma AF, Oei SL, Bleker OP. Obstetric brachial plexus injury: risk factors related to recovery. *Eur J Obstet Gynecol Reprod Biol* 2000;88:133–8.
3. Boekhuizen F, Washington J, Johnson F, Hamilton P. Vacuum extraction versus forceps delivery: indications and complications, 1979 to 1984. *Obstet Gynecol* 1987;69:338–42.
4. Crofts JF, Fox R, Ellis D, *et al.* Observations From 450 Shoulder Dystocia Simulations Lessons for Skills Training. *Obstet Gynecol* 2008;112:906–12.
5. Draycott TJ, Crofts JF, Ash JP, *et al.* Improving neonatal outcome through practical shoulder dystocia training. *Obstet Gynecol* 2008;112(1):14–20.
6. Friesen CD, Miller AM, Rayburn WF. Influence of spontaneous labor on delivering macrosomic fetus. *Am J Perinatol* 1995;12:63–6.
7. Lurie S, Ben-Arie, Hagay A. The ABC of shoulder dystocia management. *Asia Oceania J Obstet Gynaecol* 1994;20:195–7.
8. Hoffman MK, MPH; Bailit JL, Branch DW, *et al.* A comparison of obstetric manoeuvres for the acute management of shoulder dystocia. *Obstet Gynecol* 2011:117(6):1272–8.
9. Grimm MJ, Costello RE, Gonik B. Effect of clinician-applied maneuvers on brachial plexus stretch during a shoulder dystocia event: Investigation using a computer simulation model. *Am J Obstet Gynecol* 2010;203:339.e1–5.

10 Cluver C, Hofmeyr GJ. Posterior axilla sling traction – a technique for intractable shoulder dystocia. *Obstet Gynecol* 2009;113:486–8.

11 Menticoglou S. A modified technique to deliver the posterior arm in severe shoulder dystocia. *Am J Obstet Gynecol* 2006;108(30):755–7.

12 Allan RH, Bankoski BR, Butzin CA, Nagey DA. Comparing clinician-applied loads for routine, difficult and shoulder dystocia deliveries. *Am J Obstet Gynecol* 1994;171:1621–7.

13 Baxley EG, Gobbo RW. Shoulder dystocia (ALSO series). *Am Fam Physician* 2004;67:1707–14 (www.aafp.org/afp/20040401/1707.pdf).

14 Boyd M, Usher R, McLean FH. Fetal macrosomia: prediction, risks, proposed management. *Obstet Gynecol* 1983;61:715–22.

15 Diani F, Moscatelli C, Toppano B, Turinetto A. [Fetal macrosomia and mode of delivery]. *Minerva Ginecol* 1995;47:77–82. Italian.

16 Focus Group: Shoulder dystocia. In: *Confidential Enquiries into Stillbirths and Deaths in Infancy. 5th Annual Report.* London: Maternal and Child Health Research Consortium 1998;73–9.

17 Gherman RB, Chauhan S, Ouzounian JG, *et al.* Shoulder dystocia: the unpreventable obstetric emergency with empiric management guidelines. *Am J Obstet Gynecol* 2006;195:657–72.

18 Gupta M, Hockley C, Quigley MA, *et al.* Antepartum and intrapartum prediction of shoulder dystocia. *Eur J Obstet Gynecol Reprod Biol* 2010;150:134-9.

19 Gurewitsch ED, Donithan M, Stallings SP, *et al.* Episiotomy versus fetal manipulation in managing severe shoulder dystocia: a comparison of outcomes. *Am J Obstet Gynecol* 2004;191:911–16.

20 Hartfield VJ. Symphysiotomy for shoulder dystocia. *Am J Obstet Gynecol* 1986;155:228.

21 Leigh TH, James CE. Medicolegal commentary: shoulder dystocia. *Br J Obstet Gynaecol* 1998;105:815–17.

22 Lerner H. Shoulder dystocia. 2004 (http://shoulderdystociainfo.com/index.htm).

23 Magowan B. Shoulder dystocia: In: Magowan B. *Churchill's Pocketbook of Obstetrics and Gynaecology.* 2nd edn. Edinburgh: Churchill Livingstone 2000;99–5.

24 Moses S. Shoulder dystocia management. In: Family Practice Notebook.com 2000 (web-based text with regular updates) (www.fpnotebook.com/OB112.htm).

25 O'Leary J. Cephalic replacement for shoulder dystocia: present status and future role of Zavanelli manoeuvre. *Obstet Gynecol* 1993;82:847–55.

26 Overland EA, Spydslaug A, Nielsen CS, Eskild A. Risk of shoulder dystocia in second delivery: does a history of shoulder dystocia matter? *Am J Obstet Gynecol* 2009;200:506.e1–506.e6.

27 Resnik R. Management of shoulder girdle dystocia. *Clin Obstet Gynecol* 1980;23:559–64.

28 Royal College of Obstetricians and Gynaecologists. *Shoulder Dystocia.* Guideline No. 42, 2nd edn. London: RCOG; 2012 (www.rcog.org.uk/files/rcog-corp/GTG%2042_Shoulder%20dystocia%202nd%20edition%202012%20(2).pdf).

29 Sandmire HF, DeMott RK. Erb's palsy: concepts of causation. *Obstet Gynecol* 2000;95:941–2.

30 Shoulder dystocia (stuck shoulders). In: World Health Organization, Department of Reproductive Health and Research. *Managing Complications in Pregnancy and Childbirth: Guidelines for Midwives and Doctors.* Geneva: WHO 2003;S83–5. (www.who.int/reproductive-health/impac/Symptoms/Shoulder_dystocia_S83_S85.html).

ALGORITHM 32.1 Umbilical cord prolapse

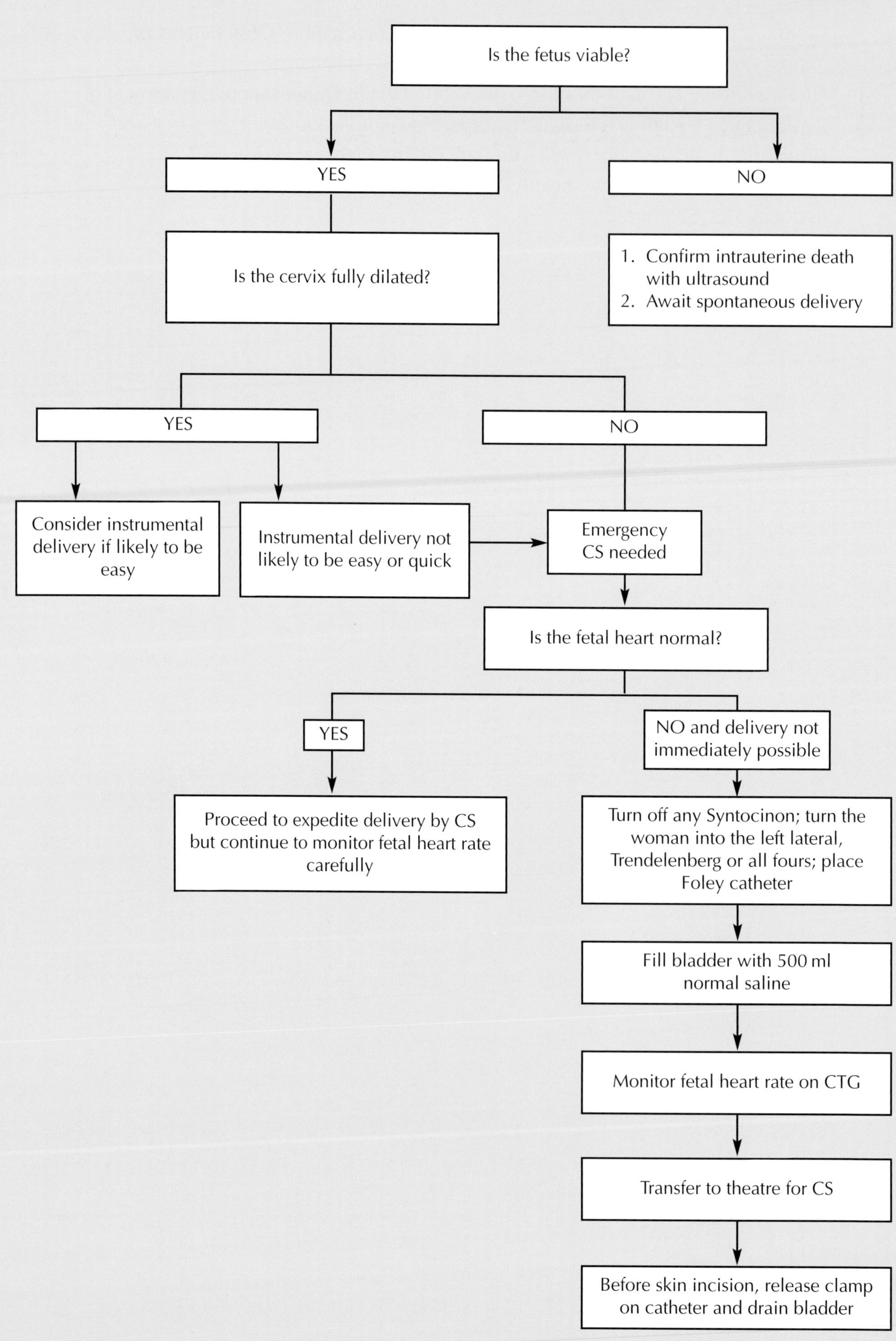

CHAPTER 32

Umbilical cord prolapse

Objectives

On successfully completing this topic, you will be able to:

- safely and efficiently manage prolapse of the umbilical cord to improve perinatal outcome whilst minimising maternal risk.

Introduction

Definition and incidence

Cord prolapse occurs when a loop of umbilical cord descends below the presenting part and the membranes are ruptured. Umbilical cord prolapse occurs in approximately 0.2% of all births.

A high percentage of mothers are multiparous. The incidence of prolapsed cord was 0.6% of all births in 1932. The reduction in frequency of the complication probably reflects reduction in family size, as well as changes in obstetric practice. These include the increased use of elective and intrapartum CS for a noncephalic, or an unengaged, presenting part and a more active approach to intrapartum management of the very preterm fetus.

Significance

In cord prolapse, the fetal perinatal mortality has been as high as 25–50% from asphyxia due to:

- mechanical compression of the cord between the presenting part and bony pelvis
- spasm of the cord vessels when exposed to cold or manipulations.

The perinatal mortality rate associated with umbilical cord prolapse has also fallen. One recent large study found a perinatal mortality rate of 91/1000. The cause of death for infants born after umbilical cord prolapse now seems to be related more to the complications of prematurity, associated congenital malformations and low birthweight, than to intrapartum asphyxia as such.

It is considered that part of the fall in perinatal mortality is due to the more rapid and frequent use of CS, once a prolapsed cord has been diagnosed. However, given the association between umbilical cord prolapse and preterm birth, improvements in neonatal intensive care are probably at least as important.

Clinical management

Aetiology

Umbilical cord prolapse tends to occur when the presenting part does not snugly fit in the lower pelvis and this, in turn, could be due to *fetal causes* such as:

- malpresentations (e.g. complete or footling breech, transverse and oblique lie)
- prematurity
- polyhydramnios
- multiple pregnancy
- anencephaly.

Or *maternal causes* such as:

- contracted pelvis
- pelvic tumours
- multiparous women with an unstable lie
- low-grade placenta praevia
- long cord
- sudden rupture of membranes in polyhydramnios.

Other risk factors

In one series, obstetric interventions (such as amniotomy, scalp electrode application, intrauterine pressure catheter insertion, attempted external cephalic version and expectant management of premature rupture of membranes) preceded 47% of umbilical cord prolapse.

Diagnosis

Clinical suspicion

A high presenting part can raise suspicions of a problem with cord presentation or prolapse especially if the fetal heart rate is showing early decelerations suggestive of cord compression.

Vaginal examination

This should be performed carefully and thoroughly to check if cord is palpable. If membranes are intact and the cord is felt this is termed cord presentation, but if the membranes are ruptured, the term is cord prolapse. The next consideration is to ascertain whether the cord is pulsating; i.e. whether the fetus is alive or dead – this must be performed gently, with minimum pressure on the cord, to avoid further compression or even spasm.

Ultrasound

An ultrasound scan can be performed to confirm a fetal heartbeat, if this facility is rapidly available. Fetal heart monitoring should be started/continued with whatever tools are to hand (Pinard/Doppler/cardiotocography). Colour flow Doppler can be useful if there is reason to suspect cord presentation.

Obstetric management of umbilical cord prolapse

Obstetric management of umbilical cord prolapse has largely been unchanged since the 1950s. The approach if the baby is alive and of a viable gestation continues to be elevation of the presenting part and rapid delivery, usually by CS (unless the cervix is fully dilated and vaginal delivery can be expedited quickly). Any oxytocin infusion should be turned off.

Early diagnosis is important and continuous electronic fetal monitoring may be of assistance as fetal heart rate changes frequently recur: the speed required to expedite delivery will vary according to whether there is a bradycardia that does not respond to the measures mentioned below, or whether the fetal heart remains normal. In either situation, if the cervix is fully dilated and the presenting part well down in the pelvis, rapid vaginal delivery can be effected.

A management plan is shown in Algorithm 32.1.

Measures that can be employed to reduce cord compression and improve the fetal heart rate

A number of manoeuvres are described to reduce the cord compression, including manual elevation of the presenting part of the cord, tocolysis, bladder filling, placing the patient in the knee–chest position and funic reduction.

Traditionally, management of umbilical cord prolapse has included knee–chest or Trendelenburg positioning and manual elevation of the presenting part of the fetus above the pelvic inlet, to relieve cord compression. Provided that delivery is not imminent and the fetus is viable, this traditional management occurs while preparations for emergency CS are made.

Measures to perform intrauterine fetal resuscitation are indicated if there is concern about the fetal heart rate: increasing the intravenous fluid rate, administering oxygen by facemask and discontinuing the oxytocin infusion are indicated. If the umbilical cord visibly protrudes through the introitus, it should be replaced in the vagina with the minimum of handling. If this is not possible it can be laid carefully between sterile gauze *soaked* in *warm,* physiological saline.

If the cord is nonpulsatile or the fetal heart is not audible the importance of prompt ultrasound assessment is vital and urgent as it has been demonstrated that fetal heart movements can be visualised in such circumstances and fetal resuscitation, as described above, should be carried out urgently.

An advance in the management of umbilical cord prolapse has been the development of bladder filling (unless rapid vaginal delivery is planned). Bladder filling was first proposed by Vago, in 1970, as a method of relieving pressure on the umbilical cord. Bladder distension raises the presenting part of the fetus off the compressed cord for an extended period of time, thereby eliminating the need for an examiner's fingers to displace the presenting part. A number 16 Foley catheter is placed into the urinary bladder. The bladder is filled, via the catheter, with physiological saline by a standard infusion set. The quantity of saline needed is determined by the fetal heart rate response and the appearance of the distended bladder above the pubis, with 500 ml usually being sufficient. The balloon is then inflated, the catheter is clamped and the drainage tubing and urine bag are attached and secured, ready for when the fluid is released prior to CS.

Bladder filling has an additional advantage in that the full bladder may decrease or inhibit uterine contractions. In a series by Chetty and Moodley, there were no cases of perinatal mortality.[1] All the babies had Apgar scores of 6 or more and the mean elapsed time from diagnosis to delivery was 69 minutes. Eight women in their study delivered after an elapsed time of 80 minutes or more.

Tocolysis may be initiated to reduce contractions and improve bradycardia by using terbutaline 0.25 mg subcutaneously. If there is no evidence of fetal distress, it may be reasonable to proceed with a regional block (but conducted in left lateral, not sitting, position). The bladder is emptied by unclamping the catheter at the time of the skin preparation.

Vaginal delivery can be conducted when umbilical cord prolapse occurs at full dilatation with either the vacuum extractor or forceps, but only if the delivery is anticipated as being straightforward and easy: this is no time to embark on a complicated or protracted instrumentation that will exacerbate cord compression and potentially worsen the fetal condition.

The evidence relating to the interval between diagnosis and delivery being associated with stillbirth and neonatal death is conflicting. Neonatal condition, assessed by Apgar scores and paired cord blood gas analysis, is more likely to be influenced by the condition of the baby during the problem, rather than the time interval itself and fetal mortality has been more consistently attributed to prematurity and congenital anomalies. Birth asphyxia is, nevertheless, important and when this condition occurs outside of hospital (approximately 25% of patients) it carries a perinatal mortality rate as high as 86.4%.

Summary

- Umbilical cord prolapse is an infrequent obstetric emergency that requires prompt recognition and rapid action.
- Perinatal outcome is improved with attention to fetal resuscitation while preparing to expedite delivery.
- Occasionally vaginal delivery can be achieved, but most patients need CS and the urgency of this depends on the condition of the baby as assessed by the fetal heart rate.

- Regular drills on an annual basis, at least, should be mandatory for staff involved in maternity services, each being aware of their specific role in such an emergency.
- It is vital to debrief staff, women and partners after such an emergent situation.

References and further reading

1 Chetty RM, Moodley J. Umbilical cord prolapse. *S Afr Med J* 1980;57:128–9.
2 Driscoll JA, Sadan O, Van Gelderen CJ, Holloway GA. Cord prolapse: can we save more babies? *Br J Obstet Gynaecol* 1987;94:594–5.
3 Fenton AN, d'Esopo DA. Prolapse of the cord during labor. *Am J Obstet Gynecol* 1951;62:52–64.
4 Ferrara TB, Hoekstra RE, Gaziano E, *et al.* Changing outcome of extremely premature infants (<26 weeks' gestation and <750 gm): survival and follow-up at a tertiary center. *Am J Obstet Gynecol* 1989;161:1114–18.
5 Goldthorp WO. A decade in the management of prolapse and presentation of the umbilical cord. *Br J Clin Pract* 1967;21:21–26.
6 Koonings PP, Paul RH, Campbell K. Umbilical cord prolapse: a contemporary look. *J Reprod Med* 1990;35:690–92.
7 Griese ME, Prickett SA. Nursing management of umbilical cord prolapse. *Neonatal Nurs* 1993:311–15.
8 Mesleh T, Sultan M, Sabagh T, Algwiser A. Umbilical cord prolapse. *J Obstet Gynecol* 1993;13:24–8.
9 Murphy DJ, MacKenzie IZ. The mortality and morbidity associated with umbilical cord prolapse. *Br J Obstet Gynaecol* 1995;102:826–30.
10 Panter KR, Hannah ME. Umbilical cord prolapse: so far so good? *Lancet* 1996;347:74.
11 Raga F, Osborne N, Ballister MJ. Color flow Doppler: a useful instrument in the diagnosis of funic presentation. *J Natl Med Assoc* 1996;88:94–6.
12 *RCOG Greentop Guideline Umbilical Cord Prolapse.* London: RCOG 2008.
13 Vago T. Prolapse of the umbilical cord. A method of management. *Am J Obstet Gynecol* 1970;107:967–9.
14 Yla-Outinen A, Heinonen PK, Tuimala R. Predisposing and risk factors of umbilical cord prolapse. *Acta Obstet Gynecol Scand* 1985;64:567–70.

ALGORITHM 33.1 Face presentation

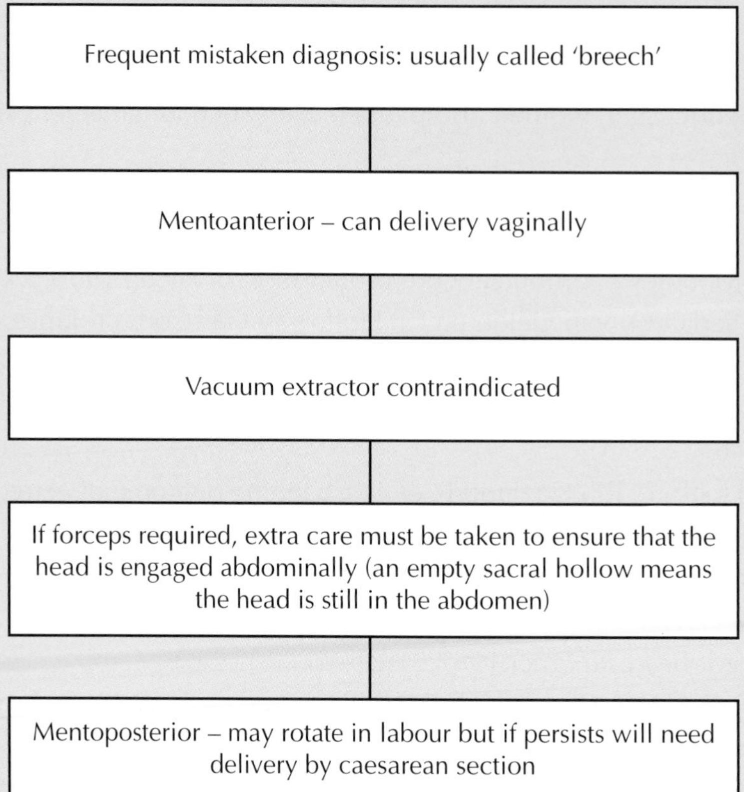

CHAPTER 33

Face presentation

Objectives

On successfully completing this topic, you will be able to:

- understand the mechanics of delivery of the baby presenting by the face
- appreciate the importance of the positioning of the face in labour and prior to delivery
- understand how to assess the situation when contemplating operative vaginal delivery.

Introduction

Face presentation occurs in approximately 1/500 to 1/1000 deliveries.

Aetiology

Predisposing causes are characteristics that reduce cephalic flexion and include the following:

- multiparity
- prematurity
- multiple pregnancy
- loops of cord around neck
- neck tumours
- uterine abnormalities
- cephalopelvic disproportion
- fetal macrosomia.

Clinical approach

Diagnosis

Primary face presentation might be detected on a late ultrasound scan. The majority of face presentations are secondary and arise in labour.

Abdominal examination

A large amount of head is palpable on the same side as the back, without a cephalic prominence on the same side as the limbs, before the head has entered the pelvis.

Vaginal examination

In early labour, the presenting part will be high. At vaginal examination (VE), landmarks are the mouth, jaws, nose, malar and orbital ridges. The presence of alveolar margins distinguishes the mouth from the anus, so distinguishing a face presentation from that of a breech. In addition, the mouth and the maxillae form the corners of a triangle, while in a breech presentation, the anus is on a straight line between the ischial tuberosities.

During VE, avoid inadvertently damaging the eyes by trauma or antiseptics.

Management

Follow the steps:

- make a diagnosis
- check for cord presentation or prolapse
- continuously monitor fetal heart rate
- examine regularly to check that progress is adequate
- give oxytocin if contractions are poor and progress is not satisfactory
- do not use scalp electrodes or perform fetal blood sampling
- if the position is mentoanterior, vaginal delivery should be possible (rotation from other positions can occur during labour)
- perform an episiotomy
- if the fetus is persistently presenting mentoposteriorly, deliver by CS.

Intrapartum considerations

Labour in face presentation

In early labour, minor deflexion attitudes are common, especially with occipito-posterior positions and multiparity. In such cases, uterine contractions often cause increased flexion. Occasionally, extension will increase, producing successively a brow presentation and finally, the fully extended face. Most face presentations are thus secondary, becoming evident only in established labour. Diagnosis is notoriously difficult. In approximately 50% of cases the diagnosis is not made until delivery is imminent.

Descent is usually followed by internal rotation, with the chin passing anteriorly thus, as with other labours, progress is assessed by dilatation, rotation and descent. If contractions are inadequate, they can be augmented with oxytocin as long as signs of obstruction have been excluded.

It must be remembered that the biparietal diameter is 7cm behind the advancing face, so that, even when the face is distending the vulva, the biparietal diameter has only just entered the pelvis. Descent is thus always less advanced than VE would suggest, even when one allows for the gross oedema that is usually present. The value of abdominal examination in such cases cannot be overstressed. However, when the chin is anterior and the occiput is posterior, it can be difficult to feel the fetal head abdominally even when it is still in the abdomen – 'the head is always higher than you think with a face presentation'. The key is feeling posteriorly on vaginal examination – check the sacral hollow, which should be filled up by the occiput – if the sacral hollow is empty, the occiput is still intra-abdominal.

Mentoanterior position

Anterior rotation of the chin usually occurs during descent and this brings the neck behind the symphysis pubis. The head is born by flexion, with the occiput following behind and causing considerable perineal distension in the process, hence the recommendation to cut an episiotomy in most cases.

With satisfactory uterine action and a mentoanterior position, spontaneous delivery or easy 'lift out' with forceps (*never* ventouse) assisted delivery will ensue in 60–90% of patients. The shoulders and body are born in the usual way.

Mentoposterior position

Even with mentoposterior positions diagnosed in labour, anterior rotation will occur in the first or second stage in most cases, so that persistent mentoposterior position or mentotransverse arrest is encountered in only 10% of face presentations.

In cases of persisting mentoposterior position, the neck is too short to span the 12cm of the anterior aspect of the sacrum. Additionally, to complete delivery, the neck would have to be extended even further, to allow the occiput to pass under the symphysis, and this is not possible as the neck is already maximally extended. Delivery in the direct mentoposterior position is thus impossible unless, as can happen with a very small fetus, the shoulders can enter the pelvis at the same time as the head. Persistent mentoposteriorly presenting fetuses are therefore delivered by CS to reduce fetal and maternal morbidity.

Vaginal manipulation in face presentations

Vaginal manipulation, including forceps delivery and the Thorn's manoeuvre to convert the mentoposterior fetal head to the occipito-anterior position, were reported historically and are contraindicated in modern obstetrics due to the high risk of fetal injury. However, it is worth noting a report by Newman *et al.* who reported on 11 cases of intrapartum bimanual conversion of mentoposterior to occipito-anterior position in orthodox Jews who refused CS delivery.[1] In the ten patients where ritodrine was administered, the manoeuvre was successful and vaginal delivery was achieved. A ritodrine bolus was administered, with concurrent upward transvaginal pressure, and the fetal head was disengaged. Bimanual fetal head flexion was then attempted using ultrasound guidance and transabdominal palpation of the occiput with gentle flexion towards the maternal pubis. Once the occipito-anterior presentation was achieved, oxytocin infusion was started. The one failure in this report was the author's initial case, in which ritodrine was not employed. Maternal and neonatal outcomes were good in all cases.

After birth, oedema and bruising of a child's face is inevitable and the parents should be warned of this in advance. In some cases, it may persist for some days and can make feeding difficult.

Summary

- Face presentation is not common but when it does occur, it is often identified late.
- Accoucheurs should be prepared for this eventuality and be aware that some patients will need CS.

Reference and further reading

1 Newman M, Beller U, Lavie O, *et al.* Intrapartum bimanual tocolytic-assisted reversal of face presentation: preliminary report. *Obstet Gynecol* 1994;84:146–52.

2 Benedetti TJ, Lowensohn RI, Truscott AM. Face presentation at term. *Obstet Gynecol* 1980;55:199–202.

3 Bhal PS, Davies NJ, Chung T. A population study of face and brow presentation. *J Obstet Gynecol* 1998;18:231:5.

4 Cruikshank DP, Cruikshank JE. Face and brow presentation: A review. *Clin Obstet Gynecol* 1981;24:333–51.

5 Cruikshank DP, White CA. Obstetric malpresentations: 20 years experience. *Am J Obstet Gynecol* 1973;116:1097–104.

6 Daw E. Management of the hyperextended fetal head. *Am J Obstet Gynecol* 1976;124:113–15.

7 Duff P. Diagnosis and management of face presentation. *Obstet Gynecol* 1981;57:105–11.

8 Mostar S, Akaltin E, Babunca C. Deflexion attitudes: median vertex, persistent brow and face presentations. *Obstet Gynecol* 1966;28:49–56.

9 Posner LB, Rubin EJ, Posner AC. Face and brow presentations: a continuing study. *Obstet Gynecol* 1963;21:745–9.

10 Schwartz Z, Dgani R, Lancet M, Kessler I. Face presentation. *Aust N Z J Obstet Gynaecol* 1986;26:172–6.

ALGORITHM 34.1 Breech and external cephalic version

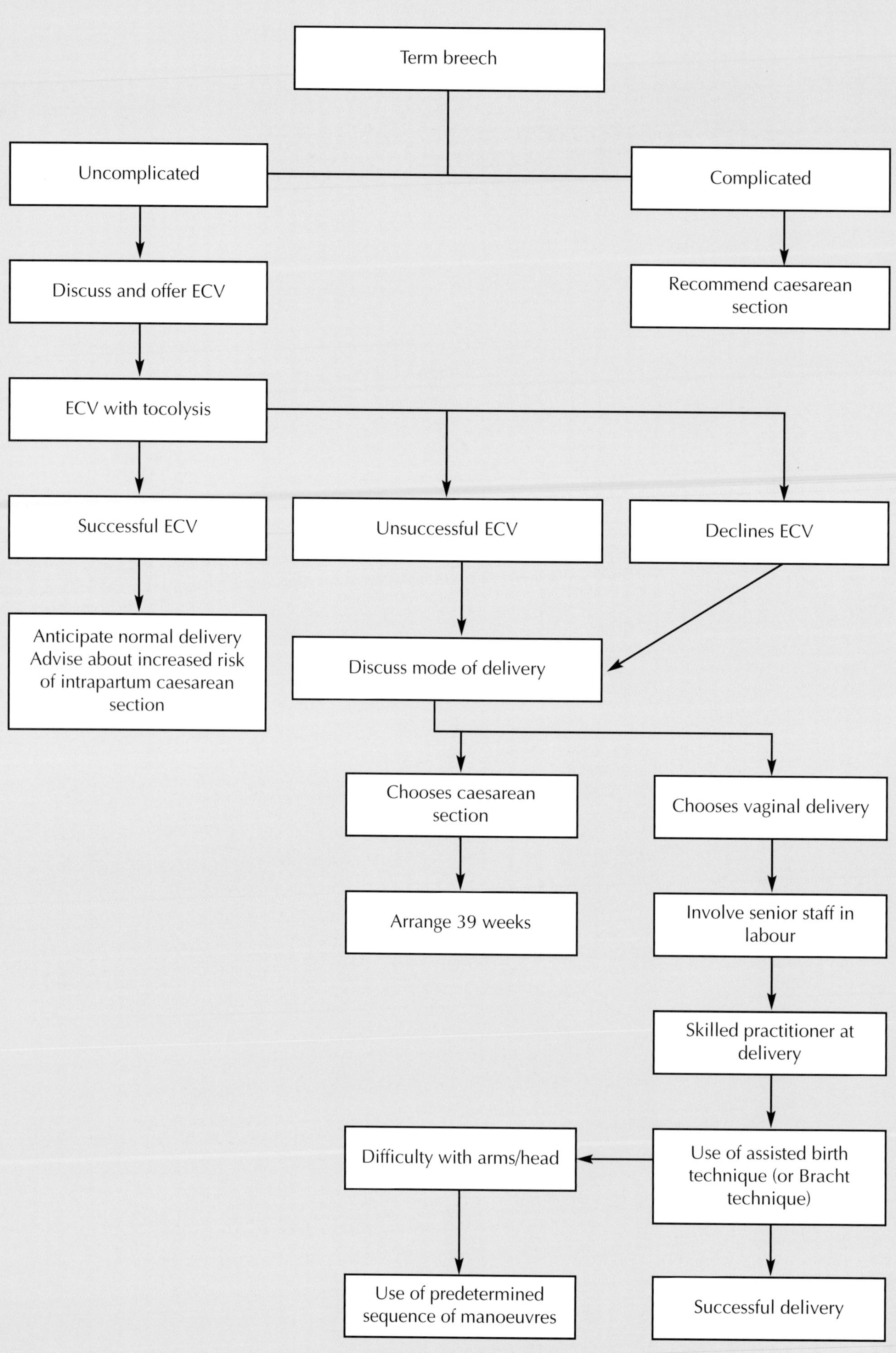

CHAPTER 34

Breech delivery and external cephalic version

Objectives

On successfully completing this topic, you will be able to:

- discuss the risks and benefits of external cephalic version
- understand the techniques of external cephalic version
- discuss the risks and benefits of vaginal breech delivery
- understand the techniques of vaginal breech birth.

Introduction

The incidence of breech presentation is about 20% at 28 weeks but has dropped to 3% by term as most fetuses turn spontaneously. Breech presentation can be a consequence of fetal or uterine abnormality, or can occur by chance. It has been widely recognised that there is higher perinatal mortality and morbidity with breech presentation, principally owing to prematurity, congenital anomalies and birth asphyxia. Breech presentation, whatever the mode of delivery, is a signal for potential fetal handicap and this should inform antenatal, intrapartum and neonatal management. CS for breech presentation has been suggested as a way of reducing the associated fetal problems and in many countries in northern Europe and North America CS has become the most common mode of delivery in this situation.

External cephalic version

External cephalic version (ECV), the manipulative transabdominal conversion of the breech to cephalic presentation, has been practised since the time of Hippocrates and through the European Middle Ages to modern times, although without much supporting evidence. In the late 1970s and 1980s, the procedure fell into disrepute but subsequent trials and the decline in the choice of vaginal breech birth has led to its wide reintroduction. It has been an RCOG audit standard for some time to offer ECV to women with a diagnosed breech presentation at term.

Efficacy

ECV at term has been subjected to rigorous scientific appraisal in a number of RCTs. There is significant reduction in the risk of CS in women where there is an intention to undertake ECV (OR 0.52, 95% CI 0.4–0.7) with no increased risk to the baby.

The perceived reduction in success rates in primigravid women has led to an examination of ECV before term. A systematic review of three older studies involving 900 women shows no reduction in CS rate (RR 1.1 95% CI 0.78–1.54). The recent Early ECV 2 Trial showed an increase in cephalic presentation at birth but no reduction in CS rate.[1] Furthermore, early ECV possibly increased the risk of premature birth.

ECV can be carried out in early labour (if the membranes are intact) with success but no randomised trials exist and studies are too small to assess safety.

ECV has been introduced successfully into practice in the UK. Although the success rate (conversion to cephalic presentation) found is less than that quoted in trials (e.g. over 80% in Africa), others have found similar success rates. Generalisation of these results in the UK would result in a significant reduction in the numbers of CS. With case selection, it is possible to achieve higher success rates and operators improve with experience. Among published US studies, an overall success rate of 65% was found.

Reversion to breech occurs after successful ECV, with between 3% and 7% being reported for term ECV. Rates of over 20% have been reported for preterm ECV.

Factors affecting success

Parity is the main factor that affects success with nulliparous success rates around one in three and multiparous success rates around two in three or greater. Amniotic fluid volume may affect success, although there is no consensus on whether there should be an absolute cut-off for attempting the procedure. Maternal weight and height affect success and fetal weight (both macrosomia and small for gestation) may be a factor. Even within the 'term' period, gestation may matter, and the degree of engagement of the fetal breech has an effect. Attempts to produce a predictive algorithm have not been helpful.

Techniques to improve success

Tocolysis and anaesthesia have been advocated to improve success rates. A Cochrane review showed a reduction in ECV failures with beta-agonist tocolysis (RR 0.74 95% CI 0.64–0.87) and a reduction in CS rate (RR 0.85 95% CI 0.72–0.99).[2] One further trial since this review confirms this efficacy. Others have used selective betamimetic treatment after failure of ECV without tocolysis, demonstrating reduction in CS rates with this approach (RR 0.33 95% CI 0.14–0.8). Sublingual nitroglycerin was not found to be effective in the systematic review and in one subsequent large study. A trial comparing betamimetic with nitroglycerine tocolysis showed better success rates with betamimetic. One trial of fetal acoustic stimulation has shown fewer failures, but this requires further study. Amnio-infusion has been advocated but there is no evidence of efficacy. Some groups have used epidural and spinal analgesia. A recent meta analysis concluded that the use of spinal or epidural with an anaesthetic dose increases the success rate of fetal version (RR 1.44).[3]

Alternative methods of producing cephalic version

Various postural methods, such as knee–elbow, knee–chest, Indian and Zilgrie positions, have been advocated. Review of clinical trials shows no increase in the rate of cephalic births.

The technique of moxibustion involves the use of burning herbs at acupoint BL 67 beside the outer corner of the fifth toenail. Although an early trial suggested an increase in cephalic presentations, a subsequent larger and better-conducted study has shown no benefit.

Complications of ECV

Systematic reviews of safety have been carried out. Transient fetal heart rate abnormalities occur in 5.7%, with persisting abnormal cardiotocography (CTG) in approximately 1/300. Placental abruption was rare, occurring in 1/1000 patients. A detailed examination of perinatal deaths in series of ECV suggests a perinatal mortality of 1.6/1000. This is not different from the perinatal mortality of pregnancies between 37 and 40 weeks.

There is a growing body of evidence that the CS rate for women who have successful ECV is around twice that of cephalic-presenting pregnancies and that the vaginal operative delivery rate may also be increased. The data are sufficiently consistent that women undergoing ECV should be informed of this.

Women's views

Most women would choose ECV to allow vaginal delivery. However, some surveys have suggested that a substantial minority of eligible women would decline ECV, opting for CS. In part, this may be a failure of education and uptake can be increased by well-constructed information packages.

Performance of ECV

There are no studies comparing different methods of performing ECV (Figure 35.1). Training is largely 'hands-on', although Burr *et al.* developed a model that has some promise.

Preparation

1. Inform the woman fully of the risks, national and local success rates and about the procedure itself.
2. Perform a CTG, which should be normal.
3. Ultrasound examination should be carried out by a practitioner with appropriate training. The examination should determine:
   - fetal position
   - position of the legs
   - liquor volume
   - head flexion.

4 It is useful to carry out an abdominal circumference measurement to exclude both small for gestation and macrosomia.

5 Written or informed and documented verbal consent should be obtained.

6 Although serious complications are rare, the practitioner should ensure that there is immediate access to an obstetric operating theatre.

7 Tocolysis, if preferred, should be given at this stage. Terbutaline 250 microgram should be given by subcutaneous injection. The woman should be warned of the adverse effects and there should be no contraindications to betamimetic drugs.

Procedure

1 Lay the woman flat and either on her side, with the fetal back upwards, or tilted using a wedge. Some practitioners also tilt the bed, placing the woman partly head down.

2 Disengagement of the fetal breech can be achieved by a number of methods, depending at present on personal preference. Most practitioners use the palmar surfaces of the fingers of both hands to gradually pull up the breech (Figure 34.1). Others use a modification of Paulik's grip to push up the breech. In some instances, an assistant may push the breech from below if a woman or circumstances demand a more aggressive attempt at ECV.

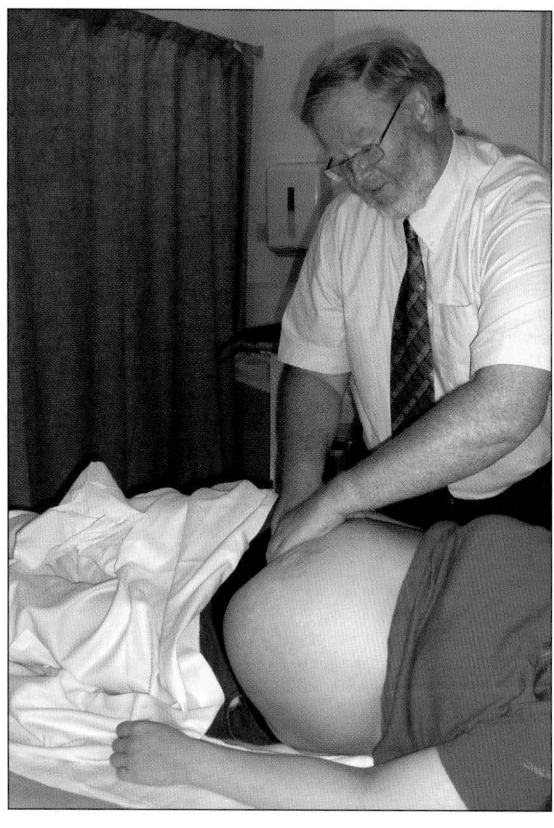

Figure 34.1 Disimpaction of the fetal breech

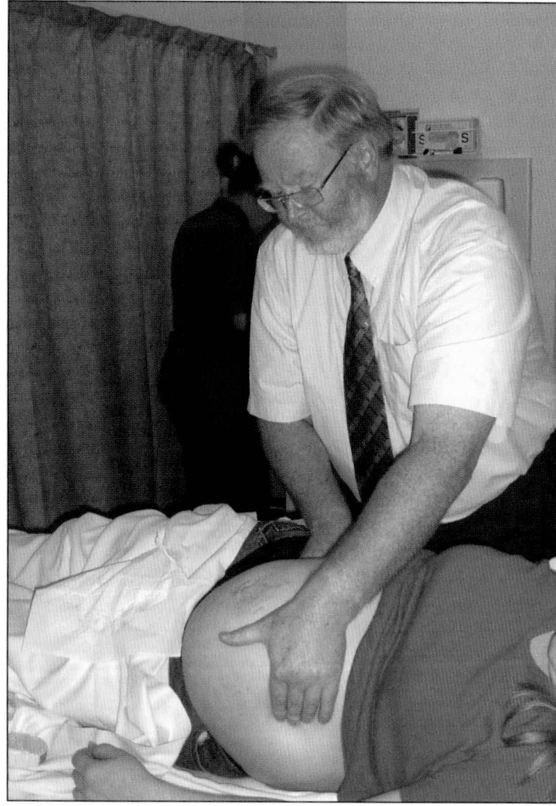

Figure 34.2 Flexion of the fetal head

3 Some use talc or various oils. There is no evidence that the use of these influences success or comfort rates.

4 Once disengaged, the breech is slowly pulled or pushed upwards and laterally to allow fetal flexion. Some practitioners rely totally on this manoeuvre, allowing the fetus to perform a forward somersault in its own time while maintaining the breech free and to the side. Others use one hand to grasp the free breech and the other to gently flex the fetal head by pressure on the occiput or nape of the neck (Figure 34.2). The hands follow the baby as he or she rotates.

5 The procedure should not be lengthy and there should be constant feedback from the woman on how uncomfortable she is. The fetal heart can be either auscultated or observed by scan if more than 2–3 minutes are needed. A maximum of three attempts can be made if the woman permits. Usually, forward somersault is the best direction but a backward somersault approach can be considered, if a third attempt is to be undertaken. The fetal heart should be observed or auscultated between attempts.

Postprocedure

- Whether successful or not, a repeat CTG should be performed.
- If the woman is rhesus negative, then blood for Kleihauer estimation should be taken and 500 units Rh immunoglobulin given.
- If successful, then spontaneous labour is awaited and advice given on bleeding and reduced fetal movements.
- If unsuccessful, then the reasons for this should be discussed. Arrangements can then be made either for a further attempt on another day, or for a discussion on the mode of delivery.

Vaginal breech delivery

The use of CS as a primary choice of delivery mode for breech presentation has been increasing in the developed world and the publication of the Term Breech Trial demonstrated clear fetal and neonatal short-term advantages for elective CS.[4] However, the two-year follow-up data showed no significant difference between the planned CS group and the trial of labour group for combined perinatal death and abnormal neurological outcomes. Furthermore, the children born in the trial of labour group reported fewer medical problems, although the significance of this is unclear. Dutch data have shown that the alteration in practice to a higher CS rate resulted in the predicted reduction in perinatal mortality, but at a cost of an increased maternal mortality rate and increased maternal morbidity in the short and long term.[5,6] The recommendation in Holland now is that the preferred mode of delivery for breech presentation is vaginally, if appropriate. Data from the French PREMODA Study suggested that with careful case selection, careful management of labour and an experienced accoucheur, the neonatal outcomes are not significantly different in the two groups. Selection of cases included assessment of the type of breech, attitude of the fetal head and estimated fetal weight.

There are maternal disadvantages to a policy of routine CS for breech. Therefore, it is imperative that clinical skills of accoucheurs should be such that the option of vaginal breech delivery is available. Currently, in the UK setting, the vast majority of women are having an elective CS for breech, although this practice is now under question.

As a consequence of these concerns and of breech presentations being diagnosed for the first time in labour (which the term breech trial did not address), vaginal breech birth will still occur and skill in delivering the breech is needed.

Many of the manoeuvres used during an assisted breech delivery or Bracht manoeuvre should be used to deliver the breech at CS and this, as well as formal manikin training, should be used to teach and maintain skills.

Conduct of labour

Where vaginal breech birth is being considered, ultrasound examination should be carried out to try to establish the type of breech presentation, the degree of flexion of the fetal head and the estimated fetal weight. If the presentation is footling (at term), if the head is hyperextended or if the estimated weight is less than 2500 g or more than 4000 g, then the woman should be advised to deliver by CS and must be made aware of the additional risks should she decide to continue with planned vaginal birth.

Currently, available data on complications of vaginal breech birth have derived from a hospital setting. There are a number of midwifery practitioners with experience of vaginal breech birth, using different techniques, but currently there are no published large case series data that can be used to incorporate these techniques into practice. This section will outline the conduct of a breech birth within a consultant led obstetric service.

Procedure

1 On admission, senior midwifery, obstetric and anaesthetic staff should be alerted and the conduct of the labour should be supervised by the most experienced obstetrician available.

2 One-to-one midwifery care with an experienced midwife should be put in place.

3 If spontaneous labour, then matters of maternal and fetal surveillance should follow the same guidance as for any labour. The breech baby is not a second-class citizen and all signs that would cause concern in a cephalic presentation should do likewise with the breech.

4 Analgesia, as requested by the woman in consultation with her midwife, should be provided. There is no evidence that epidural analgesia is of specific benefit for breech labour and delivery.

5 Labour can be accelerated using the normal doses of oxytocin where there is good evidence of poor uterine activity as a cause for poor progress in the first stage of labour. Evidence for and against augmentation is not robust and the decision to augment is best made at consultant level.

6 Where continuous electronic fetal monitoring is used and is nonreassuring, fetal buttock sampling can be carried out but discussion at consultant level should occur if this is being considered.

7 As soon as the second stage is diagnosed, a practitioner experienced in vaginal breech birth should be immediately available. The anaesthetic resident on call should be available on the delivery suite and the obstetric operating theatre free.

Conduct of the delivery

There are no recent data comparing safety or efficacy of the various techniques used in breech birth. Therefore, debates on whether classic techniques are superior to Bracht manoeuvres or whether forceps are superior to Mauriceau-Smellie-Viet (MSV) techniques are simply personal debates. The last detailed comparison of Bracht techniques versus classic techniques was carried out in 1953 and actually recommended the Bracht technique. A study in 1991 showed no difference in neonatal outcomes, comparing classic and Bracht techniques. The techniques used by midwifery practitioners are essentially derived from Bracht.

In all techniques, the avoidance of traction is the key.

Assisted breech delivery

1 Delay active pushing until the breech is distending the introitus (anus dilating).

2 Place the woman in lithotomy and perform episiotomy.

3 Initially 'hands-off'. The stool of the operator is best placed at a distance from the maternal buttocks that does not allow the operator to reach the breech. The only exception to a 'hands-off' approach is where the fetal back appears to be rotating from sacroanterior; if this occurs, then it should be corrected.

4 Allow maternal effort to expel the breech to the level of the umbilicus. The back will arch towards the maternal symphysis. There is no evidence that pulling a loop of cord down at this point is of any benefit and should be avoided, as handling of the cord produces arterial spasm.

5 If flexed, the legs will deliver spontaneously. If extended, it is legitimate to simply flex the hip by placing two fingers behind the thigh. No traction or handling of the rest of the baby is required.

6 Further expulsive efforts will continue to arch the fetal back. If the arms are flexed then they may deliver spontaneously. If not, they can be hooked down from the elbow. If this is not sufficient, two fingers can be passed over the shoulder to push the humerus across

the chest, in a manoeuvre not dissimilar to that used in shoulder dystocia. At this point, an assistant should be supporting the fetal body.

7 If the arms are extended up behind the fetal neck, then Lovset's manoeuvre should be employed. The fetus is grasped by a femoral–pelvic grip (Figure 34.3) with the thumbs parallel along the spine (avoiding the soft abdomen). There is gentle downwards traction and the body is lifted towards the maternal symphysis. The baby is rotated (back always rotating through an anterior not a posterior sweep) through 180°, bringing the posterior arm under the symphysis, where it can be hooked out by flexion of the elbow. The grip is maintained and the baby rotated back through 180° to free the other arm (again back kept anteriorly).

8 Allow descent of the head within the pelvis and await the appearance of the nape of the neck (i.e. the base of the occiput). Allowing the baby to hang can promote head extension and gentle support can be provided at this stage.

9 Delivery of the head can be achieved using forceps (ideally Pipers, but any long handled forceps will suffice; Wrigleys forceps are not suitable) (Figure 34.4) or by the technique known as MSV. With forceps delivery, an assistant is needed but with MSV, delivery can be accomplished by a sole operator. The baby is draped over one arm, with two fingers placed alongside the nose. The other hand is placed just under the occiput with the middle or index finger placed along the occiput (Figure 34.5). Both hands are used to promote flexion and delivery of the head.

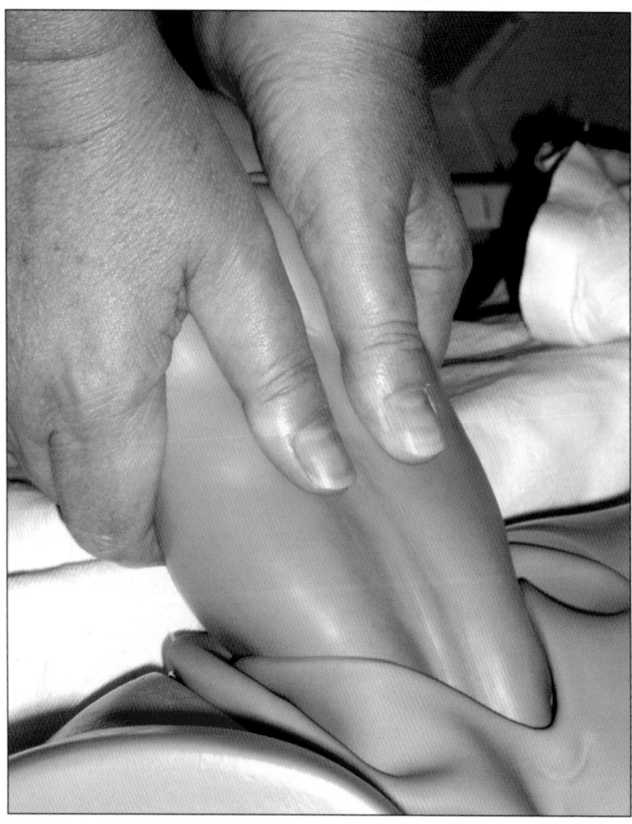

Figure 34.3 The pelvic grasp for Lovset's manoeuvre

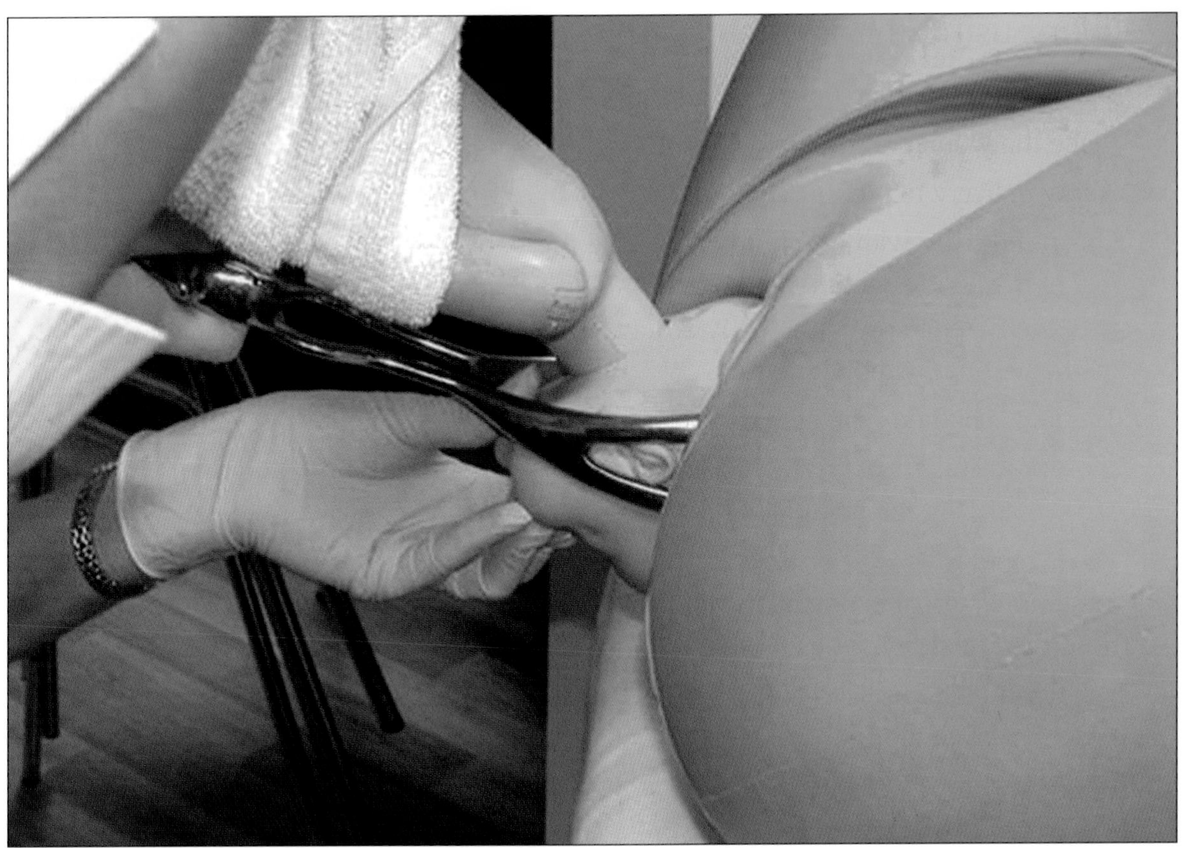

Figure 34.4 Application of forceps to the aftercoming head

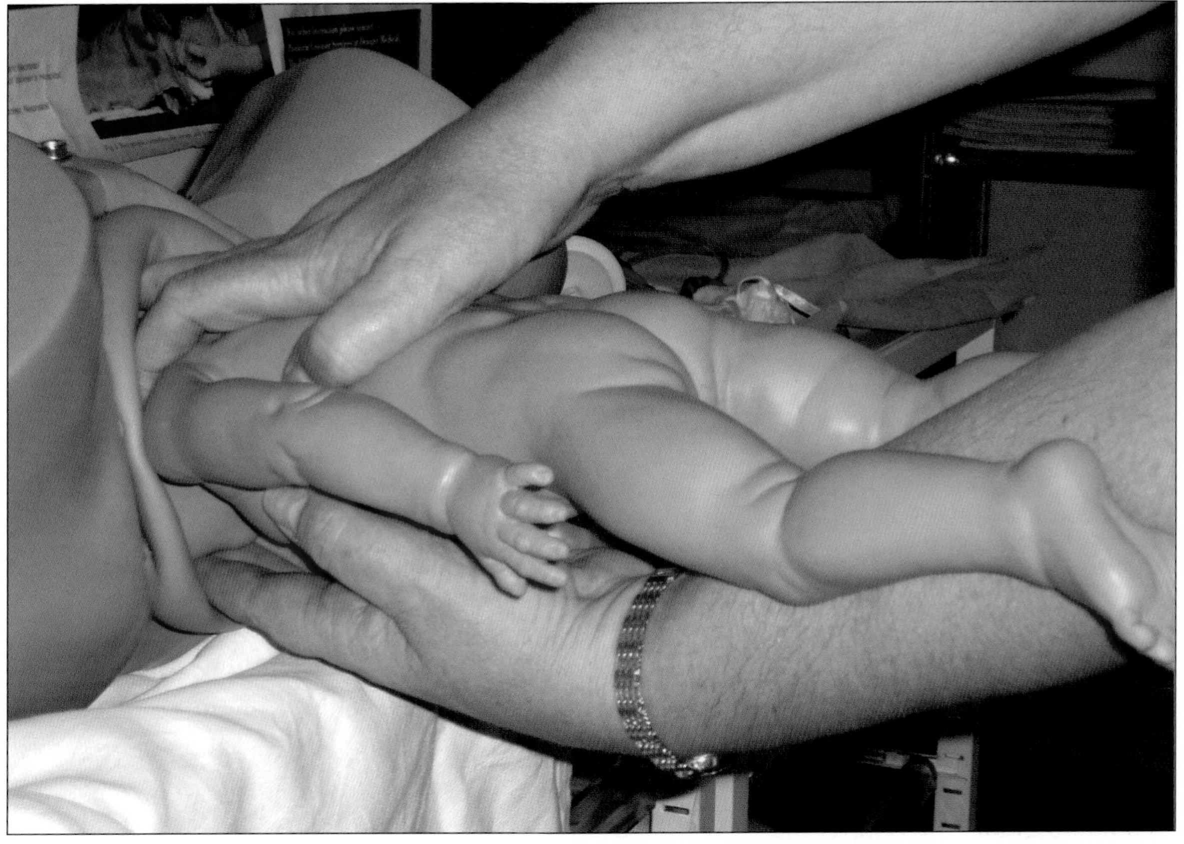

Figure 34.5 Mauriceau–Smellie–Viet manoeuvre

Delivery using the Bracht technique

1. Delay active pushing until the presenting breech is distending the introitus.
2. Place the woman in lithotomy and perform episiotomy.
3. Allow delivery to the umbilicus.
4. Grasp the baby with the thumbs pressing the baby's thigh against its stomach and the rest of the hands over the sacral and loin area (Figure 34.6). While the woman is pushing, gently rotate or lift the baby around the maternal symphysis, maintaining upwards movement but without traction.
5. The legs will then deliver and, as the upwards rotation continues, the arms will follow.
6. Most practitioners of this technique also advise an assistant providing gentle but persistent pressure on the maternal abdomen to push the head downwards.
7. Where the arms do not then follow, while a range of manoeuvres are described by practitioners of the Bracht technique, it seems simplest to revert to the manoeuvres described in the previous section.
8. With continued upwards rotation, the head may deliver spontaneously, not unlike the descriptions of the Burns-Marshall technique (Figure 34.7). If the head does not deliver then either forceps or the MSV procedure can be used.

Failure to deliver

The great fear of vaginal breech delivery is head entrapment or nuchal arms that significantly delay delivery. Most experienced obstetricians will have dealt with each of these, but experience is decreasing. Like any rare, unpredictable obstetric emergency, clinicians should have a plan or drill that they follow. There is no literature, other than case reports or small series, to guide practice.

Nuchal arms

1. Recognise nuchal arms by the fact that the shoulder is extended and the elbow flexed.
2. Try Lovset's manoeuvre.
3. If this fails, grasp the fetal feet. Rotate (swing) the fetus towards the hand of the posterior nuchal arm and above the level of the maternal symphysis. This may result in delivery of the posterior arm but, if not, it allows room for the occiput to slip below the elbow. A hand can be placed over the shoulder and behind the humerus to allow pressure on the humerus, with delivery in front of the face.
4. If the other arm does not deliver after this, then the procedure can be repeated.
5. If this manoeuvre fails, then time is important. It may be possible, with the back anterior, to insert a hand to grab the elbow of one arm and exert sufficient pressure to correct the shoulder extension, allowing reuse of Lovset's manoeuvre. If this attempt fails, then it is legitimate to force the arm across the face to deliver. Humeral or clavicular fractures are very likely, but will not cause long-term harm; perinatal hypoxia does.

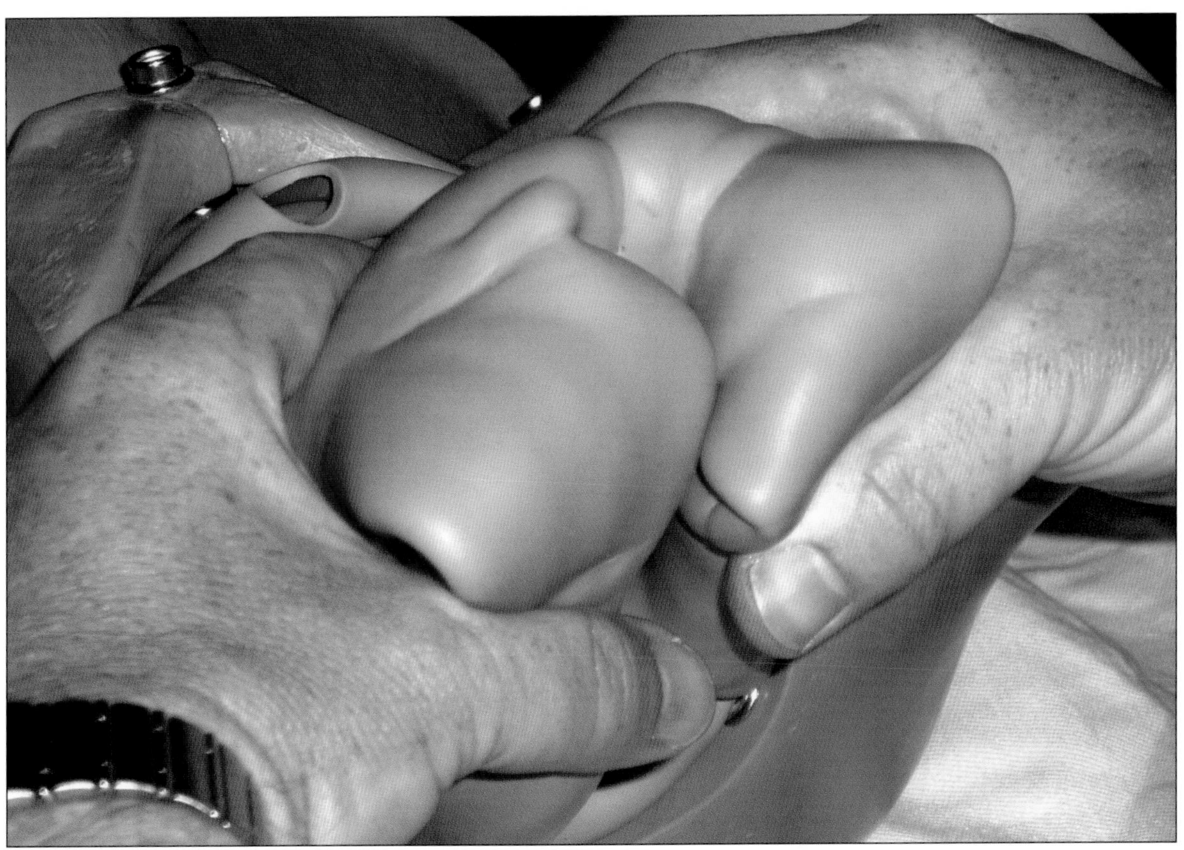

Figure 34.6 Initial placement of hands for Bracht technique

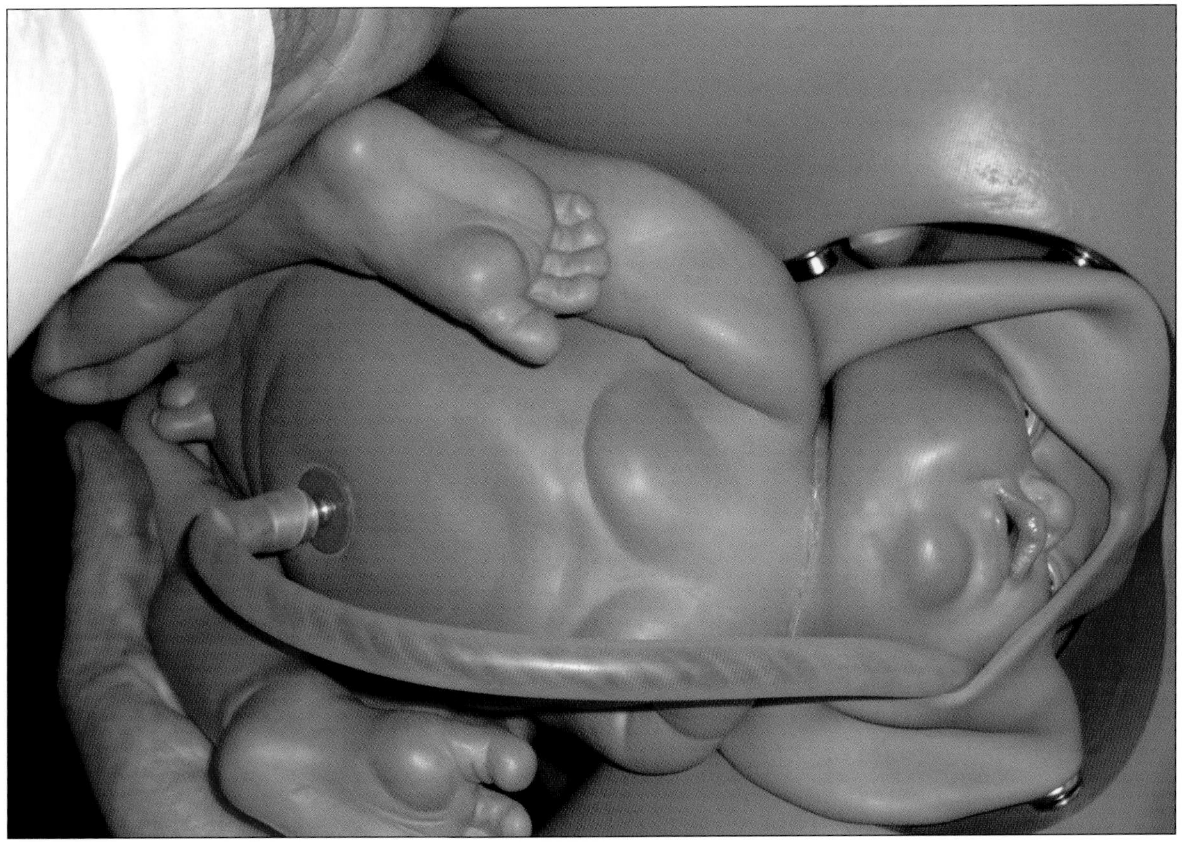

Figure 34.7 Delivery of the head by Bracht technique

Head entrapment

Intriguingly few recent texts mention how to deal with this when it occurs, merely providing advice on how to avoid it.

1 Ensure adequate midwifery and anaesthetic support; prepare for immediate CS; if expertise available, call for symphysiotomy equipment.
2 Try McRoberts' position and suprapubic pressure, as in shoulder dystocia.
3 Rotate the fetal body to a lateral position. Apply suprapubic pressure to flex head. Apply traction, then rotation back to sacroanterior and deliver by forceps.
4 Check that the cervix is still fully dilated, especially if preterm. If not, then incise at 4 and 8 o'clock.
5 Attempt midcavity forceps, if good analgesia is available.
6 Perform symphysiotomy if you have adequate training; if not, then you should now be in a position to carry out CS in the room if the baby is still alive. The baby needs to be pushed from below. The use of the ventouse has been described to assist.

Breech extraction

Breech extraction is most commonly used for the delivery of the second twin and is covered in Chapter 35. This technique is also needed for delivery of an abnormal lie at CS.

Medico-legal matters

Medico-legal concerns are increasingly rare for the singleton breech in the UK, as most women with breech presentations, who decline or fail version, choose CS. However, if proper delivery techniques are not employed at CS, trauma can result and this can lead to medico-legal issues.

Where vaginal breech delivery is to occur at any gestation, consultant or specialist input at every point in the decision process is vital. Although the literature is not supportive of absolute rules on oxytocin, continuous electronic monitoring, fetal buttock sampling and epidural analgesia, these are regarded by some practitioners as unacceptable practice. If these are being considered, the decision and discussions should be taking place at consultant level.

For UK-trained practitioners, competence is now an issue. Even consultant or specialist-level staff may have little experience or confidence at conducting a vaginal breech birth and they should ensure the availability of other colleagues if necessary.

Audit

The RCOG recommendations for audit are that:

- 'all women with an uncomplicated breech presentation at term should be offered ECV'
- maintain statistics on ECV success rates; make annual comparison with predicted rates
- all practitioners should maintain a record of competence or training in vaginal breech delivery.

Summary

- Offer and encourage ECV at term.
- There is no simple algorithm for predicting ECV success.
- Tocolysis with a betamimetic drug appears to increase ECV success rates.
- Where vaginal breech birth is chosen, ensure early involvement of consultant staff in labour.
- Assisted breech delivery or Bracht manoeuvre may be equally effective.
- Ensure that drill for nuchal arms and entrapped head is in place.
- Maintain competencies through practice at caesarean delivery for breech and through regular manikin training.
- Audit uptake and success rates of ECV.

References and further reading

1 Hutton EK, Hannah ME, Ross SJ, *et al.* The Early External Cephalic Version (ECV) 2 Trial: an international multicentre randomised controlled trial of timing of ECV for Breech pregnancies. *Br J Obstet Gynaecol* 2011;118(5):564–77.
2 Hofmeyr GJ, Gyte G. Interventions to help external cephalic version for breech presentation at term. *Cochrane Database Syst Rev* 2004;(1):CD000184.
3 Lavoie A, Guay J. Anesthetic dose neuraxial blockade increases the success rate of external fetal version: a meta-analysis. *Can J Anesth* 2010;57;408–14.
4 Hannah ME, Hannah WJ, Hewson SA, *et al.*, for the TBT Group planned caesarean section versus planned vaginal birth for breech presentation at term: a randomised multicentre trial. *Lancet* 2000;356:1375–83.
5 Verhoven AT, de Leeuw JP, Bruinse HW. Breech presentation at term: elective caesarean section is the wrong choice as a standard treatment because of too high risks for the mother and her future children. *NedTijdschr Geneeskd* 2005;149:2207–10.
6 Schutt JM, Steegers EA, Santema JG, *et al.* Maternal deaths after elective caesarean section for breech presentation in the Netherlands. *Acta Obstet Gynecol Scand* 2007;86:240–43.
7 Chan LY, Leung TY, Fok WY, *et al.* Prediction of successful vaginal delivery in women undergoing external cephalic version at term for breech presentation. *Eur J Obstet Gynecol Reprod Biol* 2004;116:39–42.
8 Chan LY, Tang JL, Tsoi KF, *et al.* Intrapartum caesarean delivery after successful external cephalic version: a meta-analysis. *Obstet Gynecol* 2004;104:155–60.
9 Cheng M, Hannah M. Breech delivery at term: a critical review of the literature. *Obstet Gynecol* 1993;82:605–18.
10 Collaris RJ, Guid Oei S. External cephalic version: a safe procedure? A systematic review of version-related risks. *Acta Obstet Gynecol Scand* 2004;83:511–18.

11 Hofmeyr GJ, Kulier R. External cephalic version for breech presentation at term. *Cochrane Database Syst Rev* 1996;CD000083.
12 Hutton EK, Hofmeyr GJ. External cephalic version for breech presentation before term. *Cochrane Database Syst Rev* 2006;CD000084.
13 Impey L, Pandit M. Tocolysis for repeat external cephalic version in breech presentation at term: a randomised, double-blinded, placebo-controlled trial. *Br J Obstet Gynaecol* 2005;112:627–31.
14 *RCOG: Greentop Guideline 20a. External Cephalic Version and Reducing the Incidence of Breech Presentation.* London: RCOG 2006.

ALGORITHM 35.1 Twin pregnancy

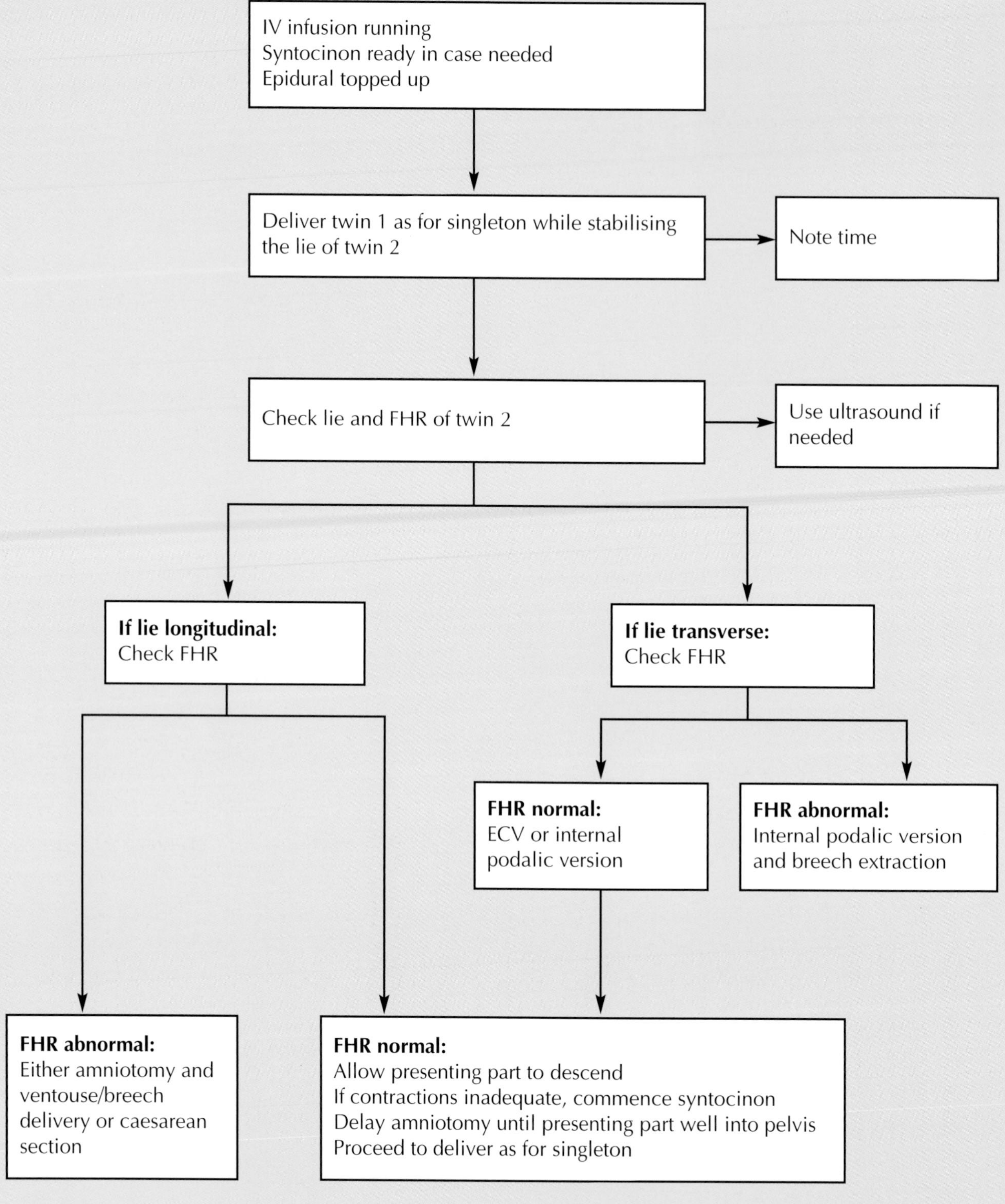

CHAPTER 35

Twin pregnancy

Objectives

On successfully completing this topic, you will be able to:

- understand how to assess suitability for vaginal delivery
- understand how to safely manage appropriate vaginal twin deliveries.

Introduction

Dizygous twinning rates vary enormously depending on age, parity, racial background and assisted-conception techniques. The incidence of twin pregnancies continues to increase, largely due to assisted reproduction techniques, giving a multiple birth rate of 16/1000 maternities in England and Wales in 2009. Monozygous twinning rates are relatively constant, with an incidence of 3.5/1000 births. Overall maternal and perinatal mortality and morbidity are higher in multiple gestations than in singletons. Premature delivery and the complications of prematurity are the main contributors to adverse outcomes. Other factors contributing to the risk are: intrauterine growth restriction; congenital anomalies; malpresentation; cord prolapse; and premature separation of the placenta.

The use of routine antenatal ultrasound assessment has facilitated the diagnosis of multiple gestations. Women with multiple fetuses who attend for antenatal care should have the chorionicity of the pregnancy determined early in pregnancy and then have serial growth scans as specified in the recent NICE and RCOG Greentop guidelines on the antenatal care of multiple pregnancies.[1,2] It is recommended that monochorionic twins are delivered after 36+0 weeks following a course of antenatal steroids, and dichorionic twins are delivered after 37+0 weeks.

A meta-analysis of the management of twin delivery did not find significant differences in outcome, in terms of mortality or neonatal morbidity, when comparing policies of planned vaginal delivery against planned CS. A cohort study of 2890 twin pairs delivered after 36 weeks of gestation found that there were no deaths in those twins delivered by CS, but nine second-twin deaths in those delivered vaginally. An international, multicentre, RCT (the Twin Birth Study) of 2400 women randomly delivered by CS and planned vaginal birth has now been completed and shows that vaginal delivery is safe.[3] However, some aspects of twin delivery remain controversial.

Presentation

Twin 1 vertex

Assess the suitability for vaginal delivery allowing for the fact that, even if twin two is cephalic prelabour, it is difficult to predict its eventual presentation at the time of delivery. If the second twin is breech, vaginal delivery is considered safe and is best delivered by assisted breech delivery or breech extraction. If the second twin is tranverse, then delivery can be either with ECV, or internal podalic version and breech extraction.

Twin 1 nonvertex

When twin one is breech, current opinion favours CS. This is the case despite a large, multicentre, retrospective study of breech first births that showed no increased risk attributable to vaginal delivery and in the context that one of the main concerns quoted about vaginal delivery in this situation is the risk of locked twins, the incidence of which is very low at 1/645. The Term Breech Trial was a singleton study and the results should not be extrapolated to twins. However, in the light of these concerns, any decision to proceed with vaginal birth should be made at consultant level. When twin one is transverse, CS is needed.

Intertwin delivery interval

The ideal time interval between the delivery of the first and second twin is not agreed. Undue haste with rupture of the membranes before the presenting part of twin two has entered the pelvis can cause problems, while undue delay is not without hazards too. In one report, umbilical cord arterial and venous pH and base excess were shown to deteriorate with increasing twin-to-twin delivery interval. There were no second twins with an umbilical pH less than 7.00 when delivered within 15 minutes of twin 1. If the intertwin delivery interval was greater than 30 minutes, 27% had an umbilical artery pH of less than 7.00. Among those with an intertwin delivery interval of greater than 30 minutes, 73% had evidence of fetal distress that required operative intervention.

Studies have previously suggested that no specific time interval needs to be set, providing that there is continuous electronic fetal heart rate monitoring of twin 2 and that this is reassuring.

ECV versus internal podalic version for transverse twin two

Both techniques are reasonable, but while many investigators report success with an attempt at ECV in the first instance, other authors have reported lower success rates with ECV with increased maternal complication rates compared with proceeding straight to internal podalic version. Nevertheless, given that ECV is less invasive, it is reasonable to consider this in the first place, if the operator is more comfortable with that technique. The experience of the operator is probably the most important factor, and more senior practitioners may choose to go straight to internal manoeuvres.

Higher multiples

Even though the incidence of triplets is rising, most obstetricians have relatively little experience of delivering triplets and even less of delivering them vaginally. Although a study from the Netherlands reported improved outcome for triplets with vaginal delivery, when compared with CS, the unit was particularly experienced at this type of delivery. For most obstetricians, the safer option would almost certainly be CS.

Previous CS

The scarce evidence available suggests that a trial of labour is a safe option in the absence of a contraindication to vaginal birth. Scar dehiscence rates have been reported to be 0–3%. Clearly, vaginal delivery is most suitable when both twins are longitudinal (both cephalic or cephalic/breech). Employing ECV or internal podalic version for the transverse lie is more controversial.

Preterm/very-low-birthweight twins

There seems to be little difference in outcome between vaginal and caesarean delivery in very-low-birthweight gestations and little difference in terms of perinatal outcome, but fetal monitoring of both twins must be accurate and continuous (see below).

Indications for CS

These include:

- conjoined twins
- monoamniotic twins
- placenta praevia
- certain congenital anomalies
- possible interlocking twins.

Intrapartum management of vaginal twin delivery

Management of stage 1

In stage 1:

- admit to delivery suite
- intravenous line
- blood tests – full blood count, group and save serum
- continuous cardiotocograph on a twin monitor
    - fetal heart rate abnormalities twin 1 take fetal blood sample
    - fetal heart rate abnormalities twin 2 perform CS.

If, at any stage, either twin cannot be monitored, then CS may be the only safe option. It is imperative that both twins are monitored and the trace should be scrutinised to ensure that this is the case (i.e. each twin has a distinct rate and both of these are different from the mother's heart rate). Equally, it is crucial to be sure which twin is which recording, as this has, on occasion, been erroneously interpreted and a fetal blood sample performed on twin 1 for a pathological trace of twin 2.

Ultrasound assessment should be performed by an appropriately trained practitioner to determine:

- presentation of each fetus
- liquor volume assessment
- placental site
- viability of each fetus
- estimation of fetal weight if not recently performed.

(Ultrasound can also guide the operator if ECV or internal podalic version is needed for twin 2 – see below.)

The use of epidural analgesia may be justified for possible intrauterine manipulations required for the delivery of the second twin. Inform:

- anaesthetist
- neonatologist
- neonatal unit.

Management of stage 2

Procedure is:

- provide appropriate analgesia
- prepare oxytocin 10 IU in 1litre Hartmann's solution, if not already receiving oxytocin infusion, in case contractions need to be stimulated between delivery of twin 1 and 2
- deliver twin 1 as if singleton
- clamp and cut cord with labelled clamp
- perform abdominal palpation to determine lie
- confirm lie, presentation and fetal heart rate of twin 2 with ultrasound scan if needed
- monitor electronic fetal heart rate continuously
- if transverse lie, perform ECV or internal podalic version (ultrasound can help with this)
- if no contractions within 5–10 minutes commence oxytocin infusion
- when lie longitudinal and presenting part in pelvis, perform amniotomy with contraction and proceed with delivery.

Management of stage 3

At stage 3:

- give Syntometrine 1 ampoule (or Syntocinon 5 IU if Syntometrine contraindicated) with the delivery of the second twin
- deliver the placenta
- consider commencing oxytocin infusion (40 IU oxytocin in 1litre Hartmann's solution), as there is a risk of uterine atony following delivery of multiple gestations.

Internal podalic version

A fetal foot is identified by recognising a heel through intact membranes. The foot is grasped and pulled gently and continuously lower into the birth canal. Keep the membranes intact as long as possible as this facilitates movement. They may break spontaneously; otherwise rupture them as late as possible once the rotation is complete. This procedure is easiest when the transverse lie is with the back superior or posterior. If the back is inferior, or if the limbs are not immediately palpable, ultrasound may help to identify to the operator where they may be found. This will minimise the risk of bringing down a fetal hand. If the foot cannot be safely reached then it may be necessary to proceed to delivery by CS.

CS for twin 2

This is often the consequence of mismanagement of the twin delivery with rupture of membranes of twin 2 before the presenting part is engaged in the pelvis. The other error is to feel the cervix after twin 1 has delivered and think that it has contracted down and delivery is no longer possible. The only reason the cervix is palpable at this stage is because the presenting part remains high. Proceeding as described above will bring the fetal pole down and the cervix will then stretch up over it.

Communication and team working

In the delivery of twins and higher multiples, team working is essential to optimise the outcome for mother and babies. Obstetricians, midwives and neonatologists should be present at the delivery. An anaesthetist should be available on the delivery suite should it become necessary to perform a CS urgently.

Summary

- Vaginal delivery of twins is often straightforward, but can be hazardous and an experienced clinician should be on hand to avoid the common pitfalls.
- Be diligent in fetal monitoring of both twins accurately.
- Do not have undue haste in rupturing the membranes of twin 2, rather wait until the presenting part is in the pelvis and contractions have recommenced.

References and further reading

1 NICE. *Multiple Pregnancy: The Management of Twin and Triplet Pregnancy in the Antenatal Period* 2011 (www.nice.org.uk/guidance/CG129).

2 *RCOG Greentop Guideline No 51. Management of Monochorionic Twin Pregnancy.* London: RCOG 2008.

3 Barrett J, Aztalos E, Wilan A, *et al.* The Twin Birth Study: a multicenter RCT of planned cesarean section (CS) and planned vaginal birth (VB) for twin pregnancies 320 to 386/7 weeks. *Am J Obstet Gynaecol* 2013;208:S4–5.

4 Adam C, Allen AC, Baskett TF. Twin delivery: influence of the presentation and method of delivery on the second twin. *Am J Obstet Gynecol* 1991;165:23–7.

5 Crowther CA. Caesarean delivery for the second twin. *Cochrane Database Syst Rev* 2000;(2):CD000047.

6 Feng TI, Swindle REJ, Huddleston JF. A lack of adverse effect of prolonged delivery interval between twins. *J Matern Fetal Investig* 1995;5:222–5.

7 Fishman A, Grubb DK, Kovacs BW. Vaginal delivery of the nonvertex second twin. *Am J Obstet Gynecol* 1993;168:861–4.

8 Gocke SE, Nageotte MP, Garite T, *et al.* Management of the nonvertex second twin: primary cesarean section, external version, or primary breech extraction. *Am J Obstet Gynecol* 1989;161:111–14.

9 Hogle KL, Hutton EK, McBrien KA, *et al.* Cesarean delivery for twins: A systematic review and meta-analysis. *Am J Obstet Gynecol* 2003;188:220–27.

10 Leung TY, Tam WH, Leung TN, *et al.* Effect of twin to twin delivery interval on umbilical cord blood gas in the second twins. *BJOG* 2002;109:63–7.

11 Miller DA, Mullin P, Hou D, Paul RH. Vaginal birth after cesarean section in twin gestation. *Am J Obstet Gynecol* 1996;175:194–8.

12 Rabinovici J, Barkai G, Richman B, *et al.* Internal podalic version with unruptured membranes for the second twin in transverse lie. *Obstet Gynecol* 1988; 71:4280–300.

13 Rao A, Sairam S, Shehata H. Obstetric complications of twin pregnancies. *Best Pract Res Clin Obstet Gynaecol* 2004;18:557–76.

14 Smith GC, Pell JP, Dobbie R. Birth order, gestational age and risk of delivery related perinatal death in twins: retrospective cohort study. *BMJ* 2002;325:1004.

15 Spinillo A, Stronati M, Ometto A, *et al.* The influence of presentation and method of delivery on neonatal mortality and infant neurodevelopmental outcome in nondiscordant low-birthweight. *Eur J Obstet Gynecol Reprod Biol* 1992;47:189–94.

16 Tchabo JG, Tomai T. Selected intrapartum external cephalic version of the second twin. *Obstet Gynecol* 1992;79:421–3.

17 Wildschut HIJ, Van Roosmalen J, van Leeuwen E. Planned abdominal compared with planned vaginal birth in triplet pregnancies. *Br J Obstet Gynaecol* 1995;102:292–6.

18 NICE. Quality Standard - Multiple pregnancy (QS46) 2013 (http://guidance.nice.org.uk/QS46).

CHAPTER 36

Complex perineal and anal sphincter trauma

Introduction

Perineal trauma resulting from childbirth remains a common problem that is associated with considerable maternal morbidity, and may have a devastating effect on family life and sexual relationships. Following vaginal birth: more than 85% of women sustain perineal trauma, up to two-thirds need suturing and up to 30% sustain obstetric anal sphincter injuries (OASIS).

Many OASIS go unrecognised, and there is considerable under-reporting with incidences quoted as low as 1–2% of vaginal deliveries. Injury increases significantly in the presence of the following risk factors that often occur in combination: birthweight >4 kg; persistent occiptoposterior position; nulliparity; induction of labour; epidural anaesthesia; prolonged second stage >1 hour; shoulder dystocia; midline episiotomy and forceps delivery. Detection rates are increased by increased awareness and training, but 'occult' AS injury (i.e. defects in the AS detected by anal endosonography) from vaginal delivery is common and most commonly due to lack of recognition, with misclassification as a second degree tear.

Definition of perineal trauma

Perineal trauma may occur spontaneously during vaginal birth or as a result of a surgical incision (episiotomy), which is intentionally made to facilitate delivery. It is also possible to have both an episiotomy and a spontaneous tear. The following classification of spontaneous perineal trauma has now been accepted by the Royal College of Obstetricians and Gynaecologists and also internationally by the International Consultation on Incontinence.

- *First degree:* Injury to vaginal or perineal skin only.
- *Second degree:* Injury to perineal muscles but not involving the AS.
- *Third degree:* AS muscles torn.

  Further subdivided into:
  - 3a: <50% thickness of external sphincter torn.
  - 3b: >50% thickness of external sphincter torn.
  - 3c: internal sphincter also torn.
- *Fourth degree*: A third degree tear with disruption of the anal epithelium.

Episiotomy

Episiotomy is a surgical incision of the perineum that increases the diameter of the vulval outlet to facilitate delivery. The mediolateral episiotomy (associated with fewer complications than the midline incision) extends from the midpoint of the posterior fourchette at an angle of 60° from the midline at approximately 8 o'clock to avoid the AS complex. Episiotomy should not be used routinely, but has a place in facilitating delivery in the following situations:

- fetal distress
- to allow access for internal manoeuvres during shoulder dystocia
- to minimise severe perineal trauma during an instrumental delivery (particularly forceps)
- to aid vaginal delivery when the perineum appears thick and inelastic
- when prolonged 'bearing down' may be detrimental to the mother's health (e.g. severe hypertension or cardiac disease).

Assessment of perineal trauma

The perineum must be examined thoroughly following the birth, with good exposure and lighting. The edges of a completely disrupted sphincter retract (following the circular pattern of the external sphincter) and are therefore not visible. Care should be taken to explore any defects or 'spaces' at either side of the anus, as the torn, free end of muscle will be found in their depths (often at 7 o'clock and 4 o'clock, respectively).

The assessment should include a rectal examination to exclude AS injury (Figure 36.1). This is of considerable importance as 'buttonhole' injuries of the rectum (Figure 36.2) can occur in isolation, even with an intact perineum. The AS should be palpated with the index finger in the rectum and the thumb on the perineum, or over the posterior fourchette, while performing a pill-rolling motion. In the absence of an epidural, the woman could be asked to contract her AS to accentuate any AS disruption.

It is essential that, prior to examination or suturing, the procedure is explained to the woman and her partner and consent obtained.

Repair of perineal trauma

1. Excessive uterine bleeding should be managed appropriately prior to commencing the perineal suturing.
2. Ensure that the wound is adequately anaesthetised prior to commencing the repair.
   (a) Local infiltration with 1% lignocaine is adequate for simple trauma, but extensive damage and difficult repairs may need more effective analgesia than the maximum dose of 20 ml will achieve. Always be careful to avoid injecting directly into a vessel.
   (b) Top up an existing epidural or administer regional anaesthesia; this is especially worthwhile for extensive trauma where access is difficult (e.g. high fornices trauma), or where the AS complex is involved.

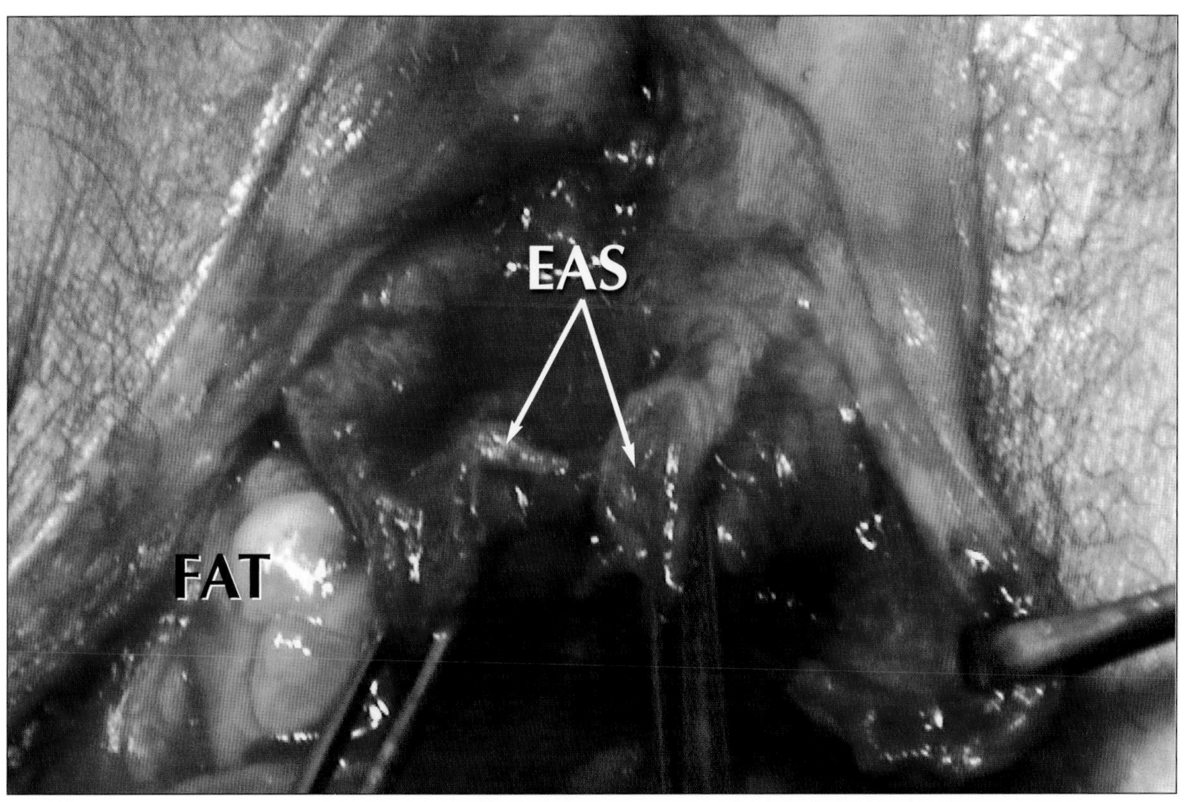

Figure 36.1 Third degree tear (Grade 3b) with the external AS (EAS) grasped by Allis forceps, the ischioanal fat is lateral to the EAS

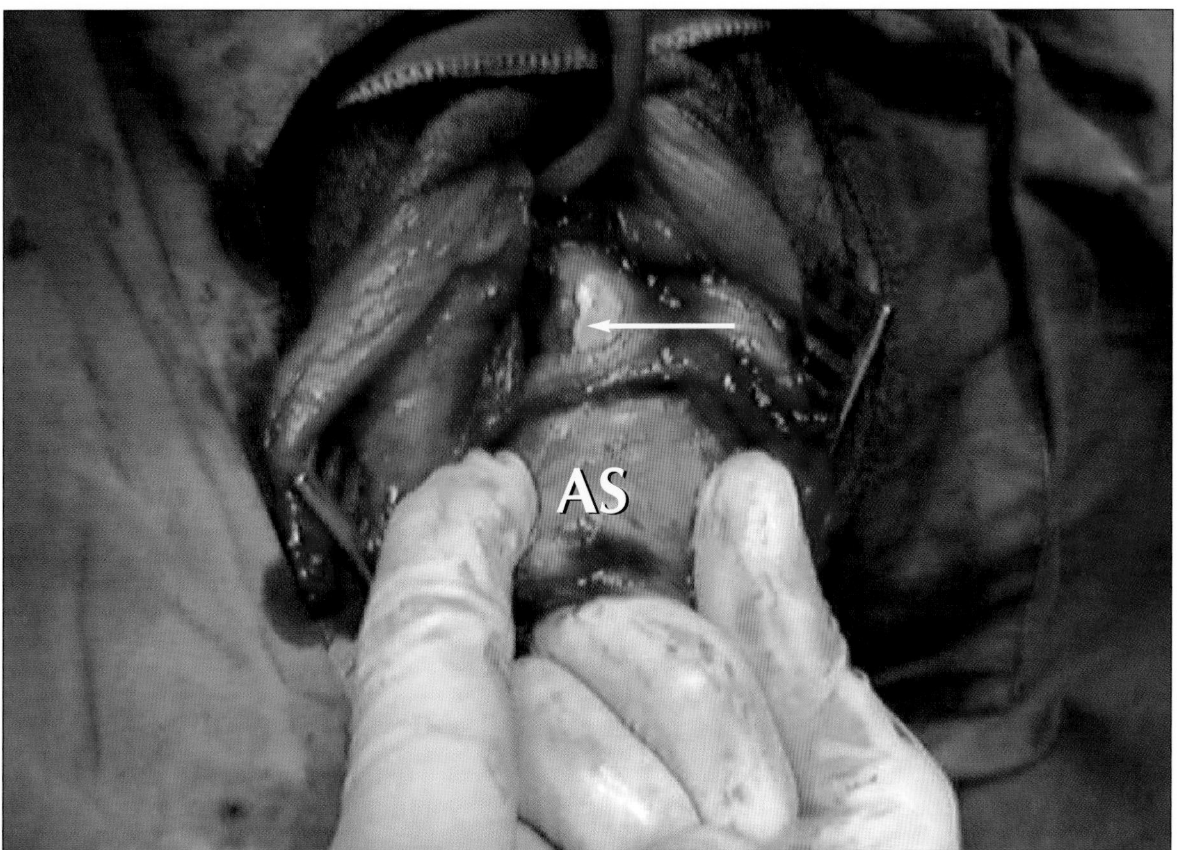

Figure 36.2 Arrow demonstrating a buttonhole tear in the rectum with an intact AS

3. A quick assessment should be made whether the operator is capable of completing the repair, as this facilitates rapid referral upwards rather than struggling for ages before admitting defeat, during which time significant blood loss may have occurred.

Current research suggests that perineal trauma should be repaired using the continuous nonlocking technique to reapproximate all layers in turn (vagina, perineal muscles and then subcuticular to the skin) with absorbable polyglactin 910 material (Vicryl rapide®).

1. Be careful to identify the apex and check the extent of the trauma; whether the trauma is unilateral or bilateral and how deep it goes. The first stitch is inserted 5–10 mm above the apex of vaginal trauma to secure any bleeding points that may not be visible, and then proceed caudally. Any large bleeding vessels should be secured individually rather than 'hiding them', as continued bleeding can occur, concealed from view, to produce an ischiorectal haematoma.
2. Check that the finished repair is anatomically correct and complete haemostasis is achieved. Perform a vaginal examination and check that the vagina is not stitched too tight.
3. A rectal examination should be performed after completing the repair to ensure that suture material has not been accidentally inserted through the rectal mucosa.
4. Check that all swabs, needles and instruments are correct and document this.
5. Following completion of the repair, the extent of the injury sustained and the suture technique and materials used must be documented in the case notes in black ink. It is also useful to include a diagram to illustrate the extent of the trauma.

Repair of third and fourth degree tears

1. A repair should be performed only by a doctor experienced in AS repair, or by a trainee under supervision. If in any doubt about diagnosis, it would be prudent to inform the consultant and await a second opinion.
2. Colorectal surgeons are not needed for straightforward third and fourth degree tears, but the height of the damage when the tear is fourth degree is vital to assess. If the tear extends beyond the anal canal into the rectum *above the levator plate* then a defunctioning colostomy may be indicated and a surgical colleague should be involved (tears of this severity are rare).
3. All third and fourth degree tears should be repaired in the operating theatre, where there is access to good lighting, appropriate equipment and aseptic conditions. The perineal repair pack should contain appropriate instruments (demonstrated in Figures 36.3 and 36.4).
4. General or regional (spinal/epidural) anaesthesia is an important prerequisite, particularly for overlap repair, as the inherent tone of the sphincter muscle can cause the torn muscle ends to retract within the sheath. Muscle relaxation is necessary to retrieve the ends, especially if it is intended to overlap the muscles without tension.

5. The full extent of the injury should be evaluated by a careful vaginal and rectal examination in lithotomy, and graded according to the classification above.

Instruments

- Weitlaner retractor (or Gilpin retractor)
- Tooth forceps (fine and strong)
- Needle holder (small and large)
- Allis forceps (4)
- Artery forceps (4)
- McIndoe scissors
- Stitch cutting scissors
- Sims speculum
  Deep vaginal side wall retractors
- Sponge holding forceps (4)
- Tampon
- Large swabs
- Diathermy

Sutures

- Anal epithelium
  Vicryl 3-0, 26mm round-bodied needle
- Internal anal sphincter
  PDS 3-0, 26mm round-bodied needle
- External anal sphincter
  PDS 3-0, 26mm round-bodied needle
- Perineal muscles
  Vicryl rapide 2-0, 5mm tapercut needle
- Perineal skin
  Vicryl rapide 2-0, 35mm tapercut needle

Figure 36.3 Instruments and sutures used for repair of AS trauma

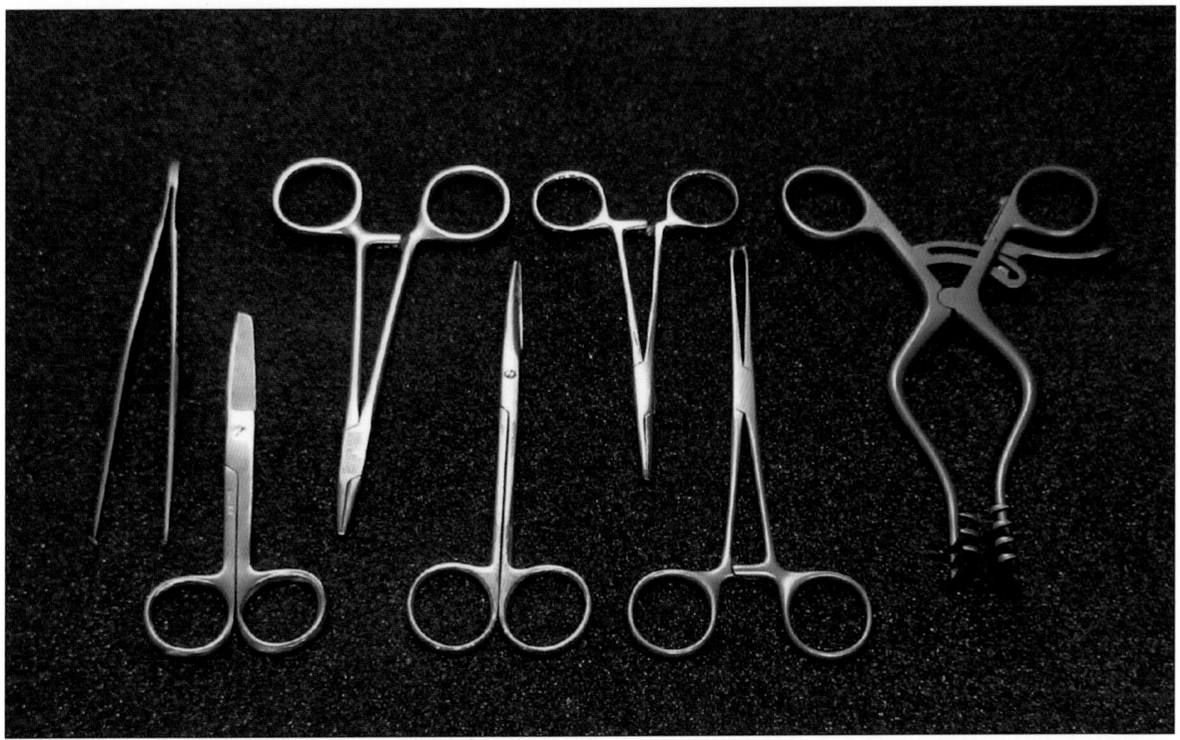

Figure 36.4 Instruments specifically used for repair of AS trauma. From left to right: tooth forceps; stitch cutting scissors; needle holder; McIndoe's scissors; artery forceps; Allis forceps; Weitlaner retractor

Step 1: suturing the anal epithelium

In the presence of a fourth degree tear, the torn anal epithelium is repaired with interrupted polyglactin 3–0 (Vicryl®) sutures with the knots tied in the anal lumen.

Step 2: suturing the AS

Prior to repairing the AS it is often worth securing the apex of the vaginal tear while access to it is facilitated by the sphincter tear, and then leave the suture with its needle protected ready to be completed later.

Where possible, the internal AS (IAS) should be identified and sutured separately from the EAS. The IAS lies between the external sphincter and the anal epithelium. It is paler (raw fish-like) than the striated external sphincter (red meat-like) (Figure 36.5) and the muscle fibres run in a longitudinal fashion rather than the circular external sphincter. A torn internal sphincter should be approximated with interrupted sutures using a fine suture material, such as 3-0 PDS or 2-0 vicryl, which cause less discomfort.

Repair of the EAS should be with either monofilament sutures, such as polydiaxanone (PDS), or braided sutures, such as polyglactin (Vicryl).

Evidence to date indicates that there is no significant difference in short-term outcome with the end-to-end (Figure 36.6) or overlap (Figure 36.7) technique and either can be used.

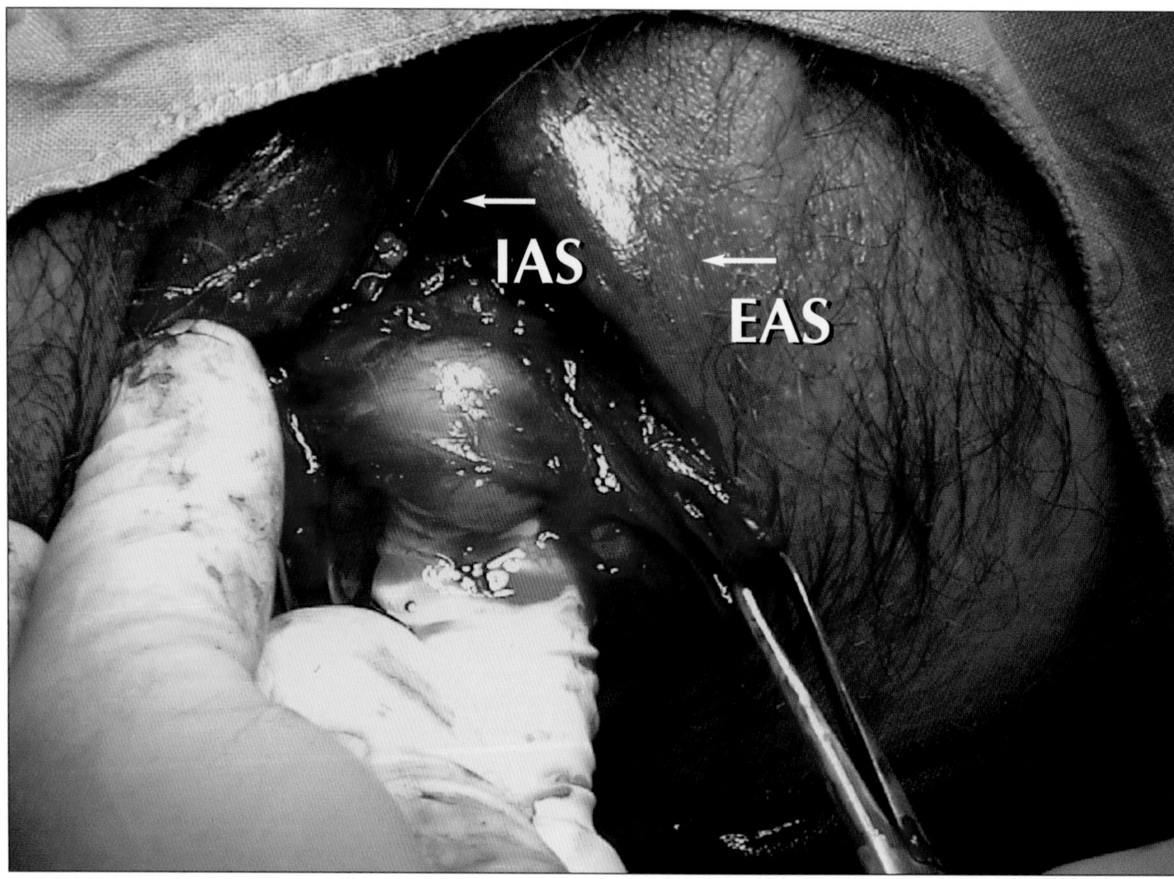

Figure 36.5 Third degree tear (Grade 3b) demonstrating intact IAS and torn ends of the EAS

If less than 50% of the EAS thickness is torn (3a tear), an end-to-end repair should be performed with mattress or figure of eight sutures to approximate the muscle ends. When more than 50% of the sphincter thickness is torn, one can perform an end-to-end repair, but if an overlap repair is going to be performed it necessitates complete division of the EAS if this has not occurred spontaneously.

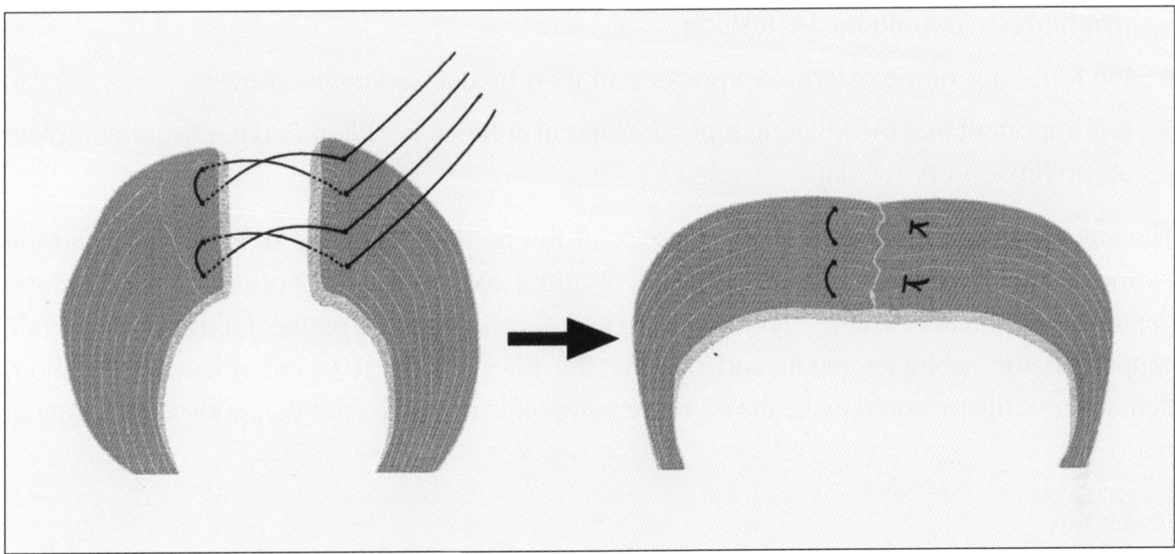

Figure 36.6 Diagramatic representation of end-to-end repair with figure of eight sutures

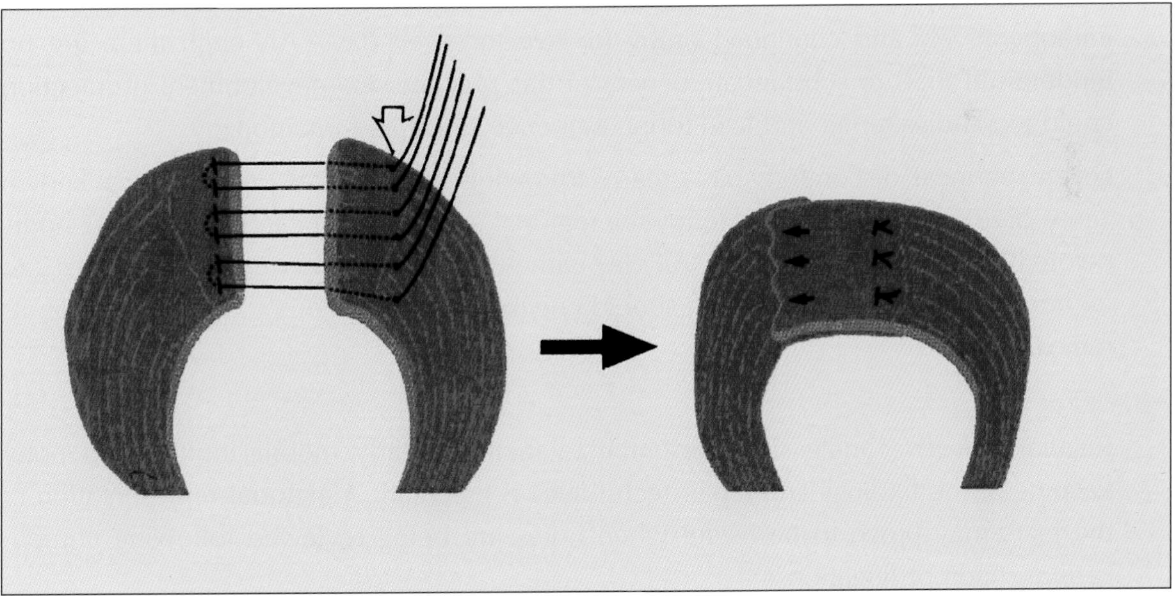

Figure 36.7 Diagramatic representation of overlap repair of EAS

The torn ends of the EAS are identified and grasped with Allis tissue forceps and, whichever technique is used, care should be taken that the ends of the knots are buried beneath the perineal muscles, particularly when using PDS in order to minimise the risk of suture migration necessitating removal at a later date. If an end-to-end repair is being performed, two figure of eight sutures are needed. For an overlap repair, more extensive dissection is needed:

- the muscle may need mobilisation by dissection with a pair of McIndoe scissors separating it from the ischioanal fat laterally (Figure 36.1)
- then the external sphincter should be grasped with Allis forceps and pulled across to overlap in a 'double-breast' fashion
- the torn ends of the external sphincter can then be overlapped as shown
- it is important that the full length of the external sphincter is identified to ensure complete approximation or overlap.

The vaginal skin is then sutured, the muscles of the perineal body are reconstructed and the perineal skin approximated (follow steps 1, 2 and 3 as for repair of episiotomy and second degree tears). Great care should be exercised in reconstructing the perineal muscles to provide support to the sphincter repair and burying the PDS sutures to avoid migration. A short, deficient perineum would make the AS more vulnerable to trauma during a subsequent vaginal delivery.

Procedure

1. As with all perineal repairs, a rectovaginal examination should be performed afterwards, to confirm complete repair and ensure that all tampons or swabs have been removed.
2. Intravenous broad-spectrum antibiotics (e.g. co-amoxiclav) should be commenced intraoperatively and continued orally for five to seven days. Although there are no randomised trials to substantiate benefit of this practice, the development of infection could jeopardise repair and lead to incontinence or fistula formation.
3. Severe perineal discomfort, particularly following instrumental delivery, is a known cause of urinary retention and following regional anaesthesia it can take up to 12 hours before bladder sensation returns. A Foley catheter should be inserted for between 12 to 24 hours and then midwifery staff should check that spontaneous voiding occurs on its removal.

After care

1. Regular, effective analgesia is essential to facilitate early mobilisation. Good note-keeping of the findings and repair techniques is essential. A pictorial representation of the tears may prove to be useful when notes are being reviewed following complications, audit or litigation.
2. As passage of a large bolus of hard stool may disrupt the repair, a stool softener (lactulose 15 ml twice daily) and a bulking agent such as ispaghula husk (Fybogel), one sachet twice daily, should be prescribed for 10–14 days postoperatively. The woman must be made to understand the extent of the tear and advised how to seek help if symptoms of infection or incontinence develop.
3. The woman should be instructed in perineal care and pelvic floor exercises before she goes home and she should be reviewed in the postnatal period.

More focused and intensive training is required to improve recognition of AS trauma. This can be facilitated by establishing hands-on workshops using purpose-built models (Figure 36.8) and fresh animal anal sphincter (www.perineum.net).

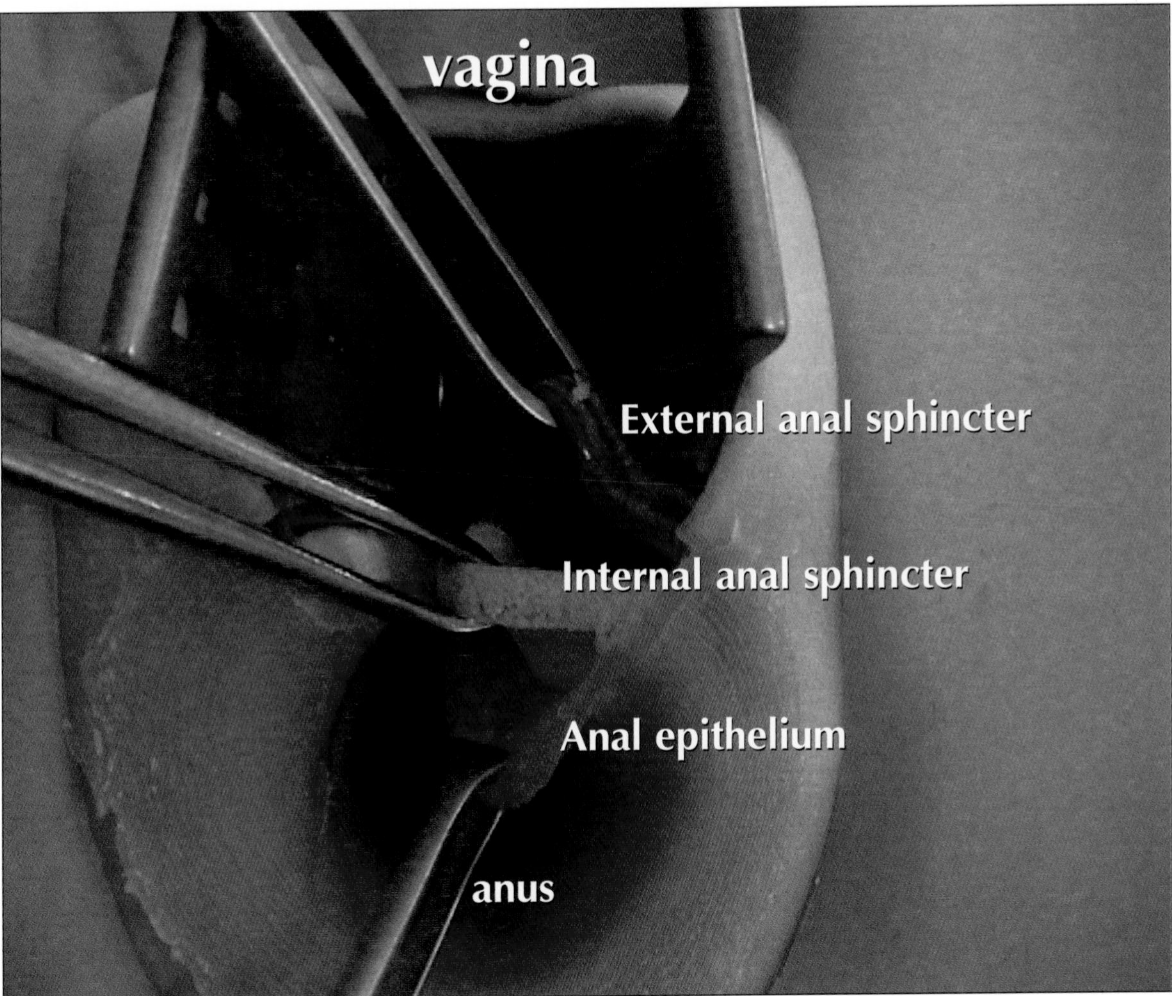

Figure 36.8 Purpose-built teaching model demonstrating AS anatomy (www.perineum.net)

Summary

- Perineal trauma is common following vaginal delivery.
- Clear explanation of the extent of the injury and consent for repair are necessary.
- Practitioner skills should be kept sharp by training.
- Third and fourth degree trauma require senior involvement.
- Meticulous technique during repair and good aftercare is necessary for a good outcome.

Further reading

1 Andrews V, Sultan AH, Thakar R, Jones PW. Occult AS injuries – myth or reality. *Br J Obstet Gynaecol* 2006;113:195–200.

2 Andrews V, Thakar R, Sultan AH, Jones PW. Are mediolateral episiotomies actually mediolateral? *Br J Obstet Gynaecol* 2005;112:1156–8.

3 Carroli G, Belizan J. Episiotomy for vaginal birth. *Cochrane Database Syst Rev* 2004;(1):CD000081.

4 Kettle C, Hills RK, Jones P, *et al.* Continuous versus interrupted perineal repair with standard or rapidly absorbed sutures after spontaneous vaginal birth: a randomised controlled trial. *Lancet* 2002:359;2217–23.

5 Norton C, Christiansen J, Butler U, *et al.* Anal incontinence. In: Abrams P, Cardozo L, Khoury, Wein A (editors). *Incontinence.* 2nd edn. Plymouth: Health Publication 2002; 985–1044.

6 Royal College of Obstetricians and Gynaecologists. *Management of Third and Fourth Degree Perineal Tears.* Guideline No. 29. London: RCOG Press 2007.

7 Sultan AH, Kamm MA, Hudson CN, *et al.* AS disruption during vaginal delivery. *New Engl J Med* 1993;329:1905–11.

8 Sultan AH, Monga AK, Kumar D, Stanton SL. Primary repair of obstetric AS rupture using the overlap technique. *Br J Obstet Gynaecol* 1999;106:318–23.

9 Sultan AH, Thakar R. Lower genital tract and AS trauma. *Best Pract Res Clin Obstet Gynaecol* 2002;16(1):99–116.

10 Thakar R, Sultan AH. Management of obstetric AS injury. *The Obstetrician and Gynaecologist* 2003;5:72–8.

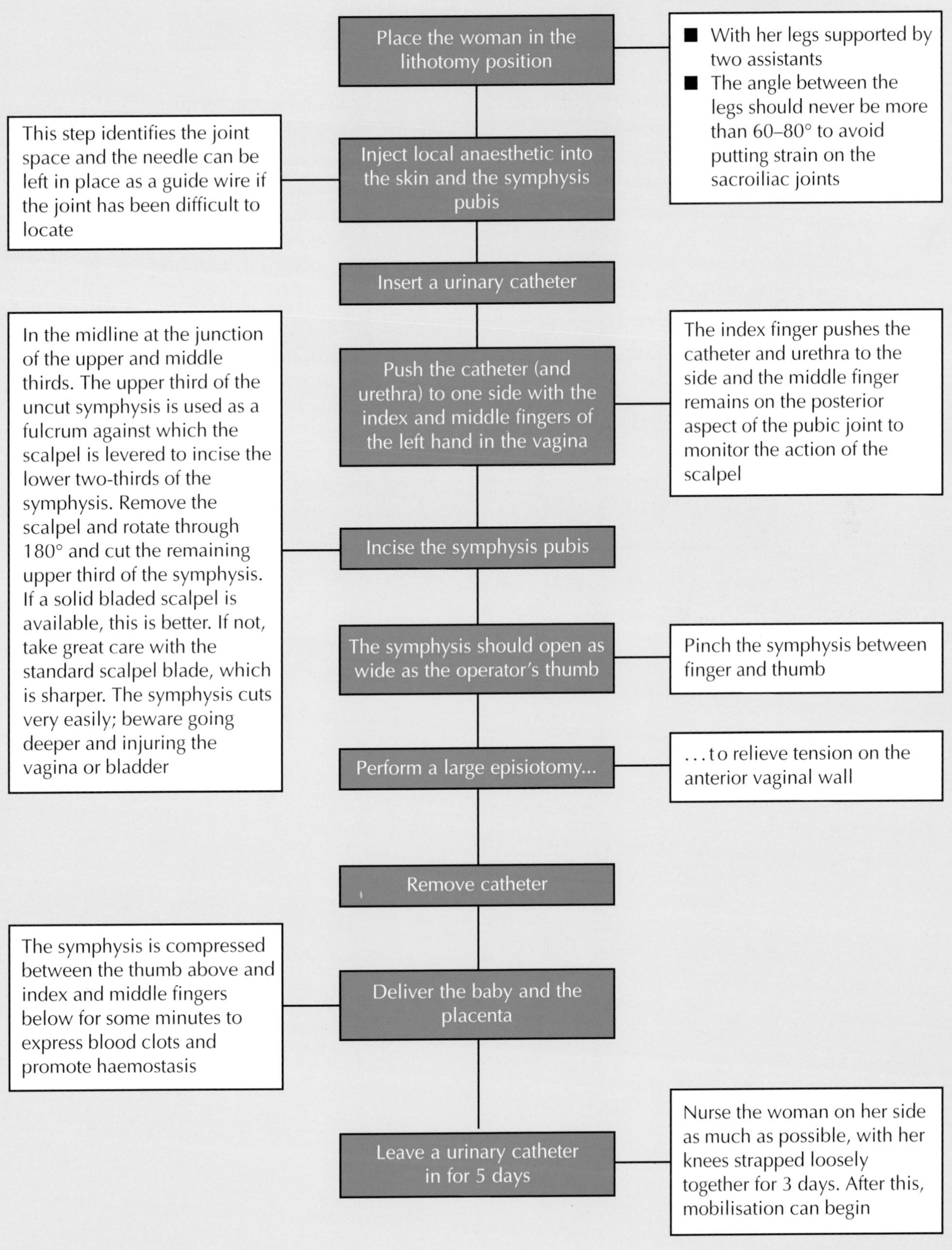
Place the woman in the lithotomy position
■ With her legs supported by two assistants
■ The angle between the legs should never be more than 60–80° to avoid putting strain on the sacroiliac joints
Inject local anaesthetic into the skin and the symphysis pubis
This step identifies the joint space and the needle can be left in place as a guide wire if the joint has been difficult to locate
Insert a urinary catheter
Push the catheter (and urethra) to one side with the index and middle fingers of the left hand in the vagina
The index finger pushes the catheter and urethra to the side and the middle finger remains on the posterior aspect of the pubic joint to monitor the action of the scalpel
Incise the symphysis pubis
In the midline at the junction of the upper and middle thirds. The upper third of the uncut symphysis is used as a fulcrum against which the scalpel is levered to incise the lower two-thirds of the symphysis. Remove the scalpel and rotate through 180° and cut the remaining upper third of the symphysis. If a solid bladed scalpel is available, this is better. If not, take great care with the standard scalpel blade, which is sharper. The symphysis cuts very easily; beware going deeper and injuring the vagina or bladder
The symphysis should open as wide as the operator's thumb
Pinch the symphysis between finger and thumb
Perform a large episiotomy...
...to relieve tension on the anterior vaginal wall
Remove catheter
Deliver the baby and the placenta
The symphysis is compressed between the thumb above and index and middle fingers below for some minutes to express blood clots and promote haemostasis
Leave a urinary catheter in for 5 days
Nurse the woman on her side as much as possible, with her knees strapped loosely together for 3 days. After this, mobilisation can begin

ALGORITHM 37.2 Destructive operations

Destructive operations are useful, although rare procedures in modern obstetric practice

In situations of fetal demise destructive operations should be considered as a first line to assist vaginal delivery rather than using the alternative abdominal approach

Obstetricians can be trained using manikins

Destructive operations can avoid unnecessary abdominal delivery and subsequent risks to the mother

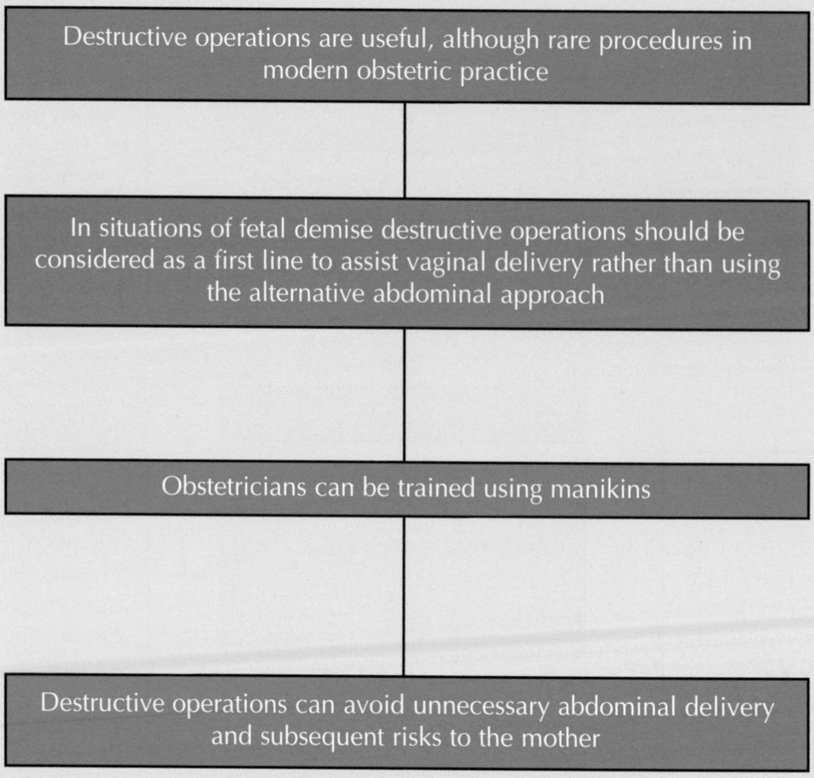

CHAPTER 37

Symphysiotomy and destructive procedures

Objectives

On successfully completing this topic, you will be able to:

- discuss the indications for symphysiotomy
- understand the technique
- understand the role of destructive operations
- understand the procedures involved in destructive operations.

Introduction

Symphysiotomy

Symphysiotomy is a relatively common procedure in the developing world, where it is used in situations of cephalopelvic disproportion when CS is not available. Symphysiotomy leaves no uterine scar and subsequent risk of ruptured uterus in future labours is not increased. Van Roosmalen illustrated the potential morbidity and mortality of caesarean sections carried out in developing country rural hospitals. Mortalities of up to 5% and an incidence of uterine scar rupture in subsequent pregnancies of up to 6.8% have been reported. Symphysiotomy has a low maternal mortality, with three deaths reported in a series of 1752 symphysiotomies. All three deaths were unrelated to the procedure.

Hartfield reviewed the cases of 138 women in whom symphysiotomy had been performed.[1] Early and late complications were few and rarely serious, if recommended guidelines were followed. He also reviewed published series of women followed up, for two years or more, after symphysiotomy and concluded that permanent major orthopaedic disability only occurs in 1–2% of cases.[2]

Pape carried out a prospective review of 27 symphysiotomies performed between 1992 and 1994.[3] Five women had paraurethral tears needing suturing, nine had oedema of the vulva or haematomas tracking from the symphysiotomy. All made a full recovery and severe pelvic pain was not a feature in any woman.

In 2001, the question of legal action against obstetricians in Ireland who carried out symphysiotomies was raised.[4] Verkuyl made the point that many symphysiotomies were performed in Roman Catholic countries because contraception was illegal, even for medical reasons, and women were spared repeated operative deliveries.[5]

Symphysiotomy is a useful technique that is occasionally required in UK practice. One report highlighted four cases where it has been used successfully in the UK.

Björkland published a comprehensive retrospective review of the literature based on papers published between 1900 and 1999; 5000 symphysiotomies and 1200 CS operations were included and the results indicated that symphysiotomy is safe for the mother and life saving for the child.[6] Severe complications are rare.

Destructive procedures

Destructive operations are also relatively common in the developing world in cases of obstructed labour, where absent prenatal care and poor intrapartum care at peripheral hospitals have resulted in fetal demise. Reported incidences range between 0.094% and 0.98% of all deliveries. A destructive procedure is an alternative to abdominal delivery that may carry considerable risk to the mother.

With the use of prophylactic antibiotics and thromboprophylaxis, CS has become safer and there is only a limited role in modern practice for destructive procedures in the developed world.

Symphysiotomy

Indications

- Trapped aftercoming head of breech due to cephalopelvic disproportion.
- Severe cases of shoulder dystocia that do not resolve with routine manoeuvres.
- In cases of cephalopelvic disproportion with a vertex presentation and a living fetus (in the developing world), when at least two-thirds of the fetal head has entered the pelvic brim; note that the use of forceps is contraindicated.
- In cases of cephalopelvic disproportion with a vertex presentation, when CS is declined by the mother.

Technique

1. Place the woman in the lithotomy position, with her legs supported by two assistants. The angle between the legs should never be more than 60–80° to avoid putting a strain on the sacroiliac joints and tearing the urethra and/or bladder.
2. Inject local anaesthetic into the skin and symphysis pubis. This step identifies the joint space and the needle can be left in place as a guide wire if the joint has been difficult to locate.

3. Insert a firm urinary catheter. Apply antiseptic solution suprapubically.
4. Push the catheter (and urethra) aside with the index and middle fingers of the left hand in the vagina. The index finger pushes the catheter and urethra to the woman's right side and the middle finger remains on the posterior aspect of the pubic joint in the midline to monitor the action of the scalpel.
5. Incise the symphysis pubis in the midline, at the junction of the upper and middle thirds. Use the upper third of the uncut symphysis as a fulcrum against which to lever the scalpel to incise the lower two-thirds of the symphysis. Cut down through the cartilage until the pressure of the scalpel blade is felt near the middle finger in the vagina.

Remove the scalpel and rotate it through 180° and the remaining upper third of the symphysis is cut. If a solid-bladed scalpel is available, this is better. If not, take great care with the replaceable standard scalpel blade, which is much sharper. The symphysis is cut through very easily; beware of going deeper and injuring the vagina or bladder or the operator's finger.

6. Once the incision is made, pinch it between finger and thumb and the symphysis should open as wide as the operator's thumb.
7. After this separation of the cartilage, remove the catheter to decrease urethral trauma.
8. Use a large episiotomy to relieve tension on the anterior vaginal wall.
9. After delivery of the baby and placenta, compress the symphysis between the thumb above and index and middle fingers below for some minutes, to express blood clots and promote haemostasis.
10. Re-catheterise and leave a urinary catheter in place for 5 days.
11. Apply elastic strapping across the front of the pelvis, from one iliac crest to the other, to stabilise the symphysis and reduce pain. The woman needs to be nursed on her side as much as possible, with her knees strapped loosely together for 3 days. After this, mobilisation can begin.

Destructive procedures

Destructive operations may be required where the fetus is dead and where a vaginal delivery is being attempted. It may be the appropriate method for delivery to minimise maternal risk, or it may be the only route by which the mother wishes to be delivered. Whenever a destructive procedure is being considered, it must only be performed with the mother's consent.

1 Initially, basic resuscitation must be carried out quickly, to avoid undue delay in delivering a dead fetus.

2 Catheterise.

3 Since urinary and genital tract infections are common, antibiotic prophylaxis should be used.

4 General or regional anaesthesia combined with sedation is ideal for the procedure.
5 The cervix should be fully dilated, although destructive surgery may be performed, by an experienced operator, when the cervix is dilated by 7 cm or more.
6 The genital tract and rectum must be carefully examined after the procedure.
7 A catheter should be left in place for at least 48 hours.

The three most common destructive procedures are:

- craniotomy
- perforation of the aftercoming head
- decapitation.

Craniotomy

Indications

Craniotomy is indicated for the delivery of a dead fetus in situations of cephalopelvic disproportion and hydrocephalus.

Method

1 The fetal head should be no more than three-fifths above the pelvic brim, except in cases of hydrocephalus.
2 Ask an assistant to steady the head from above the pubic symphysis.
3 Perforate the skull via the fontanelle, using a Simpson's perforator, with the instrument at right angles to the surface of the skull to minimise the risk of slipping. If a fontanelle cannot be palpated, the perforator should be inserted through the bone.
4 Push the blades as far as their shoulders and separate first in one direction and then in another direction, at right angles to the first.
5 Evacuate the brain and deliver the fetal head by a pull on the skull using vulsellum forceps and countertraction. It may be gentler to attach the vulsellum to a 1 kg weight (for example, a 1 litre bag of fluid) using a bandage. This will allow a slower and possibly more 'normal' delivery.
6 If the fetus is very large, reduction in the size of the shoulder girdle by cleidotomy may be required after delivery of the head. This can be achieved by cutting the clavicle at its midpoint using either scissors or scalpel.

Aftercoming head of the breech

The aftercoming head of a breech can be managed similarly by craniotomy, with perforation of the head through the base of the skull, beginning at the nape of the neck, aiming towards the vertex. If the head is deflexed, perforation of the occiput may be achieved in the region of the posterior fontanelle.

Where there is hydrocephalus and accompanying spina bifida, cerebrospinal fluid can either be withdrawn by exposing the spinal canal and passing a catheter into the canal and up into the cranium. The hydrocephalic head can be decompressed transabdominally under ultrasound control using a spinal needle.

Decapitation

Indications

Decapitation is indicated in cases of neglected, obstructed labour with shoulder presentation and a dead fetus. In an already emotionally fraught situation, the prospect of explaining the options to parents may be distressing for all. Nevertheless, in terms of minimising harm to the mother, a very early delivery remains optimal.

Method

1 If the fetus is small and the neck can easily be felt, it may be severed with stout scissors. However, for the larger fetus, and especially where the neck is not easily accessible, the Blond-Heidler decapitation tool is the safest instrument.

2 If possible, an arm is brought down and firmly pulled on by an assistant, which brings the neck lower to make it more accessible.

3 Thread the saw around the fetal neck and keep the handles attached to the ends of the saw close together. This prevents injury to the vagina and the neck is soon severed after a few firm strokes.

4 Deliver the trunk by traction on the arm, with the operator's hand protecting the vagina from laceration by spicules of bone.

5 Deliver the aftercoming head by grasping the stump with a heavy vulsellum and performing the MSV manoeuvre. It is easy to restore anatomical continuity with skin sutures to the neck.

6 The baby should be wrapped respectfully before showing to the parents.

Background

In resource-poor areas of the world, CS is often unavailable or carries significant risks. Potential problems include haemorrhage from uterine extension, generalised peritonitis and the risk of rupture of the scar in a subsequent pregnancy. Gogoi showed a much lower morbidity and mortality with craniotomy than with CS in a group of 158 women who were grossly infected.[15] Peritonitis occurred in 66% of women after CS and was nil after destructive operations, the maternal mortality in the CS group was 13/107 (12%) compared with 1/37 (2.7%) in the craniotomy group.

Marsden *et al.* described a series of four cases where the Blond-Heidler saw was used in the case of a dead baby in a transverse lie.[16] They had no complications and suggested that, in such situations, this method of delivery is more appropriate than CS, when a classic incision may often be required, which significantly increases the risk to the mother.

Reports from the developing world of maternal morbidity and mortality following destructive procedures illustrate that most problems encountered can be attributed to obstructed labour, which often necessitates their performance in the first place. It is often not easy to differentiate the complications of one from the other. Ekwempu reported on a series of 112 patients treated by embryotomy between 1974 and 1975.[17] The only complications that he could attribute to the destructive procedure were seven cases of soft-tissue (mainly vaginal and perineal) laceration. The procedures themselves have been shown to be simple with little morbidity.

There are several reports from the developing world of postoperative vesicovaginal fistula. These are often attributed to pressure necrosis in obstructed labour. However, it has been suggested that they could be secondary to the use of sharp instruments or from bony spicules exposed during the procedure. This can be avoided by regular training using dummies and appropriate case selection.

Summary

- Symphysiotomy is a useful procedure that can be used in certain emergency situations.
- It must only be performed by trained clinicians.
- Prompt decision is required to avoid fetal morbidity.
- Intrapartum and postpartum management are important to minimise maternal morbidity.
- Destructive procedures have a limited, but useful, place in the delivery of a dead fetus in the context of an obstructed labour.

References and further reading

Symphysiotomy

1 Hartfield VJ. Subcutaneous symphysiotomy: time for a reappraisal? *Aust N Z J Obstet Gynaecol* 1973;13:147–52.

2 Hartfield VJ. Late effects of symphysiotomy. *Trop Doct* 1975;5:76–8.

3 Pape GL. 27 Symphysiotomies. *Trop Doct* 1999;29:248–9.

4 Payne G. Ireland orders enquiry into barbaric obstetric practices. *BMJ* 2001;322:1200.

5 Verkuly DAA. Symphysiotomies are an important option in the developed world. *BMJ* 2001:323:809.

6 Björklund K. Minimally invasive surgery for obstructed labour: a review of symphysiotomy during the twentieth century (including 5000 cases). *BJOG* 2002;109:236–48.

7 Goodwin TM, Banks E, Millar L, Phelan J. Catastrophic shoulder dystocia and emergency symphysiotomy. *Am J Obstet Gynecol* 1997;177:463–4.

8 Menticoglou SM. Symphysiotomy for the trapped aftercoming parts of the breech: a review of the literature and a plea for its use. *Aust N Z J Obstet Gynaecol* 1990;30:1–9.

9 Spencer JA. Symphysiotomy for vaginal breech delivery: two case reports. *Br J Obstet Gynaecol* 1987;94:716–18.
10 Van Roosmalen J. Safe motherhood: cesarean section or symphysiotomy? *Am J Obstet Gynecol* 1990;163:1–4.
11 Van Roosmalen J. Symphysiotomy as an alternative to caesarean section. *Int J Gynecol Obstet* 1987;25:451–8.
12 World Health Organization, UNFPA, UNICEG, World Bank. *Managing Complications in Pregnancy and Childbirth. A guide for midwives and doctors.* Geneva: WHO 2001.
13 Wykes CB, Johnston TA, Paterson-Brown S, Johanson R. Symphysiotomy: a lifesaving procedure. *BJOG* 2003;110:219–21.
14 Greisen G. Three-year follow-up of eight patients delivered by symphysiotomy. *Int J Gynecol Obstet* 1985;23:203–5.

Destructive procedures

15 Gogoi MP. Maternal mortality from caesarean section in infected cases. *J Obstet Gynaecol Br Empire* 1971;78:373–6.
16 Marsden DE, Chang AS, Shin KS. Decapitation and vaginal delivery for impacted transverse lie in late labour: reports of 4 cases. *Aust N Z J Obstet Gynaecol* 1982;22:46–9.
17 Ekwempu CC. Embryotomy versus caesarean section. *Trop Doct* 1978;8:195–7.
18 Amo-Mensah S, Elkins T, Ghosh T, *et al.* Obstetric destructive procedures. *Int J Gynaecol Obstet* 1996;54:167–8.
19 Arora M, Rajaram P, Oumachigui A, Parveena P. Destructive operations in modern obstetrics in a developing country at tertiary level. *Br J Obstet Gynaecol* 1993;100:967–8.
20 Giwa-Osaigie O, Azzan B. Destructive operations. In: Studd J (ed.). *Progress in Obstetrics and Gynaecology Volume 6.* Edinburgh: Churchill Livingstone 1987;211–21.
21 Gupta U, Chitra R. Destructive operations still have a place in developing countries. *Int J Gynaecol Obstet* 1993;44:15–19.
22 Hudson CN. Obstructed labour and its sequelae. In: Lawson JB, Harrison KA, Berström S (eds). *Maternity Care in Developing Countries.* London: RCOG Press 2001;201–14.
23 Konje JC, Obisesan KA, Ladipo OA. Obstructed labour in Ibadan. *Int J Gynaecol Obstet* 1992;39:17–21.
24 Lawson J. Embryotomy for obstructed labour. *Trop Doct* 1974;4:188–91.
25 Maharaj D, Moodley J. Symphysiotomy and fetal destructive operations. *Best Pract Res Clin Obstet Gynaecol* 2002;16:117–31.
26 Mitra KN, John MP. Decapitation by thread saw. *J Obstet Gynaecol India* 1950;1:65–73.
27 Moir C, Myerscough P. *Munro Kerr's Operative Obstetrics.* 8th edn. London: Ballière Tindall and Cassell 1971;191:715.

ALGORITHM 38.1 Failed intubation

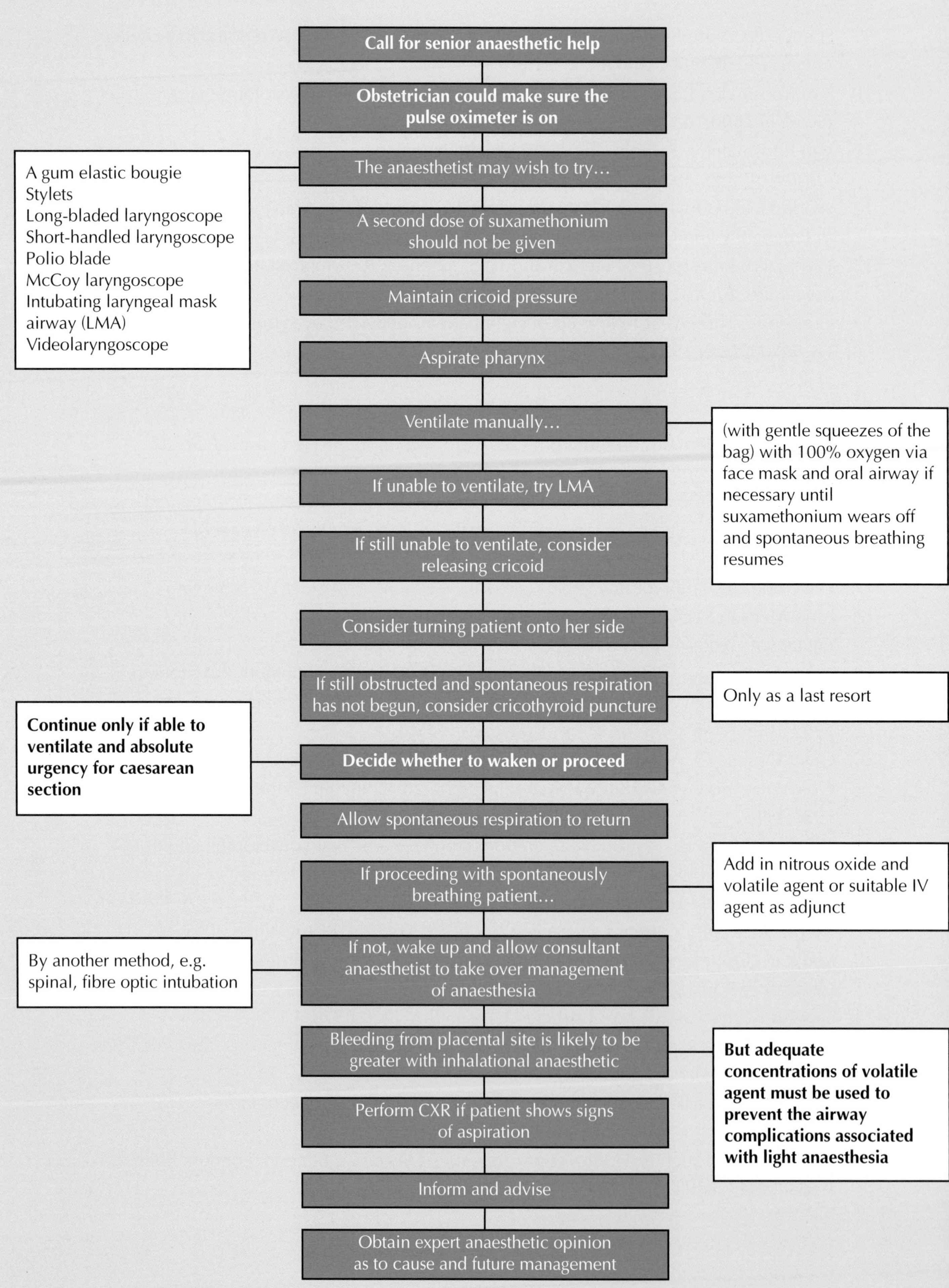

CHAPTER 38

Anaesthetic complications in obstetrics

Objectives

On successfully completing this topic, you will be able to:

- appreciate the risks posed to the pregnant women by anaesthetic drugs and techniques
- understand anaesthetic emergency problems affecting the pregnant woman.

Introduction and incidence

The proportion of women dying from complications of anaesthetics has declined markedly over the last 20 years. Deaths from airway-related problems have declined over the last ten years of Confidential Enquiry reports, but failure to ventilate the lungs is still a major concern. The risk of death from an obstetric general anaesthetic has been estimated at one in 20 000. In 2011, a large series of obstetric patients in Canada undergoing general anaesthesia confirmed that difficult intubation still occurs in 3.3% (range 1.3–16.3%) and failed intubation in one in 250 patients. The events occur almost exclusively in emergency cases and are associated with the most urgent of cases, inexperienced staff and failure to follow standard practice. Box 38.1 indicated the problems highlighted by the Confidential Enquiry reports. However improved assessment and anticipation of airway problems has led to series with fewer failed intubations.

Difficult intubations – prevention better than cure

Preparation for an intubation

1. Appropriately trained staff – anaesthetist and assistant.
2. Correct equipment checked and available to hand, including airway adjuncts for difficult airways.
3. Position of the woman optimised.

Box 38.1 Specific anaesthetic problems highlighted by Confidential Enquiry reports

Airway management especially in the obese:

- the danger of unrecognised oesophageal intubation and the importance of always using a capnograph to confirm tracheal placement
- inadequate use of intraoperative and postoperative monitoring
- the need for the proper checking of anaesthetic machines
- the need for staff to possess advanced life-support skills
- the need for staff to able to manage bronchospasm and anaphylaxis
- the contribution of isolated sites in delaying the provision of senior help and of blood products.

Other ways in which anaesthesia in some way contributed to maternal deaths include:

- issues of timely and effective communication and consultation
- failures to appreciate the severity of maternal illness
- inadequate usage of invasive monitoring
- substandard care in women who have sepsis, pre-eclampsia and haemorrhage.

Using the 25° 'back up'/ramp position makes it easier to intubate obese pregnant women and should always be used. It may be useful to employ a specific pillow that allows the obese women to be placed in the best position.

Management of failed intubation or ventilation is a core skill that should be rehearsed and practised regularly. Obstetricians should be involved in this training and need to understand how they can help. There should be an appreciation of the implications for decision-making regarding delivery. The drill for managing this situation must be clear and simple and the one offered here is based on the Difficult Airway Society guidelines.[1]

In Algorithm 38.1 for failed intubation, points which particularly apply to the obstetrician are highlighted in bold print.

It is important that the anaesthetist does not get fixated with *intubating* the trachea, since in these circumstances the goal remains *oxygenating* the lungs by whatever technique available. Case reports show that the Proseal® laryngeal mask airway has been commonly used since 2003 to obtain enough successful airway control to allow ventilation. This is a type of laryngeal mask airway that has a drainage channel, which allows early identification and drainage of regurgitated gastric contents.

A major patient management matter at the time of failed intubation is a joint assessment between obstetrician and anaesthetist about the degree of urgency of the operation and the degree of need to continue with general anaesthesia for the operation.

Other complications

Premature extubation

This problem is associated with aspiration of gastric contents and hypoxia. The woman must be fully awake, able to breathe adequately and to protect her airway, before the endotracheal tube is removed. The anaesthetist will decide whether to extubate in the left lateral or sitting position. It is advisable to leave all monitoring attached until the extubation has been successfully achieved. Potential hazards include laryngospasm on extubation. There should be early recourse to rapid reintubation rather than struggling to break the spasm. Drugs, equipment and personnel should be instantly available should this occur while still in the operating theatre.

Outside the operating theatre, mortality reports have highlighted respiratory deaths related to incorrect administration and supervision of patients receiving *opioids,* and respiratory failure from the delayed effects of *neuromuscular blockade.*

Awareness

The situation where the patient is not completely unconscious during an operation, when they were expected to be, has been particularly associated with obstetric general anaesthesia. Incidence is 0.26%; approximately double that of the nonobstetric population. Delay in intubation after a minimal dose of anaesthetic induction agent but with a muscle relaxant may lead to patient recall of the intubation. Conscious awareness with pain at the time of incision and delivery is associated with the practice of not giving opiate until after the delivery, using less than 65% nitrous oxide in oxygen and not giving adequate inhaled anaesthetic, either because of concern about the relaxant effects on the uterus with subsequent increased blood loss or because of human error.

Patient reports of awareness must always be taken seriously and reported to the anaesthetist for investigation and management, with the aim of avoiding the patient developing a post-traumatic stress disorder.

Regional blocks (epidural and spinal anaesthesia and analgesia)

The spinal cord leaves the skull within the dural tube, bathed in CSF and terminates in adults at approximately the first or second lumbar interspace.

The dural tube and CSF continue down into the upper part of the sacrum.

The epidural space is a 'potential' space that extends from the base of the skull to the sacral hiatus and contains nerve roots, fat and blood vessels. As the nerves cross the epidural space, they make connections with the sympathetic trunk before exiting laterally through the transverse foramina.

Inside the vertebral column, the dura mater is the anatomical boundary that divides the two kinds of blocks (Figure 38.1). Injection of drugs inside the dura mater is variously called

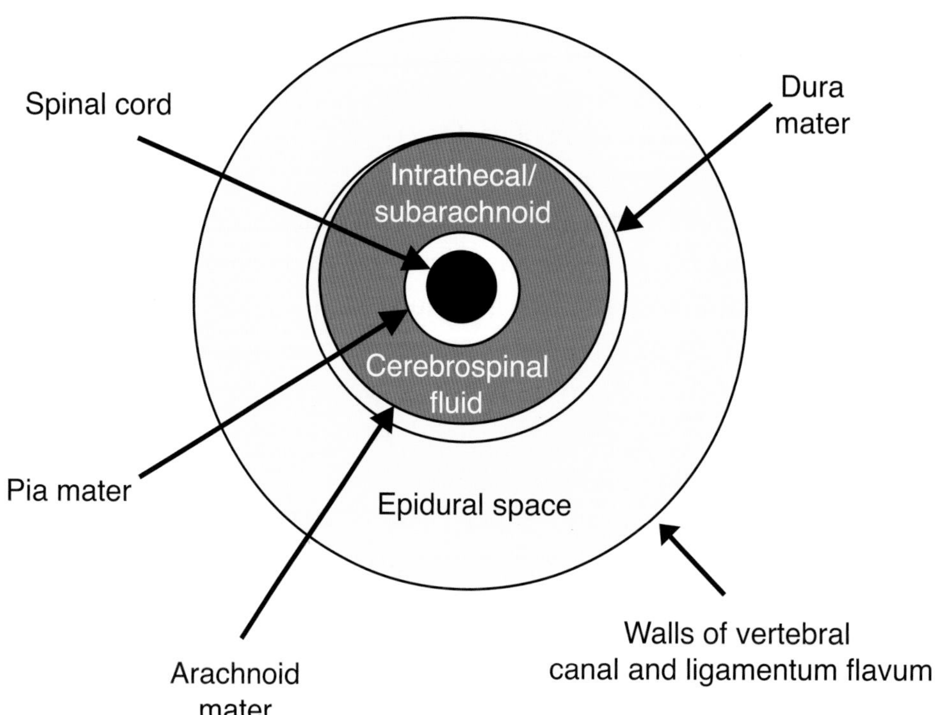

Figure 38.1 Cross-sectional diagram of spinal cord and spaces within vertebral canal

a 'spinal', 'subarachnoid' or an 'intrathecal' block. Injection of drugs outside the dura is called an epidural or extradural block.

Pain relief for labour requires sensory blockade T10–L1 (first stage) and S2, S3, S4 (second stage). Anaesthesia for CS requires motor and sensory blockade from T4 to S5.

A 'nerve' block refers to block of a single nerve e.g. pudendal whereas a 'regional' block refers to groups of nerves, as happens with a spinal or epidural injection.

During a spinal block, a small volume of concentrated drug(s) spreads rapidly within the CSF. The effect of the local anaesthetic is to block transmission of impulses along the nerves. The onset of the block is rapid because the nerves have no covering.

When local anaesthetic drugs are injected into the epidural space, the volumes of drugs required are very much greater as the volume of the space is larger. In addition the onset of effect is slower because the nerves, as they cross the epidural space, have acquired a covering of dura.

Characteristics of spinal and epidural anaesthetics

Epidural anaesthesia is conventionally used for analgesia for labour and vaginal delivery or anaesthesia for operative delivery. Conventionally, an 'epidural' refers to the placement of an epidural catheter in the epidural space so that drug can be repeatedly added to the space, or continuously infused to give analgesia for the duration of labour, irrespective of how long that is.

Epidurals are not reliably influenced by gravity or positioning and always involve larger volumes of drugs.

Occasionally, a spinal injection may be used as a method of analgesia for labour, for speed and then an epidural catheter is used for the rest of the labour. This is called combined spinal/epidural analgesia (CSE).

Spinal anaesthesia is usually used for obstetric surgery. A 'spinal' refers to a one-off injection into the intrathecal space. The effect lasts for about 2 hours, which is long enough to carry out a CS. Intrathecal infusions are not conventionally used in obstetric practice.

Epidural incremental top-ups were used more routinely for anaesthesia for CS in the past, and may still be indicated in certain patients where a slow onset of anaesthesia is desirable e.g. severe cardiac disease. For emergency caesarean sections or other operative procedures, such as retained placenta, existing epidurals can be topped up or spinal anaesthesia given. A combined spinal/epidural anaesthetic may be used for operative obstetrics, especially when the operation is expected to be prolonged, or the intention is to use the epidural catheter to deliver postoperative analgesia.

A single-shot spinal injection is expected to result in a dense, complete (no 'missed' – unanaesthetised – dermatome segments) block of rapid onset. Its downside is that it causes marked vasodilatation (owing to the effect of local anaesthetic on the thoracic and lumbar sympathetic nerves) with consequent hypotension. This predictable problem is managed with vasopressors such as phenylephrine or ephedrine. The height of the block is somewhat unpredictable and uncontrollable, but is a function of dose and patient positioning.

The desired height of block for CS is to the T2–T4 level (sternal angle of Louis). If the block is not high enough, the patient will feel pain from traction of the peritoneum that is supplied by the lesser splanchnic nerve; but above this level a spinal is described as 'high' and can cause cardiovascular and respiratory problems (see below).

When using 'heavy', i.e. hyperbaric (heavier than CSF) local anaesthetic as is used for spinals, the position of the woman affects where the local anaesthetic lies and can be used to influence the height of the block. A block that has not reached the required height can be brought higher by placing the woman in the head-down position. Similarly, a high spinal can be stopped from going higher by placing the woman head up. Gravity can be made to influence the height of the block for up to 20 minutes after the injection. Pillows under the shoulders and head virtually eliminate the spread of a spinal dose beyond the thoracic level.

Dosage calculation

Bupivacaine 0.5% contains 5 mg/ml; 10 ml therefore contains 50 mg. The calculation is as follows: 0.5% means 0.5 g in 100 ml (equivalent to 500 mg in 100 ml; divide by 100 to get 5 mg in 1 ml).

Levobupivacaine is the L-isomer of bupivacaine. It has similar properties, but is thought to have lower cardiovascular toxicity when injected accidentally intravenously. There has been a move towards using this preparation but bupivacaine is also used. The dose is the same for both isomers.

Ropivacaine is a newer local anaesthetic and also has improved safety with regard to cardiovascular complications.

Typical doses – note there is a five- to tenfold difference in volume

Spinal

A typical dose for a spinal block for CS (in the absence of pre-existing epidural) would be 2.2–2.7 ml of 0.5% hyperbaric ('heavy') bupivacaine. The hyperbaric preparation has more predictable spread and duration of action. Opioids (for example, fentanyl) are commonly added to improve the quality of the block and to provide postoperative analgesia (for example, morphine or diamorphine).

Epidural

A typical dose of bupivacaine immediately after siting an epidural for analgesia during the first stage of labour would be 6–10 ml of 0.25% or 0.125% levobupivacaine.

Subsequent management could be by top-ups, an infusion or a patient-controlled analgesia device; opioids (for example, fentanyl) are commonly added to the bupivacaine to improve the quality of the block and to minimise the local anaesthetic dose.

Complications

Complications can be grouped as follows:

- drugs used: local anaesthetics and opioids are used for both spinal and epidural techniques but local anaesthetic alone is still used occasionally; opioids are used in combination but not alone; vasopressors may have unwanted effects
- technique.

Complications of regional anaesthesia

Hypotension – defined as a greater than 20% fall in systolic blood pressure. This occurs because of block of sympathetic nerves providing tone to the blood vessels; nausea may be a heralding sign. It may occur with both epidural and spinal blocks, but more likely with a spinal since the spread of drug is faster. Hypotension may often be associated with fetal heart rate changes.

Management of hypotension

- ABC approach.
- Ensure good left lateral tilt or displacing the uterus to the left.
- Fluid loading: increase rate of crystalloid infusion; caution in pre-eclampsia.
- Vasopressor: may require bolus of vasopressor, e.g. ephedrine, in 3 mg increments intravenously approximately every 2 minutes until blood pressure recovers; caution in pre-eclampsia.

Prophylactic vasopressor infusions, i.e. started before the onset of the block, e. g. phenylephrine are commonly used with spinal anaesthesia to prevent hypotension.

Motor block

Dense motor blockade is required for operations under regional anaesthesia, but is unwanted with epidural analgesia for labour. Motor block depends on the dose of local anaesthetic used and the duration of labour.

Labour is more likely to result in instrumental delivery if there is a significant motor block as there is a loss of power to the lower limbs and abdominal muscles, which hampers the mother's attempts to push. This is an important practical point when needing maternal cooperation for an instrumental delivery.

Pressure sores are a potential complication of epidural analgesia as there is a prolonged period of relative immobility and loss of sensation to discomfort while sitting in a pool of amniotic fluid. Women should be encouraged to continue to change position throughout their labour.

Full bladder unnoticed by patient – the unopposed parasympathetic block predisposes to urinary retention, so routine monitoring is needed and catheterisation may be required.

Both motor and sensory block during labour can be minimised by reducing the dose of local anaesthetic, at the price of complete analgesia or by supplementing local anaesthetic with opioids.

Serious immediate complications

Local anaesthetic toxicity and high or total spinal can cause cardiac arrest.

Toxic effects of local anaesthetics

The maximum recommended dose of bupivacaine is 2 mg/kg nonpregnant weight in any 4 hour period. The dose for lignocaine without adrenaline is 3 mg/kg and 5–7 mg/kg with adrenaline.

Toxicity can occur from any route of injection. It is dependent on absorption and therefore is more likely from an area of high vascularity or following direct inadvertent intravascular injection. It is very unlikely to occur with spinal anaesthesia since only tiny doses of drug are used, but can occur if an epidural catheter is sited into, or migrates into, a vein.

It can also occur with the correct site of injection but an inadvertent overdose.

Toxicity is related to the membrane stabilising properties of these drugs that interfere with transmission of nerve impulses, and affects mainly the brain and heart.

Symptoms change with increasing plasma levels:

- low dose (affecting the nervous system): tingling or numbness of tongue and perioral area; dizziness; tinnitus; twitching; anxiety; confusion; convulsions and respiratory arrest
- high dose: cardiovascular depression (can be cardiac arrest) and arrhythmias; most likely rhythms are ventricular tachycardia (VT) and ventricular fibrillation (VF).

Management of local anaesthetic toxicity

Immediate:

- stop administration of local anaesthetics
- call for senior help: anaesthetic; intensive care; obstetric; paediatric
- ABC approach as for any resuscitation in a pregnant woman
- treat hypotension with IV fluids and vasopressor titrated against BP
- if in cardiac arrest, use adrenaline as dictated by the cardiac arrest protocol
- increased amounts of adrenaline may be required as there will be a profound vasodilatation.

Treat peri-arrest arrhythmias:

- local anaesthetic-induced VT and VF are often resistant to electrical defibrillation
- amiodarone 300 mg is the anti-arrhythmic drug of choice
- prolonged CPR may be required

Give antidote to local anaesthetic:

- intralipid 20% 1.5 ml/kg 100 ml over 5 minutes
- start an infusion at 0.25 ml/kg/min, followed by repeat initial bolus doses twice more at 5 minute intervals then increase infusion rate to 0.5 ml/kg/min until stable
- in most labour wards this should be stored in an emergency box in the fridge

Seizures:

- control seizures with diazepam 5–10 mg intravenously
- if this fails to quickly control fits, make sure anaesthetist present, as thiopental with intubation is required.

Check fetal heart and consider timing and method of delivery. Deliver the baby as a matter of urgency if mother's condition demands.

High spinal block

A high spinal block is a local anaesthetic block involving the spinal nerves above the level of T2. It may occur due to excessive (unpredictable) spread of an intrathecal injection of local anaesthetic (typically 2–3 ml of 0.5% bupivacaine). It may also occur following unintentional intrathecal injection of an epidural dose of local anaesthetic into the CSF via a wrongly placed catheter or via migration of the catheter from the epidural space through the dura into the CSF. Large volume epidural top-ups for CS may produce a similar picture. It is essential for an anaesthetist to aspirate an epidural catheter prior to top-up to look for blood or CSF in the catheter. A test dose to check for misplacement of a catheter should always be performed.

If there is bradycardia, hypotension, tingling or weakness in the hands or complaint of difficulty in breathing or talking, suspect a high spinal block. Check the level of sharp sensation. If there is reduced sensation at the level of the sternal notch, then this is a high spinal block.

Symptoms depend upon the height of the block:

- T1–T4: bradycardia due to block of sympathetic cardiac nerves; severe hypotension due to effect of bradycardia superimposed on the effect of vasodilatation; patient may have difficulty coughing or taking a deep breath
- C6–C8: hand paraesthesia and weakness, breathing is likely to be impaired; patient anxious, distressed and whispers
- C3–C5: diaphragmatic paralysis, with definite respiratory compromise.

Total spinal block

Intracranial spread can also occur. It produces loss of consciousness owing to the direct action of local anaesthesia on the brain. This is referred to as a 'total spinal'.

Hypotension with bradycardia occurs from the vasodilation caused by blockade of the sympathetic nervous system (T1–L2) and is exaggerated by the drug effects on the vasomotor centres in the brainstem. Hypoxia and respiratory arrest can occur because of phrenic nerve involvement and medullary depression.

Management of high and total spinal block

This should include the following:

- turn off epidural infusion, if present
- call for help, cardiac arrest team, resident anaesthetist and obstetrician and resuscitation equipment with defibrillator
- ABC principles of resuscitation of any pregnant woman.

In addition, if not yet unconscious:

- the patient may complain of difficulty in breathing because of intercostal or diaphragmatic muscle paralysis; it is not always necessary to intubate a woman who says that she has difficulty breathing; in the first instance, give high-flow oxygen, but, if her ability to breathe deteriorates, she will need to be anaesthetised and intubated to assist ventilation until the effect of the local anaesthetic block wears off.
- if the patient is already apnoeic, assist ventilation with facemask or LMA and self-inflating bag until anaesthetist arrives to protect the airway by intubation
- treat hypotension with intravenous fluids and vasopressor – if severe hypotension, adrenaline may be titrated to response
- treat bradycardia with atropine 0.6 mg intravenously

- check fetal heart and consider timing and method of delivery
- consider and exclude other causes of decreased consciousness, e.g. hypoglycaemia, epilepsy, opioid drugs, intracranial lesion
- record events and document.

Complications of opioids

These include:

- pruritus
- urinary retention
- late respiratory depression in absence of overdose, especially with long-acting opioids.

Respiratory depression should be treated by ventilatory assistance and the use of naloxone in 0.1 mg increments intravenously, titrated against response. Any woman who has had long-acting spinal or epidural opioids must be closely monitored for late-respiratory depression. Naloxone is also effective against opioid-induced pruritus.

Complications of vasopressors

Phenylephedrine is used to treat spinal-induced hypotension and can cause profound maternal bradycardia and reduced cardiac output.

Complications of technique

According to the NAP3 study of UK central neural blockade (2009) approximately 140 000 epidurals are performed each year in obstetric patients.[2] The incidence of permanent harm after obstetric central neural blockade was estimated at one in 80 000 judged pessimistically and one in 320 000 judged optimistically. Complications due to technique include the following:

- failure: complete, missed segment, unilateral block
- headache
- backache
- neurological damage
- migration of catheter causing relative intrathecal overdose
- infection.

Failure of block

Failure is unlikely with a spinal block, but when it occurs the block may need to be repeated. An epidural block can fail to provide adequate analgesia if the catheter is not correctly in the epidural space. Even if it is in the epidural space, analgesia can be inadequate as a result of a unilateral block or 'missed segment' or if the block has not spread high enough. The segment that most commonly fails to be blocked is the L1 nerve root (groin).

The remedies for unilateral or unblocked segments are to reposition the patient and to give further local anaesthetic and/or opiates or to re-site the epidural.

An epidural that is persistently providing inadequate analgesia is unlikely to provide adequate anaesthesia if topped up for CS and will need to be resited.

Headache

A puncture of the dura can cause a postdural puncture headache. The likelihood of headache is related to the size of the needle that punctured the dura and how many times it was punctured. During an epidural, there is no intention to puncture the dura, but this can occur accidentally. The incidence is 1% but may be higher among staff in training. An epidural needle (Tuohy 16G or 18G) is larger than a spinal needle (24G or 25G). The incidence of headache following dural puncture with a Tuohy needle is 70%.

Postdural puncture headache can occur following a spinal but it is less common due to the smaller needles used. The incidence is 1/150 using a needle with an atraumatic noncutting tip.

A low-pressure headache occurs secondary to the loss of CSF and traction on the meninges, which in turn causes traction on intracranial structures. A typical postdural puncture headache is frontal and or occipital and is worse in the upright position. It can come on immediately or be delayed, commonly by 24–48 hours, but may be longer. It should never need treatment with opiates as adequate relief can be achieved by lying down. Requirement for opiates should raise suspicion of some other serious and urgent intracranial pathology.

Management

- The anaesthetic team should always be informed.
- The definitive treatment is an epidural blood patch (approximately 20 ml of the woman's own blood injected under aseptic conditions into the epidural space). This may need to be repeated.
- Conservative measures may be taken initially: simple analgesics, encourage oral fluids, consider intravenous fluids, encourage caffeine intake but, if the headache is severe when standing, consider a blood patch early.
- Consider the differential diagnoses, which can include:
  - migraine
  - meningitis
  - cerebral venous sinus thrombosis
  - subarachnoid haemorrhage
  - subdural haematoma.

If any doubt exists, early access to neuroimaging and neurology opinion is necessary.

Backache

There is no evidence for an increase in long-term backache in those who have had regional blocks. Local temporary discomfort is reported at the area of needle entry.

Treat with simple analgesics and nonsteroidal anti-inflammatory drugs if no contraindication. Consider referral to a physiotherapist for ultrasound therapy.

Severe backache after delivery is highly abnormal. The differential diagnosis in a woman who has received a regional blockage would include epidural abscess or haematoma causing compression symptoms. It may also be caused by acute lumbar disc prolapse. Symptoms and signs suggestive of cord compression include motor and sensory deficit and bowel/bladder dysfunction. The patient should be investigated urgently with an MRI scan to look for surgically treatable pathology and the anaesthetic team will need to consult with a neurologist, spinal surgeon or a neurosurgeon. Urgent spinal cord or nerve root decompression may be required to avoid permanent neurological deficit.

Neurological damage

Peripheral neurological symptoms and signs in the postpartum period may be due to regional techniques or nerve compression injuries during labour and delivery.

Neuropraxia

Neuropraxia occurs due to the piercing of a nerve with a needle (intraneural injection). Damage of short duration occurs in 1 in 3000 obstetric blocks and permanent damage in about 1 in 15 000. A report of pain at the time of injection would be suggestive of neuropraxia (the injection should not have proceeded if pain was reported at the time). Peripheral nerve injury may be complicated because the fetal head may apply pressure directly on the nerves or their nutrient vessels. Obstetric neuropraxia or palsy occurs in one in 2000 deliveries. Electrophysiological studies and referral to a neurologist are indicated.

Infection (epidural abscess, meningitis or discitis)

These are serious neurological conditions and are extremely rare. Abscess formation complicates around 0.2–3.7 per 100 000 obstetric epidurals, while bacterial meningitis occurs after spinal, or combined spinal and epidural, in fewer than 1.5 per 10 000 patients. They have potentially devastating complications. Signs and symptoms include severe backache, neurological deficit including bowel/bladder dysfunction and unexplained fever. Central nervous system infection may cause bizarre behaviour and altered conscious level. Suspicion should lead to immediate investigation: CT scan or MRI and neurological consultation. Check the patient's temperature, send blood samples for white cell count and blood cultures and treat as a septic patient. Seek neurological advice immediately.

A study of 1.37 million women estimated the risk of epidural haematoma at one in 167 000. The features are similar to those of epidural abscess, but without the septic features.

Effects of complications on the fetus

Maternal compromise, such as hypoxia and cardiovascular instability, causes compromise to the fetus. Opioids may cross the placenta and the paediatrician should be informed that maternal opioids have been given. This is most likely to be a problem when opioids have been given to attentuate the response to intubation in a pre-eclamptic patient receiving a general anaesthetic. Respiratory support for the neonate may be required.

Summary

- The anaesthetist, midwife and obstetrician should work together on the labour ward and their shared care of women requires close cooperation and good communication. This is never more important than in high-risk obstetrics, obstetric emergencies and anaesthetic complications.
- Multidisciplinary input in all such situations is vital to optimise management.

References and further reading

1 Difficult Airway Society. *Guidelines.* London: Association of Anaesthetistics of Great Britain and Ireland (www.das.uk.com/guidelines/downloads.html).

2 Royal College of Anaesthetists. NAP3: Report and findings of the 3rd National Audit Project of the Royal College of Anaesthetists 2009.

3 Centre for Maternal and Child Enquiries (CMACE). Saving Mothers' Lives: reviewing maternal deaths to make motherhood safer: 2006–08. The Eighth Report on Confidential Enquiries into Maternal Deaths in the United Kingdom. *Br J Obstet Gynaecol* 2011;118(Suppl. 1):1–203.

4 AAGBI Safety guideline: *Suspected Anaphylactic Reactions Associated with Anaesthesia version 4.* 2009.

SECTION 7

Triage and transfer

CHAPTER 39

Triage

Objectives

On successfully completing this topic, you will be able to:

- understand the systematic approach advocated for prioritisation when casualties exceed resources available
- understand why prioritisation is essential in emergency situations including obstetrics.

Introduction

The word 'triage' is derived form the French *trier*, to sort or to sift as through a sieve. The word was originally used to describe the process of selecting coffee beans. Triage was first described in modern times by Baron Dominique Jean Larrey, who was Napoleon's Surgeon Marshal. He introduced a system of sorting casualties presenting to field dressing stations to ensure that soldiers with only minor wounds could be returned quickly to the battlefield with minimum treatment. In more recent times, triage has become a daily management tool within civilian emergency departments.

The aim of triage in civilian practice, wherever it is carried out, is not only to deliver the right patient to the right place at the right time so that they receive the optimum treatment but also to treat the most urgent ahead of the less urgent. Triage principles should be applied whenever the number of patients exceeds the skilled help immediately available.

Triage can be applied to acute medical and obstetric workloads. It can take place formally, as in the management of major incidents, or as a routine approach to our day-to-day practice in resuscitation rooms or on delivery suites. Triage must reflect the changing state of the patient and is therefore a dynamic, rather than a static, process; *regular reassessment of priorities across patients is vital.*

The endpoint of the triage process is the allocation of a priority. This priority is then used in conjunction with other factors to determine optimum care. Most triage systems have four categories of patients. There has to be a method of assessment to determine the category (Figure 39.1).

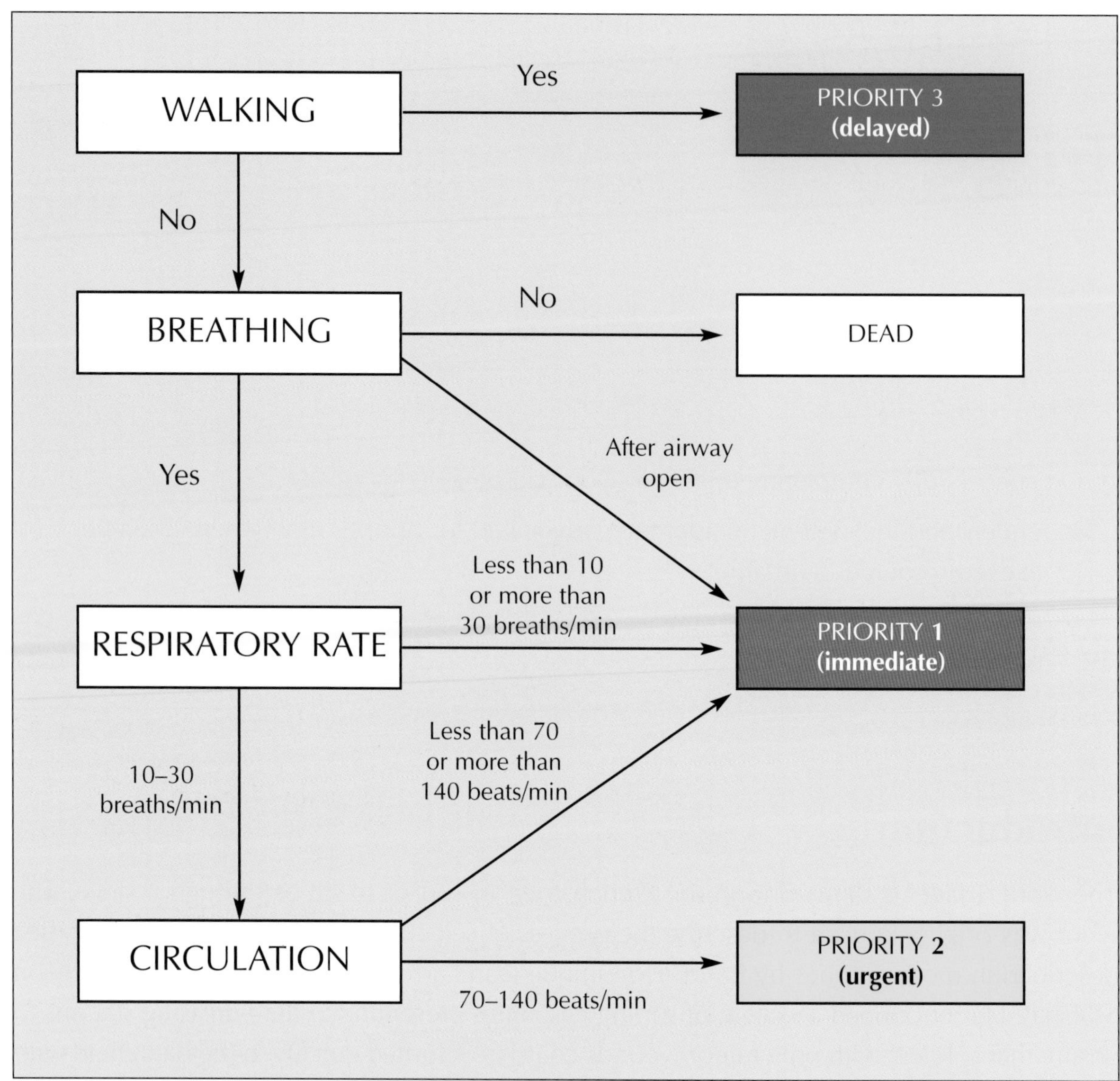

Figure 39.1 The triage sieve (reproduced with kind permission from the Advanced Life Support Group)

The triage priorities given in Table 39.1 are used in major incidents and reflect the need for clinical intervention, not the severity of injury. For example, a shocked patient bleeding from a simple scalp wound may need urgent intervention (priority red) but the injury itself may be relatively minor. By prioritising such a patient in a high category, a simple manoeuvre (application of pressure dressing) may save the casualty's life. Similarly, a patient with a large burn to the extremities clearly has a severe, possibly life-threatening anatomical injury, certainly worse than the patient with the scalp laceration. However, their prognosis may not be altered by receiving care within the first few hours rather than minutes.

If the 'P' system is in use during a major incident then the use of the fourth category is very much a decision for the senior personnel involved. The decision must be based on an overall assessment of the situation: it must take into account both the patient load and the resources

Table 39.1 Major incident triage categories (reproduced with permission from the Advanced Life Support Group)

Category	Description	Colour	Priority	Treatment
Immediate	Require immediate life-saving treatment	Red	P1	T1
Urgent	Require treatment within 6 hours	Yellow	P2	T2
Delayed	Less serious, require treatment but not within a set time	Green	P3	T3
Expectant	Cannot survive, even with treatment. Degree of treatment required is such that, in the circumstances, their treatment would seriously compromise treatment provision for others	Blue		T4
Dead	Dead	White	Dead	Dead

available. If the category is used, patients must be only considered to be within the category after assessment by senior medical personnel.

In the third-trimester pregnant woman, assessment of the fetus would immediately follow assessment of the mother.

Assessment of the pregnant woman

The principles of obstetric triage are the same, involving the ability to identify immediately life-threatening conditions and to deal with them in the correct order. The priority category is determined by the identification of problems that are likely to kill and the order in which they are likely to kill: the ABCs. In the pregnant woman, triage category is determined firstly by threats to maternal life and then presence of threats to the fetus, consider with reference to Figure 39.1:

- think ABC
- assess before treating but treat each problem before moving on
- assess mobility then assess ABC
- is the patient walking?
- if so, the patient has a patent airway, is breathing and has sufficient circulating blood volume to allow locomotion.

Move on:

- is the patient talking?
- if so, the airway is open, the patient is breathing and there is sufficient circulating blood volume to allow oxygenation of the brain.

Move on:

- is the patient breathing but unconscious?
- if so, they have a potentially urgent airway problem
- is the patient not breathing?
- open the airway
- is the patient still not breathing?
- probably dead, especially in the trauma scenario
- if the patient is breathing, check their respiratory rate
- if the respiratory rate is normal, check the circulation and the capillary refill
- assess fetal wellbeing and viability.

Scenario 1

You are the on-call SpR for obstetrics. You are on the labour ward reviewing a CTG when you hear a horn blaring, followed by a loud crash and then splintering noises. A lorry transporting an MRI scanner has crashed into the building, demolishing a wall. You run towards the affected room to find student midwife A covered in debris, walking out in a dazed way bleeding from a scalp wound. As you enter the labour room, you find that the lorry has gone through the window, the driver is still in his cab, which has stoved inwards and the windscreen has shattered. He is grasping the steering wheel and breathing very rapidly. He was not wearing a seat belt.

Mrs. B is on the bed in established labour, her legs are in lithotomy as the SHO was about to perform a ventouse delivery for prolonged second stage. The CTG machine is still running: the fetal heart appears to be normal. Mrs B is panting and saying she needs to push. The SHO is on the floor groaning, with a large piece of masonry on his pelvis. Midwife C is lying on top of Mrs B, motionless, with an obvious injury to the back of her head.

Mr B appears unscathed but grabs you on entry telling you that you must immediately deliver his baby.

Order of priority

Midwife C may have an airway problem; she may be unconscious or dead. Quickly assess her airway, breathing and the presence of circulation. If she is not breathing, after checking her airway is not obstructed, there is nothing further that can be done.

The *lorry driver* has a breathing problem, there is likely to be a chest injury, which will need early assessment. He may be trapped in the cab and may also have a circulatory problem secondary to fractured long bones. He must have early attention.

The *SHO* is groaning and therefore does not have an airway or breathing problem. He is likely to have a significant circulatory problem.

Student midwife A has a circulation problem. Her confusion may be secondary to cerebral hypoxia/hypovolaemia, or due to concussion from a blow to the head.

Mrs B appears not to have an airway or breathing problem, the midwife has shielded her from injury although her fall onto Mrs B's abdomen may cause some trauma. There is no immediate urgency to deliver the baby.

Mr B does not require any immediate medical attention.

Scenario 2

You are the SpR arriving for your shift at 0800 hours on a Sunday morning on the labour ward. The midwife in charge tells you it has been a very busy night. The previous team has recently gone to theatre with a patient who had an anterior placenta praevia and was bleeding heavily; the consultant is with them. She goes through the labour ward board with you (Table 39.2). Just as you finish the report, the support worker comes in with an urgent message from the midwife in room 7, who is unable to hear the fetal heart. The buzzer then goes off in room 1 where the midwife has recently given her patient intravenous penicillin, she is complaining of itching and is now very breathless:

Table 39.2 Triage in a labour ward

Room	Parity	VE	Epidural	Syntocinon	Comments
1	1+0	7.30 5 cm	No	No	Group B *Streptococcus* carrier
2	5+1	6.30 del.	No	No	Retained placenta: cord snapped, PPH 600 ml, continues to trickle
3	0+0	5.00 4 cm	Yes	Yes	38/40, induced for marked oedema and protein ++++, poor urine output, BP 160/95
4	2+0				Term + 14 for induction
5	0+0	7.30 9 cm	Yes	No	CTG late decelerations FBS pH 7.21 at 7.30
6	2+1	6.00 fully	No	No	
7	1+0		No	No	34 weeks c/o decreased FM and abdo pain, previous SB at 38 weeks

Order of priority

- *Room 1* has a breathing problem that could become an airway problem, as she may be having an anaphylactic reaction and needs urgent attention.
- *Room 3* could be developing a breathing and airway problem; her blood pressure is inadequately controlled, she needs early review.
- *Room 2* has a circulation problem, ensure intravenous access and crossmatched; she will need to go to theatre for a manual removal of placenta as soon as possible.

- *Room 7* may have a circulatory problem as she has probably had an abruption. She will need intravenous access, crossmatch and clotting studies.
- *Room 5* has a fetal concern; the CTG should be reviewed and a decision made if further fetal blood sampling is necessary.
- *Room 6* should have delivered and will need review if there is delay in the second stage.
- *Room 4* is not a problem and induction should be deferred until there are sufficient staff to safely care for her.

As there are several major problems requiring attention, it will be necessary to divide the resources available; if there is an anaesthetist and an SHO also coming on duty they could be sent to rooms 1 and 3. Theatre should be made aware that there are other problems so that a speedy turnaround is possible and the consultant can be freed to help as soon as the bleeding is under control.

Summary

- Triage is the key component whenever the number of casualties/patients to treat exceeds the available resources.
- More details on the process of triage are outside the scope of this manual, but are covered in the MOET course and other ALSG training courses, such as Hospital MIMMS.

Further reading

1 Advanced Life Support Group. Carley S, Mackway Jones K (editors) *Major Incident Medical Management and Support: The Practical Approach,* 3rd edn. Oxford: Blackwell Publishing 2012.
2 Advanced Life Support Group. Carley S, Mackway Jones K (eds). *Major Incident Medical Management and Support: The Practical Approach in the Hospital.* Oxford: Blackwell Publishing 2005.
3 Manchester Triage Group. *Emergency Triage,* 2nd edn. Oxford: Blackwell Publishing 2005.

CHAPTER 40

Transfer

Objectives

On successfully completing this topic, you will be able to:

- appreciate an overview of the principles of the safe transfer or retrieval of critically ill patients
- understand the systematic 'ACCEPT' approach for managing such patients.

Introduction

The aim of a safe transfer policy is to ensure that maternal and neonatal care is streamlined and of the best standard. Transfer may be necessary for maternal or fetal reasons (specialised neonatal care, or the availability of neonatal unit cots). Maternal transfer may be for an obstetric problem such as pre-eclampsia, or for a problem not directly related to the pregnancy.

To achieve successful transfer or retrieval, the right patient has to be taken at the right time, by the right people, to the right place by the right form of transport and receive the right care throughout. The added complexity in obstetrics of dealing with 'two patients' demands a highly systematic approach, that incorporates a high level of planning and preparation, prior to the patient being moved. One such approach is the ACCEPT method developed by the ALSG.

The ACCEPT systematic approach to patient transfer

A Assessment
C Control
C Communication
E Evaluation
P Preparation and packaging
T Transportation

Following ACCEPT ensures that assessments and procedures are carried out in the right order. This method also correctly emphasises the preparation that is required before the patient is transported. The component parts of ACCEPT are outlined below.

Assessment

The clinician involved in the transportation may have been involved in the care given up to that point. However, the transporter may have been brought in especially for that purpose and will have no prior knowledge of the patient's clinical history. It is the responsibility of the person undertaking the transfer to become fully appraised.

Control

Once assessment is complete, the transport organiser needs to take control of the situation. This requires the following:

- identifying the clinical team leader
- identifying the tasks to be carried out
- allocating tasks to individuals or teams.

The lines of responsibility must be established urgently. In theory, ultimate responsibility is held jointly by the referring consultant clinician, the receiving consultant clinician and the transfer personnel at different stages of the transfer process. There should always be a named person with overall responsibility for organising the transfer.

Communication

Moving ill patients from one place to another requires cooperation and the involvement of several people. Therefore, key personnel need to be informed when transportation is being considered.

People who need to know about a transfer

The neonatologists in referring and receiving units should communicate directly. Who to involve in maternal care depends on whether the mother is being transferred for an obstetric problem or a nonobstetric problem. If the transfer is for a nonobstetric problem, obstetric care also has to be continued in the receiving unit and has to be transferred to an obstetric team at the receiving unit. Consider informing the following people, as appropriate:

- the consultant responsible for current maternal clinical care
- the consultant responsible for current obstetric care if different from above
- the consultant responsible for current neonatal clinical care
- special care unit staff in transferring hospital
- the consultant responsible for the transfer of the patient (if different from above)
- the consultant responsible for maternal intensive care if appropriate
- the senior midwife in transferring unit
- the patient's relatives

- the consultant responsible for maternal clinical care in the receiving unit
- the consultant responsible for obstetric care in the receiving unit
- the consultant responsible for neonatal care in the receiving unit
- special care unit staff in the receiving unit
- the senior midwife in the receiving unit
- ambulance control or special transportation controls (when appropriate).

If anaesthetists have been involved in the obstetric care, they should communicate directly.

Communication may take a long time to complete if one person does it all. It is therefore advisable to share the tasks between corresponding teams, taking into account expertise and the local policies. Team-to-team communication is imperative. In all cases it is important that information is passed on clearly and unambiguously. This is particularly the case when talking to people over the telephone. It is useful to plan what to say before telephoning and to use the systematic summary shown below.

Key elements in any communication

- Who are you?
- What is needed (from the listener)?
- What are the relevant patient's details?
- What is the problem?
- What has been carried out to address the problem?
- What happened?
- Summary.

The second question can be repeated at the end to help summarise the situation. The response to all these questions should be documented in the patient's notes. The person in overall charge can then assimilate this information, so that a proper evaluation of the patient's requirements for transportation can be made.

Evaluation

The dual aims of evaluation are to assess whether transfer is appropriate for the patient and, if so, what clinical urgency the patient has. While evaluation is a dynamic process which starts from first contact with the patient, it is only when the first phase of ACCEPT (that is, A, C, C) has been completed that enough information will have been gathered.

Is transfer appropriate for this patient?

Transfer may be indicated for maternal reasons or in the fetal interest. The need for neonatal intensive care may be reason for in utero transfer. If the woman herself requires transfer for delivery, it is important that her condition is stabilised. Severe pre-eclampsia/eclampsia might be one reason for transfer either in the maternal or fetal interest.

The risks involved in transfer must be balanced against the risks of staying and the benefits of care that can only be given by the receiving unit.

Clinical urgency?

With the indication for transfer clear, the urgency must be evaluated. The degree of urgency for transfer, and the severity of illness, may be used to rank the woman's and fetus's transfer needs. This hierarchy also helps determine both the personnel required and the mode of transport.

Transfer categories:

- intensive
- time-critical
- ill – unstable
- ill and stable
- unwell
- well.

Preparation and packaging

Preparation and packaging both have the aim of ensuring that the patient transport proceeds with the minimum change in the level of care provided and with no deterioration in the patient's condition. The first stage (preparation) involves completion of patient stabilisation and preparation of transfer team personnel and equipment. The second stage (packaging) involves the final measures that need to be taken to ensure the security and safety of the patient during the transportation itself.

Patient preparation

To ensure best outcome for mother and fetus and to reduce the likelihood of complications during the journey, meticulous resuscitation and stabilisation should be carried out prior to transfer. This may involve carrying out procedures requested by the receiving hospital or unit (maternal or fetal). The standard airway, breathing and circulation (A B C) approach should be taken and examples of issues to address include the following:

- consideration should be given to securing a definitive airway in the patient with a high potential to fit
- hypovolaemic patients tolerate the inertial forces of transportation very poorly
- fetal wellbeing must be assessed to be certain that transfer is in the fetal interest before delivery
- steroids should be given if the woman is preterm.

All basic investigations should have been performed and the results clearly recorded in the accompanying notes, or telephoned through as soon as available. Inadequate resuscitation or missed illnesses and injuries will result in instability during transfer and will adversely affect outcome.

Equipment preparation

1 All equipment must be functioning.

2 Supplies of drugs and fluids should be more than adequate for the whole of the intended journey.

3 Particular care should be taken with supplies of oxygen, inotropes, sedative drugs and batteries for portable electronic equipment.

4 All lines and drains should be secured to the patient, the patient should be secured to the trolley and the trolley must be secured to the ambulance. The patient should be tilted to prevent aortocaval compression.

5 Specialist equipment may also be required for particular patients; for example, those patients who might be at risk of delivering (although high risk of this would preclude transfer till postdelivery) and those with spinal injuries.

6 A member of the team should be allocated the task of ensuring that all of the patient's documents, including case notes, investigation reports and a transfer form, accompany the patient.

7 The transferring personnel should know exactly the location at which they are expected.

8 The team requires a telephone and contact names and numbers to enable direct communication with both the receiving and base unit. In addition, all personnel need appropriate clothing, food if the journey is long and enough money to enable them to get home if needed.

Personnel preparation

The number and nature of staff accompanying patients during transport will reflect their transfer category. For example, the sick, pre-eclamptic patient would normally be escorted by an anaesthetist and midwife.

All staff must practise within their areas of competence. For an intensive care transfer, the Intensive Care Society recommends that the accompanying physician, 'Should have received training in intensive care and transport medicine, had involvement in previous transfers and preferably have at least 2 years' experience in anaesthesia, intensive care medicine or other equivalent specialty.' In addition, they should be accompanied by another experienced doctor, nurse, paramedic or technician familiar with intensive care procedures and with all transport equipment.

Whatever category the patient, all personnel should be competent in the transfer procedure and familiar with the equipment to be used, as well as the details of the patient's clinical condition. The team should carry accident insurance with adequate provision for personal injury, or death, sustained during the transfer.

Packaging

Drains and catheters should be fixed securely and freely draining. Drips should be fixed securely and the rate of administration closely controlled. Chest drains should be secured and unclamped with any underwater seal device replaced by an appropriate commercial drainage valve and bag system. If the patient has a simple pneumothorax, or is at risk of developing one, a chest drain should be inserted prophylactically.

Transportation

Mode of transport

The choice of transport needs to take into account several factors:

- nature of illness
- urgency of transfer
- mobilisation time
- geographical factors
- weather
- traffic conditions
- cost.

Road ambulances are by far the most common means used in the UK. They have a low overall cost, rapid mobilisation time and are less affected by weather conditions. They also give rise to less physiological disturbance.

Air transfer may be used for journeys over 50 miles, or 2 hours in duration, or if road access is difficult. The speed of the journey itself has to be balanced against organisational delays and also the need for intervehicle transfer at the beginning and end of the journey.

Care during transport

Tilt should be maintained during transfer.

Physiological problems that occur during transportation may arise as a result of the effects of the transport environment on the deranged physiology of the patient. Careful preparation can minimise the deleterious effects of inertial forces, such as tipping, acceleration and deceleration, as well as changes in temperature and barometric pressure.

The standard of care and the level of monitoring carried out prior to transfer need to be continued as far as possible during the transfer. Monitoring will include oxygen saturation, ECG and direct arterial pressure monitoring in all patients. End-tidal CO_2 monitoring should be used in all patients who are intubated.

Fetal monitoring may be appropriate.

The patient should be well covered and kept warm during the transfer. Road speed decisions depend both on clinical urgency and the availability of limited resources such as oxygen.

With adequate preparation, the transportation phase is usually incident free. However, untoward events do occur. Should this be the case, the patient needs to be reassessed using the ABC approach. Appropriate corrective measures should then be instituted. This may require a stop at the first available place. Following any untoward events, communications with the receiving unit are important. This should follow the systematic summary described previously.

Handover

At the end of the transfer, direct contact with the receiving teams must be established, so that a succinct, systematic summary of the patient can then be provided. This should be accompanied by a written record of the patient's history, vital signs, therapy and significant clinical events during transfer. All the other documents that have been taken with the patient should also be handed over. While this is going on, the rest of the transferring team can help in moving the patient from the ambulance trolley to the receiving unit's bed. The team can then retrieve all equipment and personnel and make their way back to their home unit.

Summary

- The safe transfer and retrieval of a patient requires a systematic approach.
- By following the ACCEPT method important activities will be carried out at the appropriate time.
- Specific training is available for staff undertaking transfers on the Safe Transfer and Retrieval Course (STaR) delivered by ALSG.

Further reading

1 Advanced Life Support Group. *Safe Transfer and Retrieval: The Practical Approach.* Oxford: Blackwell 2006.

SECTION 8

Human issues

CHAPTER 41

Human factors

> ## Objectives
>
> On successfully completing this topic, you will be able to:
>
> - understand the concept of human error in individuals and in teams
> - appreciate how situation awareness and good communication can help to minimise the effects of error.

Introduction

Error is inevitable, but harm is not

(Sarah Corcoran, Associate Director of Clinical Effectiveness, Central Manchester Foundation Trust, 2009)

This manual is focused on the assessment and management of the acutely ill patient. Clinicians are frequently required to utilise their knowledge and skills to care for a collapsed, or deteriorating, patient who is only one of several concurrent responsibilities.

Although the ideal of each patient being managed by a dedicated, focused, mentally and physically fit, smoothly functioning team, without interruptions or distractions, cannot be achieved, ways of working can be taught that optimise patient care.

The performance of individuals and teams working in complex, high-pressure environments is influenced by a wide range of intrinsic (personal) and extrinsic (environmental) factors. Some 20 years ago, the aviation industry began to take account of these factors, how they impact on human performance and their significance for flight safety. Today, all airline staff are required to undergo a rigorous *human factors* training programme that equips them with the tools to ensure that the safest option becomes the cornerstone of decision making. More recently, this has started to be adopted within health care as a means of improving safety and quality. The Department of Health recommends human factors training as a way of improving safety (CMO Report 2008, Safer Medical Practice).[1]

This chapter provides a brief overview of the human factors that can affect the performance of individuals and teams in the healthcare environment. The reader is encouraged to consider these factors in their everyday practice. Those attending the courses associated with this manual may receive direct feedback on their performance in this area.

Human error

Humans make mistakes. No amount of checks and procedures will obviate this fact. Consequently, it is vital to work in a way that, as well as decreasing the occurrence of mistakes, ensures that when they do occur the resulting threat to patient safety is minimised.

Error chains

Patient safety is only rarely compromised by a single mistake. Almost always a mistake or error [A] leads to harm [B] because of a series of factors that set up the conditions such that error A resulted in event B and without which event B would not have occurred. This is known as the error chain. This is the basis of the 'Swiss cheese' model (Figure 41.1).

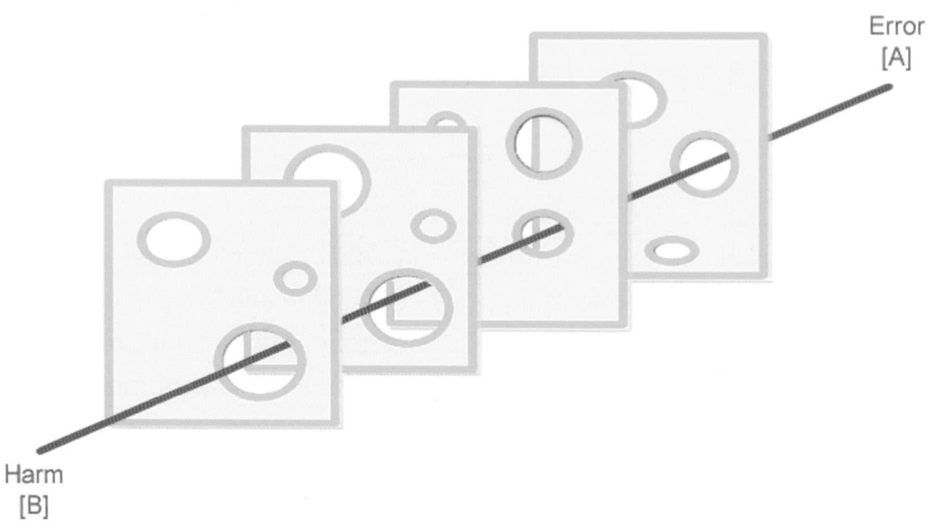

Figure 41.1 'Swiss cheese' model

Each of the slices of cheese represents barriers that should prevent A leading to B. However, such checks and balances can fail. This is represented by the holes in the slices. For A to lead to B, the holes of all the intervening slices need to line up. Simplistically viewed, the more checks that are put in place, the less likely an error is to occur. However, increasing complexity can be counterproductive, as humans will avoid or modify multiple steps to make life easier.

Consider the following critical incident:

The wrong dose of a drug has been administered to a patient by a clinician.

Why?

We know that the clinician should have checked the details of the prescription and the calculations and ensured that this all matched up with the formulation and strength of the medications they administered. People do not usually deliberately give the wrong dose and therefore it is not unreasonable to conclude that the clinician thought they had checked and matched everything as described.

So why did the error occur?

Further investigation revealed that the two drugs had been replaced in one another's normal positions in the ward trolley. The packaging of the two drugs was very similar (Figure 41.2).

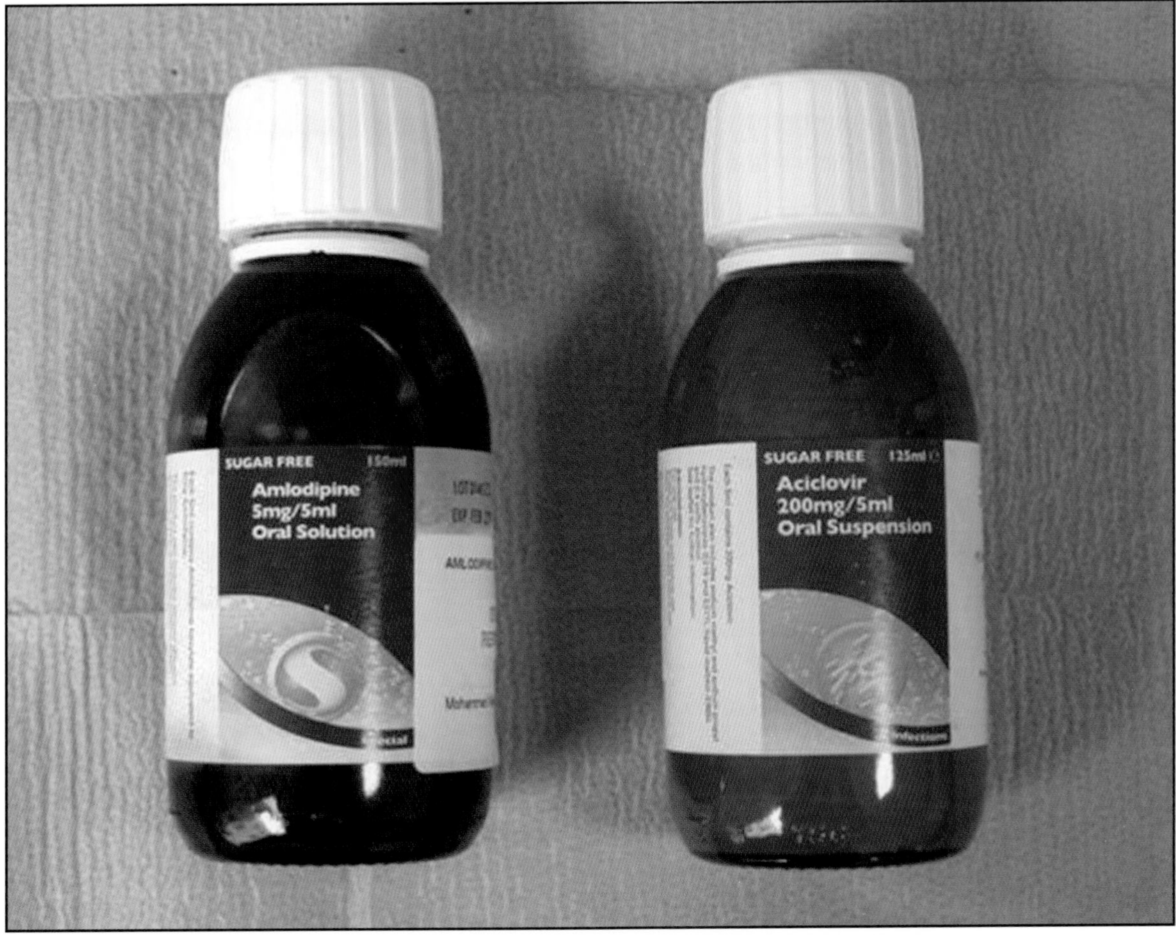

Figure 41.2 Similar package designs of two medications

The clinician picked the medication from its usual place, thought the packaging was familiar and therefore did not actively check the name and concentration of the drug. Habit can blind us to what we are doing. The problems of uniform packaging have been recognised and highlighted through a national adverse incident reporting system and recommendations made that packages for different strength medications should now look completely different. This change in practice is an example of how human factors theory is used to reduce the risk of error.

In the working environment, we may be present at the right time to observe the breaching of a barrier that would normally prevent errors occurring. It is critical that we are vigilant for these breaches and draw the attention of our colleagues to them in order to prevent the completion of an error chain. Events or conditions that are suspected of representing potential breaches in barriers preventing harm are referred to as red flags. The more red flags that arise, the greater the risk of an adverse incident occurring and therefore the greater the need to alert those involved to stop and review the situation.

Communication

Problems with communication underpin a significant proportion of critical events.

When the speaker and listener do not share the same language, the obvious solution is to use an interpreter. However there are limitations to discussions carried out through a third party. What about the matters that arise if one of the parties is communicating using their second language? Even when all parties are utilising their native tongue, nonverbal signals carry as much, if not more, information and meaning, than the words themselves. Nonverbal communication, outside the actual words we use, has been shown to contribute up to 93% of what we understand.[2] Barbour's study identified that 38% of communication relates to how words are said (volume, pitch, rhythm, etc.) and 55% body language (facial expressions, posture, etc.). When those trying to communicate come from different cultural backgrounds, both verbal and nonverbal elements can be completely misinterpreted by both parties.

Studies have shown that we understand around 61% of verbal and >50% of written communication, the remainder being miscommunicated, misinterpreted or simply misunderstood. It is not hard to see why in a busy clinical environment, when multiple tasks are being undertaken, and contact is frequently electronic or telephonic rather than face to face, miscommunication occurs so frequently. The process of communication can be described as three separate phases:

1. *The Sender* – This is the process within which the originator articulates their message in their mind, in what they perceive to be a meaningful and contextual manner.
2. *The Channel* – This is the medium of communication chosen: verbal, nonverbal or written.
3. *The Receiver* – This is the process within which the intended recipient makes sense of the information. This is easily distorted by the use of euphemisms or localised terminology.

The resulting outcome in a noisy highly pressured clinical arena is unsurprisingly one of poor information exchange. A technique to improve communication is the feedback loop. This is a process by which the receiver repeats the message back to the sender to acknowledge receipt and confirm that it has been correctly deciphered. It is quick and simple to use, easy to teach and has been shown to produce immediate benefits in busy clinical areas where requests and instructions are being passed on at breakneck speed.

To aid with communication when handing over care from one team/person to another, the SBAR tool is recommended (Box 41.1).

Box 41.1

S – Situation: a concise statement of the problem

B – Background: pertinent information related to the situation

A – Assessment: analysis and considerations of options – what you found/think

R – Recommendation: action requested/recommended – what you want to do

This formalises and structures the information transfer helping avoid assumptions of knowledge and highlighting the plan for ongoing care (recommendation). In summary, the discussion above only begins to touch on the complexity of human communication. Beyond this there are many layers of subtlety in our interactions. To try and mitigate the risk of miscommunication, it is vital that both talkers and listeners actively engage in the process.

Body language and hierarchy

All individuals should always be aware of their nonverbal signals. Messages that say 'I'm bored', 'I'm tired' or 'I don't value you' can inhibit another person from passing on a vital piece of information. The presence of a steep hierarchy can be particularly dangerous as it promotes an attitude of indifference to the input of those further down the pyramid. A culture where junior staff do not feel empowered to speak directly to senior staff, or senior staff are dismissive about concerns raised by junior staff, is inherently unsafe. If the clinical assistant walks into theatre and sees an expanding pool of blood under the operating table, they should feel able to voice their concerns. Whether or not it proves to be clinically important, their input should be positively acknowledged, as next time they might be the first to identify a critical concern.

Speaking up

A useful communication tool, utilised by the airline industry, is shown in Box 41.2.[3]

Box 41.2

Stage	Level of concern
P – Probe	I think you need to know what is happening
A – Alert	I think something bad might happen
C – Challenge	I know something bad will happen
E – Emergency	I will not let it happen

This structure can be used by any person who is concerned that they have information that might be important to others on the team. The levels *Probe, Alert, Challenge and Emergency,* are utilised sequentially to express increasing concern. If a disaster is imminent, it is entirely appropriate to use the *Challenge* or even *Emergency* stages without recourse to the initial stages. Both the speaker and the listener should recognise the level of the communication and react appropriately. In the aviation industry, reaching the level of *Challenge* on the flight deck prompts a serious review, whether or not an incident occurs.

These stages are described with examples below:

Probe: When the observer points out something they think might be a problem: 'Dr Adams, I think this woman is cyanosed.'

Alert: If there is no response to the first prompt and the situation continues. The observer strengthens their statement and suggests a course of action: 'Dr Adams, I am concerned the woman is deeply cyanosed; should we start BVM ventilation?'

Challenge: The situation requires urgent attention. One of the main protagonists needs to be directly engaged. If possible, the speaker places themselves into the eyeline of the person they wish to communicate with: 'Dr Adams – this patient is cyanosed and needs help with her ventilation now.'

Emergency: Used where all else has failed and/or the observer perceives a critical event is about to occur. If possible physical action should accompany clear verbalisation: 'Dr Adams, please move out of the way I am going to mask ventilate this cyanosed patient.'

Organisations that use this, or similar, systems sometimes make use of a code word or phrase to flag the level of concern. These may then be used to gain both the team's and a key individual's attention. For example 'Code Orange, Code Orange, please stop and listen.'

Situation awareness

People do not come to work to harm patients. When errors occur, they do so because the person making the mistake does not realise that their action will cause harm to the patient. If we have insufficient or incomplete information, we can draw the wrong conclusions about what is going on. For example, we can make a misdiagnosis. If we then intervene on the basis of that flawed diagnosis, it is not difficult to see that harm may ensue.

Good situation awareness is achieved when we have sufficient and correct information, have interpreted it correctly and correctly project the outcome of an intervention into the future, based on our current knowledge.

Consider the picture in Figure 41.3. What do you see? Around half of readers will see a young woman looking back/right and the other half will see an old woman looking forward/right (a few may see both). This is a simple example of how two people can look at the same thing yet make different interpretations.

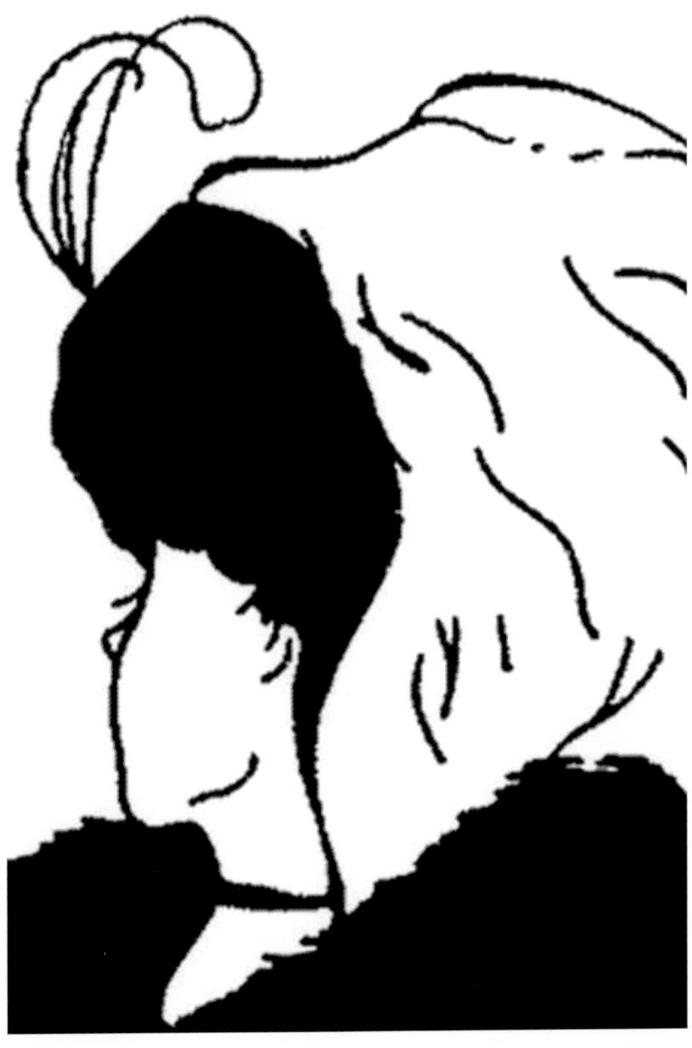

Figure 41.3 Illustration of situation awareness

The way we perceive a particular situation is affected by the information conveyed via our own sensorium, our past experience (an experienced clinician might recognise a compromised patient more rapidly than a junior), our level of alertness, our current workload and the influence of intercurrent distractions.

In psychological terms, our perception of the current situation is fitted into a model in our minds, based on our knowledge and previous experiences. We use this model to plan our next actions and anticipate the outcome of those actions. A simple example of this is a woman presenting with epigastric pain, with a previous history of severe pre-eclampsia in the last pregnancy. The clinician assessing the woman might conclude that she is suffering from gastroenteritis because of inexperience, or insufficient information (the history of previous pre-eclampsia) secondary to tiredness or distractions.

The loss of situation awareness is often triggered by the undertaking of a specific psychomotor task; an example would be the team leader who had maintained objectivity and an overall assessment of events, until he or she undertakes a specific task that greatly reduces his or her ability to receive and process information. Clinical staff have reported a complete loss of situation awareness, while undertaking complex tasks, in that they did not hear alarms or other team members alerting them to specific dangers. If it is the team leader undertaking the task and the team are also involved in busy practice, then it is not unusual for the entire team to miss critical elements of information that, if recognised, would have directly contributed to the correct diagnosis and care of the patient.

A common trap that people fall into is only seeing or registering the information that fits in with their current mental model. This is known as a *confirmation bias*. When this occurs, people favour information that confirms their preconceptions or hypotheses, regardless of whether the information is true.

For example, a clinician receives a phone call requesting them to review an acutely deteriorating patient who is known to be asthmatic. Before seeing the patient, the clinician builds up a series of preconceived expectations of what they will find. They may even formulate a management plan based upon these expectations. Once this mindset is established, it can be difficult to change. The clinician proceeds to examine only the systems affected by the presumed diagnosis. They seek to confirm their expectation by focusing on auscultation of the chest at the expense of a thorough airway assessment. On hearing bilateral wheeze their preconceived ideas are confirmed and the remainder of the assessment is completed without due attention and more as a rehearsed exercise than an open-minded exploration. They fail to notice that the patient also has a soft stridor and is hypotensive.

Alternatively, the clinician knows they have several other patients they need to get to and for this reason does not undertake a thorough assessment. The junior staff in attendance point out hypotension and signs of upper airway obstruction, but the clinician fails to recognise the significance of these signs. This occurs because psychologically they hold onto their preconceived diagnosis. In this situation they may dismiss these conflicting findings, or may even manipulate the findings to fit their preconceived mental model.

In both cases, the eventual diagnosis of anaphylaxis becomes a late consideration, or a situation that requires an objective newcomer to the team to point out the obvious.

Other examples of this loss of situation awareness relating to technical skills include the obstetrician who persists at operative vaginal delivery, with all their attention focused on successful completion of the procedure, rather than on critically assessing progress during traction; or the anaesthetist who does not recognise oesophageal intubation because, 'It felt right', or they are sure they saw the chest move.

It is vital that each individual understands the concept of situation awareness and continually questions their own thought processes and those of others around them. Remembering the possibility of the worst-case scenario helps to review things critically, to recognise warning signs early and avoid catastrophe. The whole team should also share their impressions of the current situation. There is good evidence that the situation awareness of a well-functioning team is actually greater than the sum of its individual parts. This may be in part due to the elimination of bad data. Information or comments by colleagues that are outwith one's current mental picture should be treated as a trigger to consider whether anyone's situation awareness is lacking. A discussion of the disparity should uncover the true picture. Problems occur when individuals either ignore or rationalise the errant data to fit into their current picture of the world, rather than treat it as a challenge.

Fatigue

When we are tired, we find it more difficult to absorb and process information, we react more slowly and mood can be affected. We may become impatient, uninterested and irritable. The negative impact on the ability to function individually, and as part of a team, is obvious.

Clinicians work in a highly pressured environment with the expectation that even when we know we are not functioning at 100% capacity, we will cope with a crisis. In a safe culture, staff need to feel able to say, 'I'm not fit to do this', and know they will have the support of their colleagues. While it seems obvious that we need to ensure that fatigued people are not working at the sharp end of healthcare delivery, this is not currently part of the mindset. This is a culture change we all need to embrace.

Even when prolonged or arduous shifts are avoided, circadian rhythms can produce adverse psychological and physiological changes. This is relevant as clinicians routinely work shifts, including nights, and have quick turnaround between patterns of rest/work activity. It is perhaps unsurprising to note that all of the recent major disasters attributed to human error (Exxon Valdez oil spill, Three Mile Island, Bhopal chemical plant explosion, Chernobyl) occurred on the night shift, when alertness is at its lowest point.

It is suggested that the following are caused by circadian rhythm disturbance:

- lack of concentration
- periods of inattention
- reduced vigilance
- reduction in alertness level
- slow actions
- alteration in short-term memory

- loss of critical analysis and advocacy
- interpretation errors.

Recognition of the impact of fatigue on our ability to perform carries with it important personal responsibilities. If circumstances arise that result in us being unfit for work in any way, we have the responsibility for flagging it up to colleagues and managers. They, in turn, should ensure that anyone reporting such concerns is supported and, where necessary, allowed to step down from front-line duties, until fit. If this feels overidealistic, consider the following – would you be comfortable boarding an aircraft when you knew the pilot had been up all night with his child who is critically unwell in hospital?

The discussions above are primarily focused on tiredness or fatigue due to lack of sleep. Physical or mental illness, use of medications, alcohol and personal stress can all manifest in a similar manner and require appropriate, sensitive management.

Decision making

In order to understand what factors can compromise the process of decision making, it is important to understand the factors that affect the reliability of any decision made. To reach a good decision, all aspects of a problem should be considered, all possible responses assessed and the consequences of those responses identified. The advantages and disadvantages of each course of action must be weighed up in order to draw a conclusion and make the decision. This must then be communicated to the team.

Good situation awareness is a prerequisite of this process. To achieve this, the decision maker must have all the key information. This is gathered through acquisition of data first hand (e.g. examining the patient oneself) and communication with one's team. Decision makers should be on the alert to ambiguities or conflicting information. Any inconsistent fact should be treated as a potential marker for faulty situation awareness and not dismissed as unimportant anomalies in the absence of evidence to support such a decision.

No decision-making process should be concluded until the team are satisfied they have all the information and have considered all the options. Where time is a pressure, a certain amount of pragmatism must be employed. There is plenty of evidence to confirm that experience can mitigate some of the negative effects of abbreviating the decision-making process. Those making decisions under such circumstances need to remain consciously aware of the short-cuts they have taken. They should be ready to receive feedback from their team, particularly if any member of the team has significant concerns about the proposed course of action. Practical limitations accepted, there are few situations where a delay of 1–2 minutes to share the rationale for the decision is not possible.

As discussed above, it is vital that team members feel able to raise their concerns and that the decision maker values and considers them appropriately. One only has to examine some of the high-profile medical incidents, such as the Elaine Bromiley case (see Box 41.3), to see that junior clinicians were trying to voice their (correct) concerns from a time when, if they had been heard, it may have altered the outcome.

Box 41.3

Elaine Bromiley died during a minor operation in 2005, after anaesthetists were unable to place an endotracheal tube. The doctors struggled for 20 minutes to insert the ET tube. They did not follow the standard 'Can't intubate, can't ventilate' protocol despite the appropriate kit being made available by theatre staff. During this episode Elaine Bromiley suffered irreversible brain damage and subsequently died.

When decision makers inappropriately or repeatedly disregard the opinions of others, this should be flagged up before an incident occurs.

Leadership: people, behaviours

The inevitable mix of personalities in a team will have implications for the smooth functioning of that team. In the pressured environment in which we work, latent personality traits, or even new ones, can be brought out. In extreme cases, this can manifest as aggressive or submissive affect. Depending on the individual and the team dynamics, this can be highly detrimental to the process of communication, situation awareness and decision making.

Wherever possible, the adoption of a facilitative role can serve to draw the best from all members of the team. Every opportunity should be taken to debrief teams after an episode of working together. This can be enhanced where there is opportunity for the team to practise and reflect on their interactions in a simulated environment.

Summary

- We all work in a complex, pressured clinical environment and are responsible for patient safety and so should be alert to red flags and voice concerns promptly. To do this we need to recognise and respect both our own limitations and those of the people we work with. This safety surveillance is facilitated by an understanding of the human factors at play around us.

References and further reading

1 Chief Medical Officer. *CMO Annual Report: Safer Medical Practice*. London: Department of Health 2008.

2 Koneye M, Barbour A. *Louder Than Words: Non-verbal Communication*. Columbus, OH: Merrill 1995.

3 Besco RO. *PACE: to Intervene or not to Intervene? The Co-pilot's Catch 22* (www.crm-devel.org/resource/paper/PACE.pdf).

4 www.institute.nhs.uk/safer_care/safer_care/Situation_Background_Assessment_Recommendation.html

5 Flin R, O'Connor P, Crichton M. *Safety at the Sharp End.* Farnham: Ashgate 2008.

6 Reason J. *The Human Contribution: unsafe acts, accidents and heroic recoveries* Farnham: Ashgate 2008.

CHAPTER 42

Consent matters

Objectives

On successfully completing this topic you will be able to:

- understand when and why consent is required
- appreciate the concepts of validity, capacity, autonomy and responsibility
- understand the legal status of the fetus.

When is consent required?

Consent is required before any treatment, investigation or physical contact with a patient is undertaken. Consent is also required before involving patients in research, teaching or disclosure of confidential information (which may be written, pictorial or auditory).

In England and Wales there is no statute, as in some countries, stating the principles of consent. Failure to obtain informed consent may give rise to civil or criminal proceedings as any touching of the person, no matter how well intentioned, is a trespass. However, to protect against a claim of battery, consent only in the broadest terms has to be obtained.

By contrast, a much more demanding obligation to obtain informed consent arises from a duty of care to the patient by the health professional.

Failure to provide sufficient information prevents a patient making an informed choice. If, as a result, the patient agrees to a procedure she would have refused had she been fully informed and harm arises as a result, there would be grounds for a claim of negligence (even if the harm is a recognised hazard of the procedure rather than the product of poor management).

The case of Chester versus Afshar suggests that failing to provide relevant information to a patient and ensuring that information is understood in a timely manner, could lead to a successful claim, even if the patient would have chosen the treatment had they been informed of the risk.[1] In this case, the patient developed cauda equina syndrome following discectomy (a recognised complication of this procedure). She claimed that her surgeon had not warned her of this complication. The court accepted this. She admitted that it was likely that she would have chosen to undergo surgery by the same surgeon, even if she had known, but she had been deprived of the ability to make an informed choice in the matter. The majority view, when this case was appealed in the House of Lords, was that being denied the opportunity to make a properly informed decision about whether to undergo surgery constituted the injury. The implications for English case law as a result of this ruling are profound and the NHS Litigation Authority has issued an alert on this subject.[2]

Obtaining consent should be a process begun as far in advance of a procedure as possible, but the doctor should recheck immediately prior to the procedure that the patient still consents. In obstetrics, information about potential complications and possible treatment options should be made available in the antenatal period. It is recognised that this will not be possible in the emergency situation and that those most at risk may not be accessible antenatally.[3]

The General Medical Council (GMC) suggests that obtaining informed consent is a process, not an isolated event. It suggests that, 'When providing information you must do your best to find out about patients' individual needs and priorities. You should respond honestly to any questions the patient raises.' A whole section is devoted to withholding information: 'You should not withhold information necessary for decision making unless you judge that disclosure of some relevant information would cause the patient serious harm. In this context serious harm does not mean the patient would become upset, or decide to refuse treatment.'[4]

Why is consent required? The legal and ethical considerations

The need for valid consent is not just a legal requirement but also an ethical principle that reflects respect for an individual's autonomy and is a fundamental part of good practice. This is the view of both the Department of Health[5] and the GMC.[4]

The traditional model of consent is the 'harm-avoidance model', in which the patient is informed of the risks of a procedure, described in general terms, but is otherwise excluded from the decision-making process. The patient is dealt with, 'In an authoritarian but benevolent way, (e.g. by supplying all their needs but regulating their conduct).'[6] This was considered acceptable in the case of Sidaway versus Board of Governors of the Bethlehem Royal Hospital. As the judge put it: 'When telling a patient about an operation, the doctor has to decide what ought to be said and how it should be said.'[7]

The increased emphasis on the rights of individuals has led to the requirement for a more demanding form of consent. This is the so-called 'autonomy enhancing model of consent', in which the patient must be given all the information they require to make their own fully informed decision about a proposed course of action.

Consent may be implied or express. An example of implied consent is the action of a patient holding out an arm for venepuncture to be performed. Such implied consent would usually protect against a charge of battery.

Express consent is required for a procedure carrying a 'material' risk (see below). The validity of consent does not depend on the form in which it is given: a signature on a form will not necessarily make consent valid. Equally, if consent has been validly given, the absence of a signed consent form is no bar to treatment. Written consent is considered advisable when the procedure involved is complex or risky, research or screening rather than clinical care is involved or there may be, 'Significant consequences for the patient's employment, social or personal life.'[4] It is a legal requirement for some treatments specified in the Human Fertilisation and Human Embryology Act 1990 and the Mental Health Act 1993.

What makes consent valid?

1 The patient must have sufficient information.
2 The patient must have the capacity to make a decision.
3 The patient must be allowed to make the decision voluntarily.
4 Consent is obtained by a suitably qualified and trained individual.

Sufficient information

This is an area of uncertainty with considerable changes occurring over time and between countries. Only the case in the UK will be discussed in detail.

In the UK in 1957, in the case of Bolam versus Friern Hospital it was established that a doctor's practice would be judged against that of his medical peers – the Bolam principle or 'reasonable doctor test' – and this was specifically applied to what information to give a patient.[8] This was challenged in 1985 in the case of Sidaway, when it was opined that there might be occasions when information about a particular risk was so obviously necessary that the court would decide that its omission was negligent even if this was not the opinion of a 'responsible body of medical opinion'.[9] In the cases of Bolitho and Pearce, the Bolam principle was overturned. The courts made it clear that the court itself would be the final arbiter of what was a reasonable amount of information to give a patient and not the medical profession. The reasonable doctor has been replaced by what the reasonable patient would expect to be told[10]. The situation is different in the US where, in some states, the policy of 'full disclosure' is advocated (the patient is told as much as possible).

Material risk is a risk to which a person in the patient's position would be likely to attach significance. A risk cannot be judged material on the basis of frequency alone.[11] The severity must be taken into account. The individual circumstances of the patient are also pertinent. For example, the risk of infertility following a procedure will be more significant to the primiparous woman than one who has completed her family. The type of information that patients should be told includes a description of the procedure and the incidence and severity of the risks involved (which should be mentioned even if they have not occurred in the practice of the particular doctor involved). There should be discussion on the likely or possible outcome of following or declining to follow a particular course of action and what the alternatives are (if any exist).[4]

The Association of Anaesthetists suggests that factors that might influence what the patient is told might include 'the estimated capacity' (see below) 'of the patient to want to know and to be able to understand the risks' and 'the degree of urgency of the proposed treatment'.[12]

Occasionally, a patient might wish to know very little, or request that a relative make decisions for them (commonly the partner in obstetrics). In law, no-one may make decisions on behalf of an adult. In this situation, the GMC suggests trying to explain the importance of knowing what is happening to the patient and the Department of Health considers it 'good practice' to record in the notes if information is offered but declined. A relative of an adult cannot choose to withhold information; the patient must be consulted.

In obstetrics, the problem of how much to tell the patient can be particularly demanding. Obstetric patients are usually young and fit. Younger patients want more information.[13] Women and their partners are often highly motivated to become informed. Several studies show that obstetric patients want more information than they are receiving.[14–16] There is evidence to suggest that providing more information does not increase anxiety levels in contrast to a common concern among the medical profession.[17]

Adversely influencing the opportunity to provide information that women want is lack of time: the majority of medical interventions in childbirth are unplanned, such as augmentation of labour, assisted vaginal delivery, episiotomy or manual removal of the placenta. Two-thirds of CS operations are nonelective. In a 2001 national audit, 16% of caesarean sections were considered to be category 1: when there is immediate threat to the life of the woman and her fetus and delivery within 30 minutes is considered mandatory.[18] When trauma is involved, time is invariably at a premium. Most authorities suggest that women are given information about all the obstetric complications that might arise in the antenatal period. A combination of printed material with face to face question and answer sessions appear to be the most effective way of informing patients.[19]

Capacity

For a patient to have capacity (to be competent) to make a decision concerning medical treatment the following criteria must be met:

1 The patient must be capable of comprehending the information.
2 They must be able to retain the information long enough to use it as a basis for decision making.
3 They must be able to evaluate/weigh the information as part of the decision making process.
4 They must be able to communicate their decision (not necessarily verbally).

In the UK, anyone over the age of 18 years is assumed to be competent to choose or refuse treatment unless shown not to be (for 16–18-year-olds see below). This is 'not a question of the degree of intelligence or education of the adult concerned'.[20] In order for a patient to be able to comprehend information, it must be presented in a form comprehensible to that patient (e.g.

in a language they can understand or avoiding written material in the case of illiteracy). The Department of Health warns not to underestimate the capacity to consent by a patient with learning disabilities. Extra effort should be made to present information in a form comprehensible to such patients. Furthermore, the patient need not come to a decision that is seen as rational by others: 'The patient's right of choice exists whether the reasons for making that choice are rational, irrational, unknown or even non-existent' (Lord Donaldson).[21]

No other person can consent to treatment on behalf of any adult, including incompetent ones, unless they are legally appointed with power of attorney.

Since 1969, those aged 16 or 17 years are entitled to consent to medical intervention (Section 8, Family Law Reform Act 1969). Unlike adults, however, their refusal of medical treatment may sometimes be overturned by an adult with parental responsibility. The power to overrule is based on the paramount importance of the welfare of the child. Refusal of treatment by a child or those with parental responsibility can be overruled by a court in the interests of the child's welfare. This has obvious implications in the case of children of Jehovah's Witnesses (this is not the case in Scotland, where a competent child's refusal cannot be overturned).

Children under the age of 16 years *may* have the capacity to consent to medical treatment if they are judged to have capacity by their doctor, taking into account the complexity and risk of the procedure and the child's state of health and mind. This process was known as assessing the child to be 'Gillick competent'. The doctor should ensure that all relevant considerations pertaining to their decision are documented.

In the case of obstetrics, it is worth noting that, in the UK in 2000, over 41 000 girls under the age of 18 years became pregnant, of whom 8000 were under 16 years old. A high proportion of young girls seek to terminate their pregnancy. In such circumstances, there is potential for conflict between parents and children over whether to terminate the pregnancy and it is vital to establish whether the girl is 'Gillick competent'.

Lack of capacity for consent: incompetence

The range of ability among patients follows a continuum from incompetence through to competence.[22] Where capacity is absent, so that valid consent cannot be obtained, the underlying principle guiding treatment is that of the person's best interests (the 'welfare of the child' in the case of minors). Treatment can and should be given on the legal grounds of necessity. The best interests of an individual do not refer only to their physical health but must depend on:

1 The risks and benefits of available options.
2 Whether the patient had been previously competent, evidence of previously held views, e.g. advance statement (see below).
3 Knowledge of the patient's views or beliefs.
4 Views of the patient's preferences given by a third party.
5 The treatment option that gives the patient most chance of choice in the future.

The Mental Capacity Act

This Act came into force in England and Wales in 2007 and is designed to protect people who lack capacity. It is based on five fundamental principles:

1. A person must be assumed to have capacity unless it is established that they lack capacity.
2. A person should not be deemed to lack capacity until all practicable steps to regain capacity have been taken without success.
3. A person cannot be judged to lack the capacity to make a decision merely because they make an unwise decision.
4. Any decision made under this Act for, or on behalf of, a person who lacks capacity must be made in their best interests.
5. Before the procedure is done, or the decision is made, regard must be had to whether the purpose for which it is needed can be as effectively achieved in a way that is less restrictive of the person's rights and freedom of action.

The Act requires assessment of capacity to be a two-stage process (see Box 42.1).

Box 42.1 Two-stage assessment

Stage one

Does the person have an impairment of the mind or brain, or is there some sort of disturbance affecting the way their mind or brain works? (It does not matter whether the impairment or disturbance is temporary or permanent.)

Stage two

If so, does that impairment or disturbance mean that the person is unable to make the decision in question at the time it needs to be made?

Capacity may be decision specific (the patient may have capacity to make some decisions but not others), and may fluctuate over time. Psychiatric illness does not necessarily mean lack of capacity[23,24].

The Act entitles any patient of 18 years or over with capacity to refuse specific medical treatment at a time in the future when they may lack capacity. This is known as an advance decision.

1 The individual was competent when drawing up the directive.

2 The directive expresses *refusal* of a treatment (a doctor is not obliged to undertake any particular course of action and cannot be required to undertake an illegal course of action).

3 The specific *circumstances* in which the question of treatment arises are those anticipated by the patient when drawing up the directive and the proposed treatment explicitly stated.

4 There is no evidence that the patient may have changed her mind, while she retained capacity.

Advance decisions can be verbal unless they refer to life-saving treatment when they have to be written and signed by the patient. The Act does not dictate the format of verbal advance decision and it will be up to the treating clinicians to decide if they exist and are valid at the time.

A doctor cannot choose to ignore a valid advance directive on terms of conscience or belief.

Examples of advance directives include refusal of heroic surgery or resuscitative measures in the case of progressive, debilitating disease and statements that Jehovah's Witnesses may carry, refusing the use of blood or blood products. In the case of obstetrics, the birth plan may fulfil the criteria of an advance directive. In such circumstances, what is paramount is to determine if the patient had anticipated the circumstances (e.g. more severe pain than ever previously experienced), if she had changed her mind and whether the present circumstances have rendered her currently incompetent.

If there are concerns about the validity of an advance directive, it may be necessary to consult the courts. Article 9 of the Human Rights Act 1998 (freedom of thought, conscience and religion) may have an impact in this area in the future.

Under the safeguards of the Mental Health Act 1983, patients who are mentally incapacitated may be treated compulsorily, but only for the mental disorder from which they are suffering. In 1996, a parturient with schizophrenia was forced to undergo a CS against her will on the grounds that the caesarean formed part of the treatment for her schizophrenia, not because it would save her life or that of her child.[25] The judge was of the opinion that delivery would halt further deterioration to the patient's psychiatric state; psychiatric opinion was that a live birth was necessary to make schizophrenia treatment successful and finally that the patient could not be given strong enough medication until after delivery as it might harm the fetus (but see section on rights of the unborn child).

In the case of the child who lacks capacity, the Children Act 1989 sets out who can assume parental responsibility. These include the following:

1 The children's parents if married at the time of birth or conception; this responsibility is not lost on divorce.
2 The child's mother if unmarried but not the father, unless they subsequently marry or he is granted parental responsibility by a court. However, in England and Wales for births registered from December 2003 (different dates in Scotland and Northern Ireland), an unmarried father, as long as he is named on the child's birth certificate, has parental responsibility.
3 A legally appointed guardian, adoptive parents.
4 A person in whose favour a court has made a residence order for the child.
5 A local authority if the child is under its care (usually shared with parents).
6 A local authority or person holding an authorised emergency protection order for the child.

One person with parental responsibility may give consent to essential treatment in the face of refusal by another although, if practical, such decisions should be referred to a court. In an emergency, a child who lacks capacity may be treated without consent from the person with parental responsibility.

The question of capacity and temporary incapacity is a particular dilemma in obstetrics. This has been highlighted by a series of cases in which applications were made to courts to allow emergency CS to be performed against the will of the woman. In the case of CH,[23] the surgery was allowed under the Mental Health Act 1983 because the surgery itself was deemed to be an essential part of the treatment of the mental illness. In subsequent cases, the decision whether to allow surgery was based on the question of capacity of the labouring woman. In one case, the 'pain and acute emotional stress' of labour combined with the patient's history of mental illness (she did not believe she was pregnant) were the grounds on which the judge concluded that she was incapable of weighing up the information presented to her.[25] However, in a second case, later the same day, the same judge concluded that the patient was 'unable to make any valid decision about anything of even the most trivial kind' due to the emotional stress and pain of labour. This was a woman whose obstetrician considered her to be competent and she had no history of mental illness.[26]

A third case involved a patient [MB] with a severe needle phobia who required section for breech presentation. In this case it was judged that the woman's capacity was temporarily diminished by the panic and fear induced by her needle phobia.

Factors that may temporarily erode capacity include: shock; confusion; fatigue; pain; and drugs. All these may be pertinent when considering the capacity of a woman in labour.

The Human Rights Act 1998 incorporates the European Convention on Human Rights into UK law; it is likely that it will serve to strengthen protection of individuals against treatment they refuse (Article 3, prohibition of torture; Article 5, right to liberty and security; Article 6, right to a fair trial) and emphasise their right to be fully informed[27] (Article 8, right to private and family life).

Status of the fetus

The Abortion Act 1967 gave statutory status to the principle that the fetus does not have a legal right to life. The Act sets out clearly the circumstances when termination of pregnancy is allowable, which extends far beyond the physical wellbeing of the woman. The grounds for an abortion are:

1 That the pregnancy has not exceeded its twenty-fourth week and that the continuance of the pregnancy would involve risk, greater than if the pregnancy were terminated, of injury to the physical or mental health of the pregnant woman or any existing children of her family; or

2 That the termination is necessary to prevent grave permanent injury to the physical or mental health of the pregnant woman; or

3 That the continuance of the pregnancy would involve risk to the life of the pregnant woman, greater than if the pregnancy were terminated; or

4 That there is a substantial risk that if the child were born it would suffer from such physical or mental abnormalities as to be seriously handicapped.

If, 'The termination is immediately necessary to save the life or to prevent grave permanent injury to the physical or mental health of the pregnant woman,' the pregnancy may be terminated if one registered medical practitioner is of the opinion, formed in good faith that an abortion is justified within the terms of the Act.

The fetus's lack of legal right was demonstrated in a case in which a man unsuccessfully sought an injunction preventing his wife from having an abortion.[28] This case was taken to the European Commission on Human Rights under Article 2 (right to life), but was rejected.

The Court of Appeal's ruling on the case of MB highlights not just issues of competence but also the legal status of the unborn child in relation to its mother's rights. In the judgment of the Court of Appeal, it was categorically stated that the right of a competent woman to agree to or refuse treatment takes precedence over the welfare of the fetus.[29] In a subsequent case, the Court of Appeal concluded: 'Although human, and protected by the law in a number of different ways... an unborn child is not a separate person from its mother. Its need for medical assistance does not prevail over her rights. She is entitled not to be forced to submit to an invasion of her body against her will, whether her own life or that of her unborn child depends on it. Her right is not reduced or diminished merely because her decision to exercise it may appear morally repugnant.'[30]

Voluntarily given consent

Consent will only be valid if given freely. The GMC starts the section entitled 'Ensuring voluntary decision making,' by stating, 'it is for the patient not the doctor, to determine what is in the patient's best interests.'[4] However, it accepts that the doctor may want to recommend a particular treatment. This should be acceptable if evidence-based information is presented in a dispassionate manner. It is good practice to document the discussion.

The woman's partner and sometimes other relatives, any of whom may hold strong views about her management, often accompany the obstetric patient. When considering outside influence, 'The will of the patient and the relationship of the person trying to impose their will, must be considered,' (Lord Donaldson).[21]

The same factors that may erode capacity may also undermine the woman's ability to withstand coercion (fatigue, pain, stress, etc.) Cultural factors characterising relationships between the sexes may also be a factor. In the not uncommon situation where a woman states, 'I will do as my husband decides,' it is important to try to establish the woman's wishes, preferably in the absence of the partner. The same may apply to parents, especially in the case of younger girls. In Re T, the Court of Appeal judge upheld the decision to allow a blood transfusion to a patient who was not a Jehovah's Witness but who declined blood, on the grounds that her mother, who was a Jehovah's Witness, had unduly influenced her.[21]

It should be reiterated that no-one can consent to or refuse treatment on behalf of another adult, whether competent or not (unless they have power of attorney). Thus, the partner who says, 'my wife would have wanted/not have wanted a particular intervention', has no right to impose his view. However, such a statement may alert the doctor to the existence of an advance directive that does have legal weight (see below).

Who can obtain consent?

The person providing treatment is responsible for obtaining consent. The GMC guidance states that this task can be delegated, provided that the person to whom the task is delegated is suitably trained and qualified, obtains consent in an appropriate manner and has sufficient knowledge about the proposed procedure.[4]

Summary

- Without basic consent, any physical contact with patients constitutes trespass and could result in a charge of battery or assault.
- Doctors have a duty of care to ensure that their patients give informed consent to procedures; failure to do so may constitute negligence, especially if harm ensues.
- Where informed consent cannot be obtained, doctors may legally provide care based on the principle of necessity, the basis of which is the treatment is in the best interests of the patient.
- While children under the age of 16 years may have the right to consent to treatment independently of their parents if they are deemed to have capacity ('Gillick competent'), they may not have the right to refuse treatment.
- The fetus has no legal right to life; a pregnant or labouring woman's rights are paramount, even in the face of fetal demise.
- Advance decisions, of which birth plans are examples, if valid, are legally binding.
- In general, the obstetric population wants and requires more information to inform their treatment decisions.

References and further reading

1. Chester versus Afshar [2004] UKHL 41.
2 NHS Litigation Authority. *NHSLA Risk Alert, Issue 4*. November 2004.
3 Lewis G (editor). *Why Mothers Die 2000–2002. Sixth Report of the Confidential Enquiries into Maternal Deaths in the United Kingdom*. London: RCOG Press 2004.
4 General Medical Council. Consent: patients and doctors making decisions together. GMC 2008 (www.gmc-uk.org/guidance/ethical_guidance/consent_guidance_index.asp).

5 Department of Health. *Reference Guide to Consent for Examination or Treatment.* London: DoH 2001 (www.doh.gov.uk/consent/refguide.htm).
6 Switankowsky IS. *A New Paradigm for Informed Consent.* Lanham, MD: University Press of America 1998.
7 Sidaway versus Board of Governors of the Bethlehem Royal Hospital and Maudsley Hospital and others [1965] AC 871, HL at 871.
8 Bolam versus Friern Hospital Management Committee 1957.
9 Sidaway versus Board of Governors of Bethlehem Royal Hospital 1985 AC 871.
10 Bolitho versus City & Hackney Health Authority 1997, Pearce versus United Bristol Healthcare Trust 1999.
11 Rogers versus Whitaker 1992.
12 Association of Anaesthetists of Great Britain and Ireland. *Information and Consent for Anaesthesia.*1999 (www.aagbi.org).
13 Farnhill D, Inglis S. Patients' desire for information about anaesthesia: Australian attitudes. *Anaesthesia* 1993;48:162–4.
14 Kelly GD, Blunt C, Moore PAS, Lewis M. Consent for regional anaesthesia in the United Kingdom: what is material risk? *Int J Obstet Anesth* 2004;13:71–4.
15 Plaat F, McGlennan A. Women in the 21st century deserve more information: Disclosure of material risk in obstetric anaesthesia. *Int J Obstet Anesth* 2004;13:69–70.
16 Pattee C, Ballantyne M, Milne B. Epidural analgesia for labour and delivery: informed consent issues. *Can J Anaesth* 1997;44:918–23.
17 Inglis S, Farnhill D. The effects of providing preoperative statistical anaesthetic risk information. *Anesth Intensive Care* 1993;21:799–805.
18 Royal College of Obstetricians and Gynaecologists Clinical Effectiveness Support Unit. *The National Sentinel Caesarean Section Audit Report.* London: RCOG Press 2001.
19 Webber D, Higgins L, Baker V. Enhancing recall of information from a patient education booklet: a trial using cardiomyopathy patients. *Patient Educ Couns* 2001;44:263–70.
20 Re C (Adult: Refusal of treatment) 1994.
21 Re T (Adult: Refusal of treatment) 1992.
22 Maybury M, Maybury J. *Consent in Clinical Practice.* Oxford: Radcliffe Medical Press 2003.
23 Tameside and Glossop Acute Services Trust versus CH.
24 www.medicalprotection.org/uk/uk-factsheets/mental-capacity-act
25 Norfolk and Norwich NHS Trust versus W 1996.
26 Rochdale NHS Trust versus C 1997.
27 Hewson B. Why the Human Rights Act matters to doctors. *BMJ* 2000;321:780–1.
28 Paton versus trustees of British Pregnancy Advisory Services 1979.
29 Re MB (Adult medical treatment) 1997.
30 Re S (Adult refusal of treatment) 1992.
31 Sedgwick P, Hall A. Teaching medical students and doctors how to communicate risk. *BMJ* 2003;327:694–5.

Index

ABC(DE) approach 17
- cardiopulmonary resuscitation 111
- neonatal resuscitation 146
- unconscious patient 191

abdominal emergencies 228, 229
abdominal pain 32, 229
- algorithm 228
- clinical management 235
- examination 234
- history taking 231
- investigations 234
- location and likely causes 232
- pathophysiology 230

abdominal pathology, maternal deaths 229, 230
abdominal trauma 179
- diagnostic aids 183
- fetal assessment 184
- penetrating injury 181
- primary survey and resuscitation 181
- secondary survey 184
- spinal injuries 207

abortion
- maternal deaths 13
- *see also* termination of pregnancy

Abortion Act 1967 13, 488
ACCEPT approach, patient transfer 459
ACE inhibitors 245
activated partial thromboplastin time (APTT) 134, 135
activated protein C, recombinant (drotrecogin alfa) 61
acute coronary syndromes 243
adrenaline (epinephrine)
- for anaphylactic shock 49, 49, 49
- in CPR 114
- for neonatal resuscitation 151
- in sepsis 59

adult respiratory distress syndrome (ARDS) 57
advance directives 307, 486
advanced life support (ALS) 110, 114
- algorithm 108

Advanced Life Support Group (ALSG) 3
aftercoming head of breech
- destructive operations 432
- forceps delivery 361, 362, 402, 403
- symphysiotomy 430

age, maternal mortality and 10
air transfers 464
airway
- assessment 86
- burns injury 221, 223
- definitive 91
- maintenance 90
- problems 86
- suctioning *see* suctioning, airway
- surgical 95, 101

airway devices
- nasopharyngeal 90
- oropharyngeal (Guedel) 90, 91, 98, 98
- supraglottic 95

airway management 85
- advanced techniques 91
- basic life support 111
- neonatal resuscitation 146, 152
- practical procedures 98
- primary survey 17
- problems contributing to maternal deaths 438
- sepsis 58
- techniques 88
- unconscious patient 191

airway obstruction 85, 86
- burns 221
- causes 86
- clearance 88
- diagnosis 87
- spinal injuries 206

all-fours position, in shoulder dystocia 376
ambulances, road 464
aminophylline 49
amiodarone 114
amniotic fluid embolism (AFE) 121
- algorithm 120
- clinical manifestations 122
- diagnosis 124
- incidence 121
- management 125
- maternal deaths 13, 121
- neonatal outcome 127
- recurrence risk 126
- symptoms and signs 123, 124
- uterine trauma 181

AMPLE history 182
amputations, traumatic 217
anaemia, newborn baby 155
anaesthesia
- awareness during 439
- caesarean section 440, 440
- complications 436, 437
- major obstetric haemorrhage 306
- manual removal of placenta 329
- maternal deaths 13, 437, 438
- perineal repair 418, 420
- pre-eclampsia/eclampsia 285
- rapid sequence induction 93, 306
- *see also* regional anaesthesia

anal sphincter injuries, obstetric (OASIS) 417
- assessment 418, 419, 419
- classification 417
- occult 417
- postoperative care 424

repair 420, 421, 421, 422
training 425, 425
anaphylactic shock 43, 48
angiotensin-receptor antagonists 245
antenatal care
diabetes mellitus 253, 254
psychiatric illness 270
anti-D (Rh) immunoglobulin 182, 399
antibiotics 8
prophylactic 424
in sepsis 59, 60
anticoagulation
citrate, blood products 72
during labour and delivery 135
postnatal 136
prosthetic heart valves 247
pulmonary embolism 134, 135
anticonvulsant mood stabilisers 272
antidepressants 272, 274
antihistamines 49
antihypertensive drug therapy 276, 283, 293
antiplatelet drugs 244, 245
antipsychotic drugs 272, 273
anxiety 33, 267, 267
aortic dissection 246
aortic rupture
spontaneous 173
traumatic 175
aortocaval compression 116
see also supine hypotension syndrome
apnoea
neonatal resuscitation 146
primary 140, 141, 141, 143
terminal 140, 141, 141, 142, 142, 143
appendicitis, acute 232, 236
arrhythmias
local anaesthetic toxicity 443, 444
non-shockable 114
shockable 114
Arrow Peripheral Emergency Infusion Device (EID) 66
Arrow Rapid Infusion Catheter (RIC) 66, 67
arterial blood gases (ABG) 34, 35
guiding fluid replacement 77
pulmonary embolism 131
arterial embolisation, major haemorrhage 304
asphyxia, birth
pathophysiology 140, 141
shoulder dystocia 370
see also fetal distress
aspiration of gastric contents 92, 95
aspirin 245
assisted vaginal delivery *see* operative vaginal delivery
asthma 32
asystole 114
ATOMFC mnemonic, thoracic injuries 172
augmentation of labour
breech presentation 401
uterine rupture risk 341
automated external defibrillator (AED) 107, 113
autoregulation, organ perfusion 40
AVPU assessment 192
awareness during anaesthesia 439

B-Lynch brace suture 304, 304
backache, after regional blocks 448
bacteraemia 52
bag mask ventilation, neonatal resuscitation 148, 149
balloon tamponade, intrauterine 303
base excess 34, 35
basic life support 109, 110
algorithms 106, 107
Battle's sign 198
benzodiazepines 261
best interests principle 485
beta-blockers 245, 284
bicarbonate
neonatal resuscitation 151
standard 34, 35
bipolar illness 267, 271
bladder filling, umbilical cord prolapse 386
bladder function, spinal cord injury 207
Blond–Heidler saw 433
blood
coagulation defects *see* coagulopathy
components for transfusion 72, 74
crossmatching 73
blood gases, arterial *see* arterial blood gases
blood loss
classification 45, 46
clinical signs 46, 47, 76, 76
difficulties in recognising 41, 45, 70, 298, 299
hypovolaemic shock 41
see also haemorrhage; hypovolaemia
blood pressure (BP)
automated recording systems 278, 280
control, in pre-eclampsia 282
defining pre-eclampsia 277
measurement 280
observations 26
see also hypertension; hypotension
blood products 72, 74
blood transfusion
amniotic fluid embolism 126
autologous 75, 122
citrate anticoagulation 72
indications 73
introduction 9
patients refusing 296, 307
risks 73
sepsis 60
blood volume, circulating 41
Boas's sign 234
body language 472, 473
Boerhaave syndrome 175
Bolam principle 483
Bolitho versus City & Hackney Health Authority 483
brachial plexus injuries 370
Bracht technique, breech delivery 401, 404, 405, 405
bradycardia
high/total spinal block 445
in spinal injuries 206
brain contusions 196

brain injury
  assessment 193
  open 197
  primary 190
    diffuse 195
    focal 196
  secondary 190
    prevention 191
brain lacerations 197
brain tumours 263
breathing
  agonal 112
  basic life support 112
  in neonatal resuscitation 148
  newborn baby 140, 145, 146
  rescue 112
  in sepsis 58
  unconscious patient 192
  see also ventilation
breathing problems
  burns injury 223
  high/total spinal blocks 445, 445
  spinal injuries 206
breathlessness 31, 32, 62
breech delivery, vaginal 199
  conduct of delivery 401
  conduct of labour 400
  failure 404
  head entrapment 406, 430
  nuchal arms 404
  see also aftercoming head of breech
breech extraction 319, 406
breech presentation 395
  algorithm 394
  audit 406
  caesarean section 319, 395, 399
  external cephalic version 395
  medico-legal issues 406
  twin pregnancy 412
  vaginal delivery *see* breech delivery, vaginal
Bromley, Elaine 478, 479
bronchodilators 49
bupivacaine
  dose 441, 442, 443
  hyperbaric 442
burns 221
  algorithm 220
  delivery of fetus 225
  depth 225
  electrical 226
  immediate first aid 222
  pathophysiology 221
  primary survey and resuscitation 223
  secondary survey and definitive care 225
  severity 224
  shock 44

C-reactive protein (CRP) 57, 235
caesarean section (CS) 313
  in abdominal trauma 185
  anaesthesia 440, 440
  audit standards 321
  autologous blood transfusion 122
  avoiding problems 311, 314
  breech presentation 319, 195, 399
  in developing countries 433
  difficult 317
  failed vaginal breech delivery 406
  forced 487, 488
  macrosomic babies 372
  pelvic fractures 214
  periarrest/perimortem 117
  placenta praevia 319
  postoperative management 311
  prerequisites for 310, 313
  previous
    induction of labour after 340
    placenta accreta 325
    twin delivery 413
    uterine rupture 340
  second stage of labour 317, 347
  supervision 317
  thromboprophylaxis 320
  twin delivery 411, 415
calcium channel blockers 245
calcium chloride 115
calcium gluconate 287
calcium infusion, during blood transfusion 72
capacity to consent 484
  patients lacking 485
  temporary lack 488
  two-stage assessment 486
capillary refill time (CRT) 45
capnography 94, 113
caput, ventouse delivery and 351, 356
carbon dioxide (CO_2)
  build-up, airway obstruction 85
  end-tidal monitoring 94, 113
carbon monoxide inhalation 222, 223
carboprost, major obstetric haemorrhage 303
cardiac arrest
  amniotic fluid embolism 122, 123
  appropriate response to 249
  caesarean delivery during 117
  hyperkalaemic, crush injuries 215
  incidence 109
  local anaesthetic toxicity 443, 444
  management 110
  non-shockable rhythms 114
  reversible causes 114
  shockable rhythms 114
  see also cardiopulmonary resuscitation; collapse, maternal
cardiac disease 242
  acquired 242
  congenital *see* congenital heart disease
  fluid administration 81
  inherited 249
  ischaemic 243
  maternal deaths 14, 241
  service provision 247
  valvular 246

cardiac drugs 245, 245
cardiac massage, open 117
cardiac obstetric clinics, joint 248
cardiac surgery 244
cardiac tamponade 173
Cardiff wedge 203
cardiogenic shock 42, 48
cardiomyopathy
  peripartum 242
  in pregnancy 242
cardiopulmonary resuscitation (CPR) 109
  advanced life support 110, 114
  algorithms 106
  basic life support 109, 110
  caesarean delivery 117
  communication and teamwork 119
  defibrillation 113, 114
  discontinuing 118
  fetal outcome 118
  logistics 119
  medico-legal issues 118
  physiological changes in pregnancy affecting 116
  positioning of pregnant woman 110
  starting 112
cardiotocography (CTG)
  abdominal pain 234
  pre-eclampsia/eclampsia 282
cell salvage 75, 122
central venous pressure (CVP) monitoring
  guiding fluid management 78
  line placement 69
  in pre-eclampsia 80, 290
  in sepsis 59
Centre for Maternal and Child Enquiries (CMACE) 7
cephalic replacement, shoulder dystocia 377
cephalopelvic disproportion, symphysiotomy 430
cerebral malaria 263
cerebral perfusion 190
cerebral perfusion pressure (CPP) 190
cerebral thrombosis 257
cerebral venous sinus thrombosis 257, 262
cerebrospinal fluid leaks 198, 258
cerebrovascular accident (CVA) 257
cervical collars 202, 209
cervical spine immobilisation 202, 202, 208
  airway management and 88
  cervical collar application 209
  headblocks and tape 210
  manual in-line 208, 208
cervical spine injuries 202
chest, flail 173
chest compressions 112
  neonatal resuscitation 149, 150
chest drains 176, 178
  complications 178
  insertion 176, 178
  for transfers 464
chest injuries *see* thoracic injuries
chest pain 243
chest radiograph (CXR) 132
chest wound, sucking 173
Chester versus Afshar 481
child protection cases 269, 270
children, capacity to give consent 485, 487, 489
chin lift/head tilt 88, 89, 111
chlorpheniramine 49
cholecystitis, acute 232, 234, 236
chorioamnionitis 232
circadian rhythm disturbances 477
circulating volume *see* volume, circulating
circulation
  abdominal trauma 182
  basic life support 112
  burns 222, 224
  neonatal resuscitation 149
  newborn baby 140, 141, 145
  sepsis 58
  unconscious patient 192
citrate anticoagulation 72
clarithromycin 60
clavicular fractures
  intentional 378
  shoulder dystocia 370
  vaginal breech delivery 404
clindamycin 60
co-amoxiclav 60
coagulation screen, pre-eclampsia 281
coagulopathy
  amniotic fluid embolism 122, 122, 123, 123, 125, 125
  burns patients 225
  major obstetric haemorrhage 298
collapse, maternal
  ABC approach 19
  amniotic fluid embolism 123, 123
  peripartum, causes 124
  see also cardiac arrest; shock
colloids, synthetic 72
colonic pseudo-obstruction 233, 237
colour, newborn baby 145, 146
combined spinal/epidural analgesia (CSE) 441, 441
communication
  in CPR 119
  in domestic violence 166
  feedback loop technique 473
  hierarchy and 473
  in major obstetric haemorrhage 300
  nonverbal 472, 473
  PACE strategy 474, 474
  parents of newborn baby 156
  problems 472
  SBAR tool 28, 29, 473
  transfers 460
  in trauma 161
compartment syndrome 217
computed tomography (CT)
  abdominal emergencies 235
  abdominal trauma 183
  fetal radiation doses 36
computed tomography pulmonary angiogram (CTPA) 131
concussion 195

Confidential Enquiries into Maternal Deaths (CEMD) 7
confirmation bias 476
confusion, causes and management 257
congenital heart disease 242, 247
  inheritance 249
  psychotropic drugs and 273
conscious level
  assessment 192, 194
  causes of decreased 189
  hypovolaemia 45
  observations 26
  see also unconscious patient
consent 481
  capacity to 484
  implied and express 482
  lack of capacity to 485
  legal and ethical aspects 482
  operative vaginal delivery 349
  patients declining blood/blood products 307
  requisites for valid 483
  responsibility for obtaining 490
  status of fetus and 488
  sufficient information for 481, 483
  voluntariness 489
  written 482
contraception, in heart disease 250
convulsions *see* seizures
cord *see* umbilical cord
coronary angiogram 244
coronary artery bypass surgery 244
coronary artery dissection 243
corticospinal tract 204
corticosteroids
  anaphylactic shock 49
  antenatal, pre-eclampsia 288
  sepsis 61
CPR *see* cardiopulmonary resuscitation
craniotomy 432
cricothyroidotomy
  needle 95, 101, 102
  surgical 95, 96, 103
Crohn's disease 230, 232
crossmatching, blood 73
crush injuries 215
cryoprecipitate 74, 75
  amniotic fluid embolism 126
crystalloids 71
Cushing's response 192
cyanosis, newborn baby 155

D-dimers 134
dalteparin 134
decapitation, fetal 433
decision making 478
deep venous thrombosis (DVT) 130
  diagnosis 132
  pelvic vessels 233
  treatment 134
defibrillation 113, 114
delivery
  in burns injury 225
  at caesarean section 315, 317
  during CPR 116, 117
  heart disease 249
  in pre-eclampsia 288
depression 267
  antenatal 267
  postnatal 268, 269
dermatomes 205
destructive operations 428, 430, 431
developing countries
  destructive operations 430, 433
  maternal deaths 15
  symphysiotomy 429, 430
dextrose (glucose) solutions 71, 151, 252
diabetes mellitus 250
  classification 250
  emergencies in pregnancy 251
  gestational 250, 255
  maternal deaths 241
  prevention of shoulder dystocia 373
  service provision 252
diabetic ketoacidosis 32, 252, 259
  algorithm 240
diabetic nephropathy 250
diabetic retinopathy 250
diagnostic peritoneal lavage (DPL) 184
diaphragm, traumatic disruption 174
diarrhoea 32
diazepam 292, 444
  rectal 261
diffuse axonal injury 195
dilated cardiomyopathy 242
discitis 448
dislocations 216
disseminated intravascular coagulation (DIC) 57
  see also coagulopathy
distress 33
documentation
  domestic abuse 166
  major obstetric haemorrhage 300
  operative vaginal delivery 363
  shoulder dystocia risk factors 373
  trauma 161
domestic abuse 163
  communication and teamwork 166
  diagnosis 165
  maternal deaths 15, 159, 164
  medico-legal issues 166
  pregnancy and 164
  recognition 164
  useful contacts 166
Domestic Violence Crime and Victims Act 2004 166
Doppler ultrasound
  deep vein thrombosis 132
  guiding fluid management 79
  pre-eclampsia/eclampsia 282
drains, after caesarean section 316
drotrecogin alfa 61
drugs
  administration errors 471, 471
  CPR 115

neonatal resuscitation 151
drying, newborn babies 144, 144
duodenal ulceration 230

Ebstein's anomaly 273
echocardiography 133, 244
eclampsia 277
algorithm 276
complications 279
definition 277
emergency box 292, 292
epidemiology 278
fetal assessment 282
headache 257
management 291
maternal deaths 11, 278
postpartum care and follow-up 293
principles of management 278
prophylaxis 286
see also pre-eclampsia
ectopic pregnancy, maternal deaths 13
ECV *see* external cephalic version
Ehlers–Danlos syndrome type IV 246
electrical burns 226
electrocardiogram (ECG) 133, 243
electronic fetal monitoring *see* cardiotocography
embolisation, arterial, for major haemorrhage 304
Emergency Infusion Device (EID), Arrow Peripheral 66
encephalopathy 259
endometritis 60
endotracheal intubation 92, 93
checking tube placement 94
in CPR 112
difficult 437
extubation 97
failed 436, 438, 479
in neonatal resuscitation 152
oxygenation during difficult 94
premature extubation 439
enoxaparin 134
epidural abscess 448
epidural anaesthesia (block) 439
characteristics 440
complications 262, 442
doses 441
failure 446
major obstetric haemorrhage 306
top-ups 441, 444
twin vaginal delivery 414
epidural blood patch 262, 447
epidural haematoma 448
epidural space 439, 440
epilepsy 258, 260
maternal deaths 15
status epilepticus 260
epinephrine *see* adrenaline
episiotomy 418
forceps delivery 357, 361, 362
shoulder dystocia 374
ventouse delivery 354
Erb's palsy 370
ergometrine 9
cardiac disease 249
major obstetric haemorrhage 303
pre-eclampsia 289
error chains 470, 470
escharotomy 225
ethical principles, consent 482
ethnic minority groups
maternal mortality 10, 10
sepsis 54
etomidate 307
external anal sphincter (EAS), repair techniques 422, 423, 423
external cephalic version (ECV) 394, 395
complications 397
efficacy 396
second twin 412
technique 397, 398, 398
extradural haemorrhage 196
extubation 97
premature 439

face presentation 389
diagnosis 390
management 361, 388, 390
FAST (focused assessment sonography in trauma) 183
fatigue (of clinicians) 477
feedback loop 473
femoral vein access 69
fetal death
destructive operations 431
placental abruption 305
shoulder dystocia 370
trauma 159
see also perinatal mortality
fetal distress
amniotic fluid embolism 126
trauma-related haemorrhage 181
see also asphyxia, birth
fetal head
aftercoming, of breech *see* aftercoming head of breech
bobbing, shoulder dystocia 373
fractures, pelvic trauma 185, 214
impaction, at caesarean section 317
position, operative vaginal delivery 349, 350, 355
fetal head entrapment
caesarean section 319
vaginal breech 406, 430
fetal lie, at caesarean section 315, 318
fetal outcomes
amniotic fluid embolism 127
cord prolapse 386
peri-cardiac arrest caesarean section 118
shoulder dystocia 370
fetal wellbeing and viability, assessment 20
abdominal trauma 184
pre-eclampsia/eclampsia 282
unconscious patient 193
fetus

complications of maternal diabetes 251
effects of regional blocks 449
legal status 488
radiation dose 35, 36
fibroids 232, 318
flail chest 173
fluid administration *see* intravenous fluid administration
fluid balance, pre-eclampsia 282, 285, 289
fluid loss 41
see also blood loss
fluid overload, pre-eclampsia 290, 291
focused assessment sonography in trauma (FAST) 183
forceps delivery 356
aftercoming head of breech 361, 362, 402, 403
face presentation 361, 391
failed ventouse delivery 362
indications 348, 349
method 357, 358, 359
postpartum care 363
rotational 358
safety rules 346, 356, 357
shoulder dystocia risk 371
foreign bodies, intracranial 197
four Hs 115
four Ts 115, 302
fracture-dislocations 216, 218
fractures 214
assessment 216
fetal *see* clavicular fractures; humerus, fractures
immobilisation 215
open 216
fresh frozen plasma (FFP) 73, 74
sepsis 60
furosemide (frusemide) 290

Gaskin manoeuvre 376
gasping
asphyxiated neonate 140, 142
cardiac arrest 112
gastric contents, aspiration of 92, 95
genital tract trauma 9, 371
gestational diabetes 250, 255
Gillick competence 485
Glasgow Coma Scale (GCS) 194, 194
glucagon 251, 252
glucose (dextrose) solutions 71, 151, 252
glucose tolerance test (GTT) 255
glycaemic control, peripartum 253
glyceryl trinitrate (GTN) *see* nitroglycerin
Group A beta-haemolytic *Streptococcus* 13, 53, 60
Guedel oropharyngeal airway 90, 91
insertion 98, 98

haematocrit 46, 301
haemorrhage
amniotic fluid embolism 122, 123, 124, 125, 125
cell salvage 75
compressible 47
difficulties in recognising 41, 45, 70, 298, 299
fluid therapy 70, 79
hypovolaemic shock 41
intra-abdominal *see* intra-abdominal haemorrhage
intracranial 196
limb injuries 214
major obstetric *see* major obstetric haemorrhage
non-compressible 47
pelvic trauma 185, 214
see also blood loss; hypovolaemic shock
haemostasis, at caesarean section 316
haemothorax, massive 173
haemotympanum 198
Hagen–Poiseuille equation 65
handover
after transfer 465
SBAR tool 473
Hartmann's solution 71
Haultain's technique 336
head, fetal *see* fetal head
head bobbing, shoulder dystocia 373
head injury
assisted ventilation 96
classification of severity 195
fetal assessment 193
pathophysiology 190
primary survey and resuscitation 191
secondary survey 193
types 195
head position, neutral, newborn baby 146, 147
head tilt/chin lift 88, 89
CPR 111, 113
headache 31, 256
causes and management 257, 261
investigations 260
postdural puncture 258, 261, 447
red flag features 31, 256
heart disease *see* cardiac disease
heart rate
in hypovolaemia 44, 76
neonatal resuscitation 150
newborn baby 145, 146
heat loss, preventing
newborn babies 144, 144
preterm babies 152, 153
HELLP syndrome 277, 293
diagnosis 281
HELPERR mnemonic 378
heparin, unfractionated, pulmonary embolism 134, 135, 135
hepatic failure, in sepsis 57
herpes zoster 234
hierarchy, and communication 473
human error 470
drug administration 471, 471
human factors 469
Human Rights Act 1998 487, 488
humerus
fractures 370, 404
intraosseous access 67, 68
Huntingdon's procedure 336
hydralazine 276, 284, 284
hydrocortisone 49, 61, 126
hydrostatic repositioning, inverted uterus 335

hydroxyethyl starch 72
hyperbaric oxygen therapy 223
hypercarbia 85
hyperkalaemia, crush injuries 215
hypertension
- diabetes mellitus and 250
- management 282
- pre-eclampsia 277, 279

hypertensive disease 277
- definitions 277
- maternal deaths 11
- *see also* eclampsia; pre-eclampsia

hypertrophic obstructive cardiomyopathy (HOCM) 242
hypoglycaemia, diabetic 251, 259
hypotension
- amniotic fluid embolism 122, 123
- head injury 192
- high/total spinal block 445
- hypovolaemia 45
- regional anaesthesia 41, 442
- in sepsis 55
- supine *see* supine hypotension syndrome

hypotensive resuscitation, in pregnancy 160
hypothermia
- intravenous infusion-related 70
- newborn baby 144

hypovolaemia
- major obstetric haemorrhage 298
- newborn baby 151, 155
- recognition 41, 45
- signs 44, 47, 76
- *see also* blood loss

hypovolaemic shock 40
- absolute 41
- clinical presentation 44, 299
- principles of treatment 47
- relative 41

hypoxia 269
- amniotic fluid embolism 122
- fetal 140
- susceptibility of pregnant women 116
- *see also* airway management

hysterectomy
- major obstetric haemorrhage 305
- placenta accreta 327, 328
- uterine rupture 342

induction of labour
- after previous caesarean section 340
- macrosomic babies 373
- uterine rupture risk 341

infection
- complicating regional blocks 448
- continuum of clinical response to severe 52
- diabetes-related risks 250
- headache and confusion 257
- identifying source 60

influenza A/H1N1 62
information, sufficient for consent 481, 483
instrumental vaginal delivery *see* operative vaginal delivery
insulin therapy
- diabetes mellitus 253, 255
- diabetic ketoacidosis 240
- sepsis 61

intensive care transfers 463
intercostal drains *see* chest drains
internal anal sphincter (IAS), repair 422
internal podalic version (IPV) 412, 415
interpreters 165, 248, 472
interventional radiology, major obstetric haemorrhage 304
intestinal obstruction 230, 232, 233, 238
intestinal pseudo-obstruction 233, 237
intra-abdominal haemorrhage
- assessment 231
- maternal deaths 230
- traumatic 181, 182, 185

intracerebral lacerations 197
intracranial haematomata 196
intracranial neoplasms 263
intracranial pressure (ICP) 190, 191
- raised 190, 192, 258

intralipid infusions 444
intraosseous (IO) access 66, 67
intraperitoneal (abdominal) pain 232
intrauterine tamponade 303
intravenous access 64, 65
- algorithm 64
- burns 224
- ultrasound-guided 69

intravenous cannulae
- flow rates under gravity 65, 66
- large-bore, types 66, 67

intravenous cut down 70
intravenous fluid administration 70
- advanced monitoring techniques 78
- algorithm 64
- amniotic fluid embolism 126
- burns 224
- guidance 76, 77
- haemorrhage 70, 79
- head injury 192
- neonatal resuscitation 151
- pre-eclampsia/eclampsia 80, 284, 285, 285, 289
- pressure devices 71
- sepsis 58, 80

intravenous fluids 71
- warming 70

ischaemic heart disease 243

jaw thrust 88, 89
- CPR 112
- newborn baby 147, 148
- pocket mask 99, 99

Jehovah's Witnesses 307
- advance directives 307, 487
- antenatal and intrapartum care 308
- cell salvage for 76
- obtaining consent 307

jet ventilation 102
joint injuries 216

ketamine 306
Kiwi omnicup 351
Kjelland forceps 349, 358, 360
Kleihauer test 182, 399

labetalol 276, 283
lactate, blood 34, 56
laparoscopic cholecystectomy 236
laparotomy
 abdominal trauma 183, 185
 intestinal obstruction 238
 uterine rupture 342
laryngeal mask airway (LMA) 95, 438
 insertion 99, 100
 sizes and inflation volumes 101
lateral tilt position *see* left lateral tilt position
latex sensitivity 43
leadership 479
left lateral tilt position 41, 42
 CPR 110, 116
 major obstetric haemorrhage 301
 spinal immobilisation and 203
legal issues *see* medico-legal issues
levobupivacaine 441, 442
life, signs of 110
life-threatening illness, recognition 25
lifeless person, apparently 19, 110
lignocaine (lidocaine) 443
limb injuries
 life-threatening 214, 215
 limb-threatening 215
limb weakness, unilateral, unconscious patient 193
linezolid 60
lithium 271, 273
lithotomy position 217
liver
 pain 233
 rupture 230
liver failure 230
Lloyd Davies position 217
local anaesthesia
 perineal repair 418
 symphysiotomy 430
local anaesthetics
 antidote 444
 doses for epidural/spinal blocks 441
 hyperbaric 441, 442
 toxicity 443
log-rolling 204, 204
 procedure 210, 211, 211
loin pain 233
lorazepam 273
Lovset's manoeuvre 402, 402
low-molecular weight heparin (LMWH)
 cardiac disease 245, 247
 during labour and delivery 135
 postnatal 136
 pulmonary embolism 134, 135
lumbar spine immobilisation 203
lung function
 burns patients 222
 changes in pregnancy 116

macrosomia, fetal 251
 elective caesarean section 372
 induction of labour 373
 shoulder dystocia risk 371
magnesium sulphate
 adverse effects 287, 288
 anaphylactic shock 49
 CPR 115
 doses 287
 eclampsia 276, 291
 pre-eclampsia 286
 uterine inversion 335
magnetic resonance imaging (MRI)
 abdominal emergencies 235
 neurological emergencies 260
 placenta accreta 326
Magpie trial 277, 283, 286
major obstetric haemorrhage 297
 algorithm 295
 anaesthetic management 306
 causes 298
 communication and documentation 300
 definition 298
 diagnostic tests 301
 four Ts-based management 302
 guidelines 299
 maternal mortality 11, 12, 297
 monitoring 302
 patients refusing blood/blood products 296, 307
 placenta accreta 328
 placental abruption 305
 practical management 299
 recognition 299
 resuscitation 300
 specific causes 305
 surgical interventions 303
malaria, cerebral 263
Marfan's syndrome 173, 246
mask, pocket 99, 99
maternal deaths 3, 7
 abdominal pathology 229, 230
 amniotic fluid embolism 13, 121
 anaesthetic complications 13, 437, 438
 cardiac disease 14, 241
 coincidental 15
 confidential enquiries 7
 direct 11, 11
 domestic violence 15, 159, 164
 indirect 14, 14
 lessons from the past 8
 major obstetric haemorrhage 11, 12, 297
 pre-eclampsia/eclampsia 11, 278
 psychiatric disorders and suicide 14, 269
 risk factors 10
 sepsis 13, 52
 substandard care 15, 25
 thromboembolism 12, 129
 trauma 9, 9, 159
 uterine rupture 9, 341

worldwide 15, 16
maternal mortality, trends 8
Mauriceau-Smellie-Viet (MSV) manoeuvre 401, 402, 403
MBRRACE-UK (Mothers and Babies – Reducing Risk through Audit and Confidential Enquiries across the UK) 7, 8
McRoberts' manoeuvre 374
mean arterial pressure (MAP) 190, 191
meconium aspiration 147
medico-legal issues
breech delivery 406
domestic abuse 166
perimortem caesarean section 118
refusal of blood/blood products 307, 307
shoulder dystocia 378
see also consent
meningitis 257, 262, 448
Mental Capacity Act 2007 486
Mental Health Act 1983 487, 488
mental health problems *see* psychiatric illness
mental state, altered 45, 259
mentoanterior position 391
mentoposterior position 391, 392
MEOWS (modified early obstetric warning systems) 26
charts 26, 27
escalation procedure 30
immediate midwifery measures 29
observations 26
SBAR tool 28, 29
triggering 28
methicillin-resistant *Staphylococcus aureus* (MRSA) 54, 60
methotrexate, placenta accreta 328
metronidazole 60
midazolam 261
migraine 257
Mini-Trach 104
misoprostol, major obstetric haemorrhage 303
MIST mnemonic 181, 215
modified early obstetric warning systems *see* MEOWS
monitoring
electronic fetal *see* cardiotocography
intravenous fluid administration 78
in major obstetric haemorrhage 302
in pre-eclampsia 282
pregnant woman 20
during transfers 464
mood stabilisers 271
motor block, regional anaesthesia 443
mouth to mouth ventilation 112
moxibustion, in breech presentation 397
multiple organ failure 58
multiple pregnancy 411
higher order 413
see also twin pregnancy
musculoskeletal trauma 213
algorithm 212
limb-threatening 215
primary survey and resuscitation 213
in spinal injuries 207
myocardial contusion 174
myocardial infarction (MI) 243
myometrial necrosis/abscess 60

naloxone 152, 155, 446
nasopharyngeal airway 90
necrotising fasciitis 60
needle cricothyroidotomy 95, 101, 102
needle thoracocentesis 176
neonatal adaptation syndrome 272
neonatal resuscitation 139
algorithm 138
assessment 144
births outside delivery room 155
communication with parents 156
discontinuation 156
equipment 142, 143
pathophysiology 140
poor initial response 154
preterm babies 152
response to 152
strategy 143
nerve injuries, traumatic 218
neurogenic shock 206
neurological assessment
spinal injuries 204
unconscious patient 193
neurological disease 15, 241
neurological emergencies 256
neurological level, spinal cord injury 205
neurological sequelae
amniotic fluid embolism 127
peri-cardiac arrest caesarean delivery 118
regional blocks 448
shoulder dystocia 370
neurological signs, lateralising, unconscious patient 193
neuromuscular blockade, complications 439
neuropraxia 448
newborn babies
assessment 144
diabetic mothers 251, 255
drying/keeping warm 144, 144
normal physiology 139
resuscitation at birth *see* neonatal resuscitation
nifedipine 276, 284
nitrates, organic 245
nitric oxide 54
nitroglycerin (glyceryl trinitrate; GTN)
caesarean section during labour 312, 318
external cephalic version 396
retained placenta 329, 329
uterine inversion 335
nonverbal communication 472, 473
noradrenaline (norepinephrine) 59
nuchal arms, vaginal breech delivery 404

obesity
maternal mortality and 10
sudden unexpected cardiac death 242
thromboembolism risk 130

uterine rupture risk 340
observations of vital signs, systematic 26
obstetric injury, maternal deaths 9, 9
obstructed labour
destructive operations 430, 433, 433
maternal deaths 9
see also shoulder dystocia
occipitolateral positions, ventouse delivery 353
occipitoposterior positions
forceps delivery 358
ventouse delivery 353, 355
occipitotransverse position, forceps delivery 358
oesophageal disruption 175, 230
Ogilvie's syndrome 237
olanzapine 272
oliguria, in pre-eclampsia 289
operative vaginal delivery (OVD) 347
audit standards 364
cord prolapse 356, 386
documentation and debriefing 363
epidural blocks leading to 443
indications 348
postpartum care 363
prerequisites for 344, 349
safety issues/choice of instrument 349
shoulder dystocia risk 371
supervision 363
training and simulation 348
trial of 361
see also forceps delivery; ventouse delivery
opioids/opiates
burns 224
complications 446
effects on newborn 155
epidural/spinal blocks 442
incorrect use 439
oral anticoagulants, venous thromboembolism 135, 136
oropharyngeal (Guedel type) airway 90, 91
insertion 98, 98
O'Sullivan's technique, uterine inversion 335
ovarian cyst rupture/torsion 233
oxygen administration 85
burns 223
CPR 112, 113
difficult endotracheal intubation 94
neonatal resuscitation 149
via needle cricothyroidotomy 102, 103
oxygen saturation, monitoring
burns 223
newborn baby 145, 146
pre-eclampsia 282
preterm babies 154, 154
see also pulse oximetry
oxytocin (Syntocinon)
cardiac disease 249
major obstetric haemorrhage 303
pre-eclampsia 285, 289
retained placenta 329
twin delivery 414, 415
uterine rupture and 341
PACE structure, communication 474, 474
packed red cells 72, 74
$PaCO_2$ (PCO_2) 34, 35
pain relief
burns 224
labour 440, 440
Pajot's manoeuvre 357
pancreatitis, acute 230, 234, 236
panic attacks 273
PaO_2 35
paraplegia 205
parents
consent for child 485, 487, 489
newborn baby 156
Patwardhan's procedure 320
Pearce versus United Bristol Healthcare Trust 483
pelvic fractures/injuries 185, 214
penetrating injuries
abdomen 181
skull 197
peptic ulceration 232, 233, 233
percutaneous coronary intervention (PCI) 244
perforation, of a viscus 232, 233, 238
perinatal asphyxia *see* asphyxia, birth
perinatal mortality
cord prolapse 383, 386
maternal diabetes 251
uterine rupture 340
see also fetal death
perineal trauma 417
aftercare 424
assessment 418, 419, 419
classification 417
fourth degree tears 417, 420
operative vaginal delivery 363, 363
repair 418
third degree tears 417, 419, 420, 422
peripartum cardiomyopathy 242
peripheral venous access 65
alternatives to 66
peripheral venous cannulae
flow rates under gravity 65, 66
large bore 66, 67
peritoneal lavage, diagnostic 184
peritonitis 230, 232, 238
pH, arterial blood 34, 35
phenylephedrine 446
Piper forceps 361, 402
piperacillin–tazobactam 60
placenta
adherent 325
at caesarean section 315, 319
manual removal 329
retained *see* retained placenta
placenta accreta 325, 330
algorithm 323
diagnosis 326
management 326
placenta increta 325
placenta percreta 325
placenta praevia, caesarean section 319

placental abruption 305
    clinical presentation 231, 232
    traumatic 159, 180, 182
plasma, fresh frozen *see* fresh frozen plasma
Plasmodium falciparum 263
plastic bags, for preterm babies 153
platelets
    for sepsis 60
    for transfusion 74, 75
pneumonia 32
pneumothorax
    chest drain insertion 176
    needle thoracocentesis 176
    newborn baby 155
    open 173
    tension 172
pocket mask 99, 99
polyhydramnios 251
porphyria, acute intermittent 259
Portex Mini-Trach 104
positioning, pregnant woman
    compartment syndrome due to 217
    CPR 110, 116
    major obstetric haemorrhage 301
    operative vaginal delivery 349
    on spine board 203
postdural puncture headache 258, 261, 447
posterior axillary traction, shoulder dystocia 377
posterior columns, spinal cord 204
postnatal depression (PND) 268, 269
    well at-risk women 271
postpartum care
    cardiac disease 249
    diabetes mellitus 255
postpartum haemorrhage
    placental abruption 306
    shoulder dystocia 371
    see also major obstetric haemorrhage
postural supine hypotension *see* supine hypotension syndrome
pre-eclampsia 277
    algorithm 276
    antepartum/intrapartum management 282
    complications 279
    definition 277
    epidemiology 278
    fetal assessment 282
    fluid management 80, 284, 285, 285
    headache 277
    management principles 278
    maternal assessment 279
    maternal deaths 11, 278
    monitoring of clinical signs 282
    planning delivery 288
    postpartum care and follow-up 293
    postpartum fluid management 80, 289
    seizure prophylaxis 286
    symptoms and signs 279
preconceptual care
    cardiac disease 247
    diabetes mellitus 253
    psychiatric illness 270
pressure sores 443
preterm babies
    caesarean delivery 320
    plastic bags for 153
    resuscitation at birth 152
    twin 413
primary survey 17
prolonged labour, maternal deaths 9
Proseal laryngeal mask airway 438
prosthetic heart valves 247
proteinuria
    measurement 281
    pre-eclampsia 277, 279, 282
pseudomembranous colitis 230
psychiatric illness 259, 267
    after delivery 268
    alerting neonatal paediatrician 273
    chronic severe, management 271
    consent issues 486, 487, 488
    implications for obstetric practice 270
    labour ward crises 272
    managing well at-risk women 271
    maternal deaths 14, 269
    in pregnancy 267
puerperal psychosis 259, 268, 269
    well at-risk women 271
puerperal sepsis 8
    see also sepsis
pulmonary angiography 133
pulmonary artery balloon tipped flotation catheters 78
pulmonary contusion 174
pulmonary embolism (PE) 129
    algorithm 128
    clinical presentation 32, 131, 131
    incidence 129
    management 132
    massive 131, 134
    pathophysiology 130
    see also venous thromboembolism
pulmonary hypertension 32
pulmonary oedema 32, 290
pulse, observations 26
pulse oximetry 20, 28, 85
    preterm babies 154
    see also oxygen saturation, monitoring
pulse pressure, narrowed 45
pulseless electrical activity (PEA) 114
pupillary responses, unconscious patient 192, 193
pyelonephritis 233
pyrexia 30

quadriplegia 205

RADAR 165
radiation dose, fetus 35, 36
radiographs
    abdominal pain 235, 237
    fetal radiation doses 36
    musculoskeletal trauma 215, 216
radiology, pregnant woman 35

rape 164
Rapid Infusion Catheter (RIC) 66, 67
rapid sequence induction 93, 306
recognition, serious illness 25
record keeping *see* documentation
rectum, buttonhole tears 418, 419
red-cell concentrates 72, 74
red flag symptoms 30
referred pain 232, 234
regional anaesthesia 439
  complications 442
  doses 441
  failure 446
  hypovolaemic shock 41
  major obstetric haemorrhage 306
  perineal repair 418, 420
  pre-eclampsia 285
  see also epidural anaesthesia; spinal anaesthesia
renal failure, in sepsis 57
renal function, pre-eclampsia 281, 289
renal replacement therapy, sepsis 61
respiration *see* breathing
respiratory depression, opioid-induced 446
resuscitation 18
  see also cardiopulmonary resuscitation; neonatal resuscitation
retained placenta 329
  algorithm 324
  management 329
reverse Woods' screw manoeuvre 376
rhabdomyolysis, traumatic 215
Rhesus (anti-D) immunoglobulin 182, 399
Ringer's lactate 71
ritodrine 335, 392
road traffic accidents 15, 159, 180, 180
ropivicaine 442
Rubin I manoeuvre 375
Rubin II manoeuvre 375
rule of nines 224
ruptured uterus *see* uterine rupture
Rusch balloon 303

salbutamol 49
saline, normal 71
SBAR tool 28, 29, 473
scalp wounds 197
schizophrenia 267, 272, 487
seat belts 180
secondary survey 18
seizures 260
  amniotic fluid embolism 123
  eclamptic 291
  local anaesthetic toxicity 444
  management 260
  prophylaxis in pre-eclampsia 286
selective serotonin reuptake inhibitors (SSRIs) 272, 274
sepsis 51
  after burns 225
  algorithm 50
  causes 53
  clinical features 55, 56
  confusion 258
  epidemiology 54
  fluid resuscitation 58, 80
  management 57
  maternal deaths 13, 52
  microbiology 53
  monitoring and investigations 56
  pathophysiology 54
  severe 52
  starting treatment 57
  terminology 51, 52
septic shock 43, 47
  definition 52
septicaemia 52
serious illness
  clinical symptoms and red flag features 30
  MEOWS 26
  recognition 25
  structured approach 19
severe sepsis 52
sexual abuse 154
shift working 477
shock 39
  algorithm 38
  anaphylactic 43, 48
  cardiogenic 42, 48
  clinical presentation 44, 299
  distributive 42
  fluid replacement 64, 70
  hypovolaemic *see* hypovolaemic shock
  intravenous access 64, 65
  neurogenic 206
  obstructive 44
  pathophysiology 39
  pitfalls in recognition 45
  principles of treatment 47
  septic *see* septic shock
  types 40
shoulder dystocia 369
  definition and incidence 369
  early detection 373
  fetal mortality and morbidity 370
  management 368, 373
  maternal morbidity 371
  mechanism 372
  medico-legal aspects 378
  prevention 372
  risk factors 371, 371
  symphysiotomy 377, 430
  training and teaching 372
shoulder pain 234
shoulder presentation, caesarean section 320
Sidaway versus Board of Governors of Bethlem Royal Hospital 482, 483
sigmoid volvulus 233, 238
situation awareness 475
skin care, spinal cord injuries 207
skin colour, newborn baby 135, 136
skull fractures 198
sling technique, shoulder dystocia 377
socio-economic classification, maternal mortality and 10

sodium bicarbonate 115
sodium chloride solution, 0% 71
spinal anaesthesia (block) 439
    characteristics 440
    complications 262, 442
    doses 441
    failure 446
    high and total 444
spinal/spinal cord injuries 201
    algorithm 200
    assessment 203
    immobilisation techniques 202
    practical procedures 208
    principles of treatment 206
    recovery and rehabilitation 207
spine board 203
spinothalamic tract 204
splenic artery rupture/aneurysm 230, 233
squames, fetal 123, 124
statins 245
status epilepticus 260
steroids *see* corticosteroids
Streptococcus pyogenes (group A *Streptococcus*) 13, 53, 60
structured approach to emergencies 3, 17
subarachnoid haemorrhage 197, 257
subdural haemorrhage 196
substance misusers 269, 269, 270
substandard care 15, 25
suctioning, airway 88
    meconium aspiration 147
    newborn baby 147
sudden adult death syndrome (SADS) 242
suicide 14, 159, 269
supine hypotension syndrome 41, 116, 203
supraglottic airway devices 95
suprapubic pressure, in shoulder dystocia 375
surfactant 153
Surviving Sepsis Campaign 61
Swiss cheese model 470, 470
symphysiotomy 429, 430
    algorithm 427
    failed breech delivery 406
    indications 430
    shoulder dystocia 377, 430
    technique 430
Syntocinon *see* oxytocin
Syntometrine 289, 415
    see also ergometrine; oxytocin
systemic inflammatory response syndrome (SIRS) 52

tachycardia
    hypovolaemia 44, 76
    major obstetric haemorrhage 302
tamponade, intrauterine 303
team leader, situation awareness 476
teams
    CPR 119
    decision making 478
    leadership 479
    situation awareness 477
teicoplanin 60
temperature control
    neonatal resuscitation 144
    preterm babies 152, 153
    spinal cord injuries 207
tendon reflexes 280
terbutaline
    during caesarean section 318
    cord prolapse 386
    external cephalic version 398
    uterine inversion 335
Term Breech Trial 399, 412
termination of pregnancy
    consent issues 485, 488
    heart disease 248
    maternal deaths 13
thoracic injuries
    algorithm 180
    initial assessment and management 172
    life-threatening 172
    potentially lethal 174
    practical procedures 176
    secondary survey 174
    types 171
thoracic spine immobilisation 203
thoracocentesis, needle 176
thromboembolism *see* venous thromboembolism
thrombolysis
    acute myocardial infarction 244
    pulmonary embolism 135
thrombophilia 130
thromboprophylaxis, caesarean section 320
tibia, intraosseous access 67, 68
tinzaparin 134
tocolysis
    during caesarean section 318
    cord prolapse 386
    external cephalic version 396, 398
    face presentation 392
tracheobronchial disruption 175
transfer 459
    ACCEPT approach 459
    handover 465
    in pre-eclampsia/eclampsia 289
transportation 464
trauma 159
    abdominal 179
    causes 159
    deaths 9, 9, 159
    documentation and communication 161
    head *see* head injury
    musculoskeletal 213
    obstetrician's/midwife's role 160
    spine and spinal cord 201
    thoracic 171
triage 453
    pregnant woman 455
    priorities and categories 453, 454, 455
    scenarios 456
trial-of-instrumental delivery 361
triplet pregnancy 413

troponin 244
tryptase, serum 43
turtle sign 373
Twin Birth Study 411
twin pregnancy 411
  algorithm 410
  external cephalic version 412
  internal podalic version (IPV) 412, 415
  intertwin delivery interval 412
  mode of delivery 411
  presentations 412
  vaginal delivery 411, 412, 413

UK Obstetric Surveillance System (UKOSS) 13
ulcerative colitis 232
ultrasound
  abdominal emergencies 235
  abdominal trauma 183
  cord prolapse 385
  fetal assessment 20
  guided intravenous access 69
  placental site assessment 326
  second stage of labour 350
  twin pregnancy 411, 414
  see also Doppler ultrasound
umbilical cord
  clamping 144, 144
  presentation 384
umbilical cord prolapse 383
  aetiology 384
  diagnosis 384
  management 382, 385
  operative vaginal delivery 356, 386
unconscious patient 189
  algorithm 188
  amniotic fluid embolism 123
  changes in vital signs 195
  fetal assessment 193
  primary survey and resuscitation 191
  secondary survey 193
  treatment principles 190
  see also conscious level; head injury
unresponsive patient
  ABC approach 19
  cardiopulmonary resuscitation 110
unstable lie, at caesarean section 318
urine output
  guiding fluid replacement 77
  monitoring 28
  pre-eclampsia 282, 289
uterine artery, ligation 304
uterine atony
  amniotic fluid embolism 126
  major obstetric haemorrhage 302
uterine contractions 232, 317
uterine inversion 332, 333
  management 334
  symptoms and signs 334
uterine rupture 339
  algorithm 338
  laparotomy findings 342
  management 342
  maternal deaths 9, 341
  perinatal outcome 340
  practice and training issues 341
  risk factors 339, 340
  in shoulder dystocia 371
  traumatic 159, 180
uterus
  B-Lynch brace suture 304, 304
  balloon tamponade of bleeding 303
  closure, at caesarean section 316
  incision, at caesarean section 315
  manual displacement 110, 111, 116
  manual replacement of inverted 335
  packing, to control haemorrhage 303
  pain, acute presentation 232
  trauma 180, 320

vacuum extraction *see* ventouse delivery
vaginal delivery
  breech presentation 399
  destructive operations 431
  operative *see* operative vaginal delivery
  pre-eclampsia/eclampsia 288
  twins 411, 412, 413
valproate, sodium 272, 273
valvular heart disease 246
vascular access 64, 65
vascular accidents, intra-abdominal 233
vascular injuries 217
vasodilatation, hypovolaemic shock 41
vasodilators 284
vasopressors 59, 441, 442
  complications 446
vena cava occlusion 116
  see also supine hypotension syndrome
venous cut down 70
venous thromboembolism (VTE) 129
  burns patients 225
  maternal deaths 12, 129
  pathophysiology 130
  prophylaxis at caesarean section 320
  risk factors 130
  treatment 134
  see also deep venous thrombosis; pulmonary embolism
ventilation 85
  assessment 87
  assisted (artificial) 96
  basic life support 112
  efficacy in pregnancy 116
  management 96
  mouth to mouth 112
  in neonatal resuscitation 148, 149
  preterm babies 153
ventilation/perfusion (V/Q) scan 131, 131
ventouse cups
  metal (hard) 351
    anterior 353, 354
    posterior 353, 355
  positioning 351, 352

selection of appropriate 353
silicone rubber (soft) 351, 353, 353
ventouse delivery (vacuum extraction) 351
avoiding failure 355
first stage of labour 356
forceps for failed 362
indications 348, 349
method 353
postpartum care 363
safety rules 345, 351, 352
shoulder dystocia risk 371
umbilical cord prolapse 356
ventricular fibrillation (VF), CPR 113
very-low-birthweight twins 413
vesicovaginal fistula 434
violence, domestic *see* domestic abuse
volume, circulating 70
classification of lost 46
recognition of hypovolaemia and 41
replacement *see* intravenous fluid administration
see also hypovolaemia

warm, keeping *see* heat loss, preventing
white blood cell (WBC) count 57, 235
Woods' screw manoeuvre 376
Wrigley's forceps 319

X-rays *see* radiographs

Zavanelli manoeuvre 377